ANCIENT MEDICINE

# Ancient Medicine

*From Mesopotamia to Rome*

Laura M. Zucconi

William B. Eerdmans Publishing Company
Grand Rapids, Michigan

Wm. B. Eerdmans Publishing Co.
4035 Park East Court SE, Grand Rapids, Michigan 49546
www.eerdmans.com


Published 2019
Printed in the United States of America

25 24 23 22 21 20 19 1 2 3 4 5 6 7

ISBN 978-0-8028-6983-8

**Library of Congress Cataloging-in-Publication Data**

Names: Zucconi, Laura M., author.
Title: Ancient medicine : from Mesopotamia to Rome / Laura M. Zucconi.
Description: Grand Rapids : Eerdmans Publishing Co., 2019. |
Includes bibliographical references and index.
Identifiers: LCCN 2019005484 | ISBN 9780802869838 (hardcover : alk. paper)
Subjects: LCSH: Medicine—Religious aspects—History.
Classification: LCC BL65.M4 Z829 2019 | DDC 610.938—dc23
LC record available at https://lccn.loc.gov/2019005484

*To Dr. George Robert Zucconi*

# *Contents*

# *Foreword*

Medicine seems to us to be a liminal practice. In modern societies health is easily acquired and medical practice easily sequestered into sanitized, brightly lit spaces that are scented with antiseptic and bounded from the ordinary world. This conception could not be further from the ancient world, in which broken limbs never fully healed; aging brought wisdom, impaired vision, and hearing loss; and the population as a whole was vulnerable to a whole host of diseases deemed minor today.

Medicine in the past, therefore, was not only, at certain points in time, a distinct *techne* or profession, but it was also the domain of the priest, the magician, and the cook. It was conducted in sanctuaries as well as around the hearth. The biting awareness of the frailty of human existence rendered healthcare a central component of the human experience. But even as all ancient peoples were forced to think about the tenuousness of good health, they did not always do so in the same way. We often, erroneously, think of Hippocrates as the founder of medicine and push to the side those medical practices that predate him while dismissively labeling them as "superstition" or "magic."

Part of the problem is that few modern scholars possess the linguistic, archaeological, and historical skill sets to evaluate ancient cultures, let alone differentiate or even adequately distinguish one from another. The small steps between regions and cultures that would have been traversed on a daily basis by ancient people are less easily followed by modern scholars, whose areas of expertise are balkanized into specializations based on linguistic competency and geographical region. The experience of an ancient farmer living on the border is inaccessible to those who do not have the linguistic abilities or breadth of knowledge to speak of Egyptian, Mesopotamian, Persian, and Roman medicine.

More problematic is the sense that many scholars of the ancient world have limited interest in understanding medicine beyond the exalted status played by Hippocrates and his Greek- and Latin-speaking heirs. A whole subfield of medical literature published in the hallowed pages of the *JAMA* and the *Lancet* is devoted to tracing the evolution of thought from Hippocrates to the present with hardly a sideways glance at the practices of the ancient Levant.

It is into this complicated web of geographical, social, and historical boundaries that *Ancient Medicine: From Mesopotamia to Rome* steps. Laura Zucconi's work performs a welcome and desperately needed intervention in a field of literature in which experts in Greco-Roman religion are unable to speak to specialists in Hittite medicine. She adeptly navigates the difficult waters of sources, textual traditions, material culture, and ancient theories and distils the medicine of the ancient world into easily digestible chunks. Noting, in the traditions of the pseudo-Hippocratic texts *Airs, Waters, and Places*, that medical theory is deeply connected to geography and lived experience, she introduces cultures, regions, and medical praxis in a way that is accessible even to someone who knows almost nothing about the ancient world and even less about medicine.

*Ancient Medicine* does more, however, than fill the sizeable gap in scholarly histories of medicine and is not content, as we should not be either, with rounding out traditional histories of medicine so that Persians, Hittites, Canaanites, and Egyptians are represented alongside figures like Hippocrates and Galen. Zucconi takes seriously the underlying logic of the various thought-worlds she examines. Rather than derisively dismissing what we might call unsuccessful treatment methods as historical curiosities, she seeks to understand the rationale underpinning the medical practices she examines.

She reveals the astonishing fact that ancient medicine was a rich tapestry of practices that varied widely across the ancient Mediterranean. Rather than striving to uncover the seeds of modern medical practice as if they were discoveries accidentally stumbled upon by ancient practitioners, we should examine ancient medical thought on its own terms, in the variegated ways in which it was practiced and theorized and the multiplicity of contexts in which it was performed. As the book builds, we learn not only about medicine but also about cosmology, community, institutionalized religion, philosophy, the rhetorical boundaries that divorce medicine from magic and religion, and the role of warfare in propelling, supporting, and crafting healing practices. Even as her chapters create ever-expanding pools of knowledge, there is nothing simplistic here: just as Jupiter is not merely

Zeus renamed, Zucconi reminds us, so too the medicine of the Romans is not merely a recapitulation of Greek and Egyptian healthcare.

As the related fields of disability studies and history of medicine have grown up alongside one another, it is rare that the work of the accomplished historian has been successfully infused with the observations of the critical theorist. In the introduction to her book Zucconi proves that she is as methodologically thoughtful as she is historically and philologically qualified. It takes rare ability and a mature historical consciousness to provide such a nuanced and rigorous view of medicine in the ancient world. Though Zucconi complicates our beloved cultural image of Hippocrates as the father of medicine, we will be wiser for it and thank her for serving as our guide.

*December 5, 2018*

Prof. Candida Moss
Cadbury Professor of Theology
School of Philosophy, Theology & Religion
University of Birmingham

# *Acknowledgments*

Writing the acknowledgments for a work of this scope is a rather daunting task, since so many in the last seven years have contributed in a variety of ways to its completion. I would like to mention a few by name, with my apologies to any whom I may overlook; any mistakes in this work are all my own. Candida Moss, Joel Baden, Rebecca Raphael, and JoAnn Scurlock, for not only their own work in the field of ancient medicine, health care, and disability, but also for their time and friendship in helping guide my research. My colleagues Drs. Lisa Rosner, William Lubenow, and the rest of the history faculty at Stockton University, for their mentorship, support, encouragement, and lively debates. I am indebted to Wolfson College and the McDonald Institute for Archaeological Research at the University of Cambridge for their research support and providing a home away from home. The editors Allen Myers and Trevor Thompson at Eerdmans Publishing graciously and patiently allowed me to run with the idea of a history of ancient medicine. On a more personal note, I am forever grateful for the friendship and wing nights with Margaret Lewis and Mike Lague, for Nishtha Madan's welcoming family, and finally for Manish Madan standing in my office doorway making sure I finish (despite also distracting me with fabulous Bollywood suggestions).

# *Abbreviations*

| | |
|---|---|
| *AJSL* | *American Journal of Semitic Languages and Literatures* |
| *ANRW* | *Aufstieg und Niedergang der Römischen Welt* |
| BAM | *Babylonisch-assyrische Medizin* |
| *CML* | *Corpus Medicorum Latinorum* |
| CTH | *Catalogue des textes hittites* |
| DK | Diels and Kranz, *Die Fragmente der Vorsokratiker* |
| *GV* | *Griechische Vers-Inschriften* |
| *IGR* | *Inscriptiones graecae ad res romanas pertinentes* |
| KTU | *Die keilalphabetischen Texte aus Ugarit* |
| KUB | *Keilschrifturkunden aus Boghazköi* |
| *MAMA* | *Monumenta Asiae Minoris Antiqua* |
| *Nat. Fac.* | Galen, *On the Natural Faculties* |
| *PDM* | *Papyri Demoticae Magicae* |
| *PGM* | *Papyri Graecae Magicae* |
| *PHP* | Galen, *On the Doctrines of Hippocrates and Plato* |
| *UP* | Galen, *On the Utility of the Parts* |

# 1. Introduction

Roy Porter's *The Greatest Benefit to Mankind*, a seminal work on the history of medicine, devotes only six of the nearly seven hundred pages to medical practice that predates classical Greece.[1] He devotes thirty pages to Greco-Roman medicine. Porter includes a chapter on faith and medicine but limits it to the Judeo-Christian-Islamic religions. Other popular books simply begin their history with Hippocrates.[2] These works essentially ignore the rich history of medical practices across the ancient Near East and Mediterranean as well as the fundamental relationship between medicine and the theological concepts of the regions' different cultures. This work seeks to fill the gap not only by examining more in depth the medical culture of Mesopotamia, Egypt, Greece, and Rome but also by expanding the analyses to the Levant, the Anatolian Peninsula, and the Iranian Plateau. Numerous studies on ancient medicine exist but treat each area in isolation rather than showing how a given area represents a local manifestation of a wider ancient medical culture.

## Medical Anthropology

Another problem with the studies on the history of medicine is the tendency to highlight those practices that directly led to modern techniques and theories as an inevitable evolution of the field. When briefly addressing the ancient world, practices that became an "evolutionary dead end," so to speak, are mentioned more as a curiosity about how far the discipline has

1. Roy Porter, *The Greatest Benefit to Mankind: A Medical History of Humanity* (New York: W. W. Norton, 1999).

2. William Bynum, *A History of Medicine* (Oxford: Oxford University Press, 2008); Paul Strathern, *A Brief History of Medicine* (New York: Carroll & Graf, 2005).

come or an example of nonscientific thinking. The reason for this lies in the prominence of reduction and causation ideologies in medicine itself.

Causation tries to determine the single entity that created the disease, whether a germ or a gene. Once the cause is known, treatments can target it to stop the disease and promote healing. Closely tied to this is the reductionist view, which separates the pathogen from the patient; the bacteria or virus is the problem, not the person. Even genetic disorders are isolated as a particular gene causing difficulty. This aids in the targeting approach to therapy. Attention is then focused on the disease agent; the patient becomes secondary.

Since the clinical practice of medicine relies on reduction/causation, the history of the field has reflected and supported that process. The key figures in that history, besides the disease itself, are the ones who have correctly identified a cause and reduced it to develop targeted treatments. Yet this method ignores another important player in the history of medicine, the patient. Additionally, reduction/causation makes medicine synonymous with only the natural world, subject to investigation by the scientific method. Any medical system making use of the supernatural was dismissed. Yet more recent studies on the history of medicine now investigate the relationship between the disease, the patient, and the healer, with a focus on how the patient and healer function within a cultural context. This anthropological approach allows scholars to understand the way people view health and illness as connected to the supernatural world as well as the natural one. The history of medicine is no longer only a narrow, natural-world point of view but a wider, integrated perspective on human interaction.

This present study attempts to incorporate key concepts of medical anthropology to highlight the rational thought process behind ancient medical practices that reconcile natural phenomena with cosmological perspectives; particular attention is paid to how ancient societies understood the role of humans in that cosmology. This is not a unique approach for studies focusing more exclusively on ancient cultures, such as the work of JoAnn Scurlock on Mesopotamia.[3] But it has not been applied to a more comprehensive study of ancient medicine across cultures.

3. JoAnn Scurlock, *Sourcebook for Ancient Mesopotamian Medicine* (Atlanta: Society of Biblical Literature, 2014); JoAnn Scurlock, *Magico-Medical Means of Treating Ghost-Induced Illnesses in Ancient Mesopotamia* (Boston: Brill, 2006); JoAnn Scurlock and Burton R. Andersen, *Diagnoses in Assyrian and Babylonian Medicine: Ancient Sources, Translations, and Modern Medical Analyses* (Urbana: University of Illinois Press, 2005); JoAnn Scurlock, "Physician, Exorcist, Conjurer, Magician: A Tale of Two Healing Professions," in *Mesopotamian Magic: Textual, Historical, and Interpretative Perspectives*, ed. Tzvi Abusch and Karel van der Toorn (Groningen: Styx, 1999), 69–79.

## Health

Central to medical anthropology is the concept of health, which at first seems rather simple and intuitive; all know when they are healthy as opposed to when they feel sick. Yet the actual definition of health can vary. The standard medical explanation is the ability to function optimally in terms of physiology, psychology, or culture.[4] More anthropological definitions see health as a balance between people, nature, and the supernatural,[5] while some keep it simply to "the absence of disease."[6] The common element in all of these definitions is their reliance on cultural norms. This is true even for the apparent scientific "absence of disease," since disease itself is culturally defined. Modern Western clinical medicine uses numerical measurements to define the norm, such as the ratio of height to weight, blood pressure, or hemoglobin count. Health then is how well one fits into a statistical range in a variety of categories. But this focuses on just the biochemical factors. Norms can be applied in psychodynamic, behavioral, and social models, as found in the practice of psychiatry.

Because health relies upon one's ability to fit into culturally defined categories, we can analyze health within two spheres, the personal and the communal. The personal sphere is how an individual perceives his or her own status, while the communal sphere is how other people perceive someone's status. Many take a dualistic approach to the personal sphere, dividing it between the mind and the body, although this minimizes or completely disregards the intimate connection between the two. A person's interaction with work, family, and religion comprises the communal sphere. Although these spheres allow for an ease of analysis, they should not be used as exclusive categories but recognized as intertwining at certain points. The exact form of blending the personal and communal spheres can vary by culture. Modern Western bio-medicine values the personal bodily sphere, whereas the biblical world of Job gives priority to the communal religious sphere.

4. Thomas Stedman, *Stedman's Medical Dictionary* (Baltimore: Lippincott Williams and Wilkins, 2012), 789; World Health Organization, "Constitution," in *The First Ten Years of the World Health Organization* (Geneva: WHO, 1958), 449.

5. Cecil G. Helman, *Culture, Health, and Illness* (Boston: Butterworth Heinemann, 2007), 84.

6. Christopher Boorse, "Health as a Theoretical Concept," *Philosophy of Science* 44 (1977): 555.

## Disease and Illness

A corollary to health is disease or illness. But this concept also has a variety of definitions dependent on cultural norms. Most people, like clinical physicians, use the terms disease and illness interchangeably. Medical anthropologists work with separate definitions for disease and illness. Disease means a deviation from an official norm, such as physiochemical parameters as declared by an accepted authority, such as a board-certified physician. Illness, in contrast, is the perception of a disruption in the personal or communal sphere, or even both, linked to a somatic symptom. This may also need to be recognized by an accepted authority such as a physician but can also be done by other types of authorities, such as a priest or even a parent. ("You're too sick to go to school today.")

The actual presence of a physical ailment is less a concern in medical anthropology. The issue is how one perceives him- or herself and the extent to which the community agrees with that perception. When the communal and personal spheres agree, a person can assume the sick role.[7] Assuming the sick role allows a person to avoid obligations within the communal sphere. The sick role also has certain responsibilities, mainly seeking out help and the restoration of health from an accepted authority. The sick role is ideally a temporary state. The disruption to the communal sphere, and possibly the personal sphere, will eventually be removed, thus reintegrating the person into society and reestablishing community cohesion. Even without the removal of the physical disruption, restoration can occur by shifting the sick role to a new categorization, such as "disabled," that allows one to reintegrate with the community in a different fashion. Such restoration of health depends upon the patient and the healer agreeing to an explanatory model of illness.

## Explanatory Model of Illness or Cultural Concepts

In medical anthropology, an explanatory model of illness is not simply disease etiology, but the conjunction of physiology, disease etiology, and therapeutic measures. One model does not explain every case of illness. It cannot, since the disease etiology itself may vary, whether it is bacteria, virus, gene, allergen, an imbalance of humors, or even a god or ancestral spirit. In mod-

7. Helman, *Culture, Health, and Illness*, 85.

ern Western bio-medicine, the somatic aspect is emphasized, so the disease agent's impact on the accepted understanding of proper physiology guides the types of treatments used to alleviate physical symptoms. The more the body is returned to proper physiological function, the better the cure. In the ancient Near East and Mediterranean, the focus is on community cohesion both among people and within the supernatural realm. Physiology reflects those relationships, so treatments target their restoration, with the success of cures depending on the person's reintegration within the human and supernatural communities.

Physiology plays an important role in the explanatory model of illness, but that term tends to conjure a rather clinical image of the body, as used in Western bio-medicine. The importance of physiology for the history of medicine really is how a person conceptualizes the structure of the body, that is to say its anatomy, as well as its function. Collectively, this is better known in medical anthropology as body image. A part of this body image is an understanding of the boundaries of the physical body and how it interacts with the environment. For many people, their body image is formed by various elements of culture, such as the media, socio-economic status, and religion. As we shall see, ancient cultures often had the belief that their anatomical parts could form distinct relationships on the basis of their religious understanding of the formation of humans. Symbolic anatomy is a common form of conceptualizing the structure of the body. It links body parts to cosmological forces, such as the gods, as a way of understanding how various relationships affect the body and health. For some cultures, the anatomy's ability to form such relationships makes it more a case of symbiotic rather than symbolic anatomy; organs such as eyes are not fully under control of the individual but exist as independent entities that tacitly agree, symbiotically, to work with the individual.

How the body actually functions can take a variety of forms as well, but two of the most ubiquitous are the balance and plumbing models. The balance model explains that the body properly functions as long as certain substances or forces within it are kept in balance. Treatment measures then aim to restore the balance. The plumbing model sees the uninterrupted flow of substances/forces through the body as the basis of health. Restoration of health revolves around unblocking that movement. The ideas of symbolic anatomy, balance, and plumbing can easily work in conjunction in a single explanatory model of illness.

Although a general principle such as community cohesion underlies the explanatory model of illness, one must keep in mind that the exact form of expression for community cohesion will vary when analyzing the medical practices across a spectrum of cultures. Because the ancient documents relating to medical practices frequently, but not exclusively, mention the gods and other supernatural entities as key to disease etiology and treatment, this study looks at the prominent theology for each culture as a way to understand their particular forms of an explanatory model of illness.

As the chapters examine the different cultural concepts governing issues of physiology and anatomy, a pattern can be discerned as the ancient Near East and Mediterranean transform into a Hellenistic worldview. Guiding principles such as community cohesion now must integrate with a growing sense of individualism. This can be traced to the popularity of later Roman works such as Galen's *De Locis Affectis*. Modern scholarship such as *Medicine and Space* analyzes this swinging pendulum, with essays on the tendency in late antiquity through the Middle Ages, to look at physiology as simply understanding form following function, while the early modern period begins to redevelop theories of organs and systems working together.[8]

## Healers

Most societies have a multiplicity of healers from which patients can choose; this is known as medical pluralism. Different factors such as economics, location, and especially an explanatory model of illness can determine the types of healers consulted. Yet patients experiencing one episode of illness may seek aid from more than one type of healer. A friend may be consulted at the onset of symptoms, but their persistence can lead to seeking out a more powerful or authoritarian healer, what anthropologists term the hierarchy of resort. Each "rung" on the hierarchy may have a different explanatory model of illness or concentrate on a particular aspect within a culturally dominant explanatory model.

Typically, scholars divide the hierarchy of resort into three broad categories of Professional, Popular, and Folk, based on not only the explanatory model of illness but also factors such as remuneration and education. The professional healer is sanctioned by other authority structures in society, religious and political ones being the most frequent. The professional healer may even be a part of one of these, such as a priest. Often, there is an internal

8. Patricia A. Baker, Han Nijdam, and Karine van 't Land, eds., *Medicine and Space: Body, Surroundings, and Borders in Antiquity and the Middle Ages* (Leiden: Brill, 2011).

hierarchy of specialists within this professional category. These healers tend to concentrate in urban centers, near the other power structures.

In contrast, the popular healer is a nonprofessional and nonspecialist, such as a family member, and usually the first to be consulted. The patient recognizes the healer's authority in health matters as drawing from naturally accruing wisdom and experience. The folk healer is a nonprofessional specialist with ties to religious structures that are not part of the dominant culture. This term is often a catch-all in studies where the popular and professional labels do not easily apply. It also betrays a colonial perspective that marginalizes authority not directly linked to preferred power structures. The overlap of these different categorizations for healers, especially as they cross cultural boundaries, has recently undergone more nuanced studies, at least in terms of Greco-Roman medicine.[9]

The classification of ancient healers into these categories is difficult. Most textual sources come from an elite class that attest to what could be called the professional healer. Some archaeological evidence may indicate popular or even folk medicine, but we lack the necessary type of evidence to make a discernment. Additionally, a clear division between folk and professional itself is questionable and only serves to replicate a distinction between a secular biomedical system, favored by Western powers over what is considered "ethnomedicine" in colonized areas.[10] To avoid these anachronistic complications, this study does not strictly delineate a specific hierarchy of resort for the different ancient Near Eastern and Mediterranean cultures. The terms for healers in their original languages are retained as much as possible, eschewing the typical translations such as "magician" and "physician." Exceptions to this rule occur when the texts use a term for a magician/sorcerer that is commonly understood as such in a nonmedical context. Similarly, "physician" is used for the Greek *iatros*. There is also an attempt to note the contexts in which a patient may move between the various types of available healers, without assigning a hierarchical status to them but noting that many are intimately connected to established power structures.

9. William V. Harris, ed., *Popular Medicine in Graeco-Roman Antiquity: Explorations* (Leiden: Brill, 2016).

10. Byron J. Good, *Medicine, Rationality, and Experience: An Anthropological Perspective* (Cambridge: Cambridge University Press, 2008).

### Patients

Anthropological and even historical studies on modern medical cultures benefit from the availability of information generated by the patients themselves in order to illuminate the social-cultural contexts, especially power structures in the patient-healer relationship. Such accounts are rare for the ancient world, with the exception of a few letters, usually from the elite classes, attesting to their experiences. More often, the patient's perspective must be gleaned from literary descriptions or comments about them by attending healers such as Hippocrates, Galen, and Soranus.[11] These sources also carry an inherent bias toward an elite understanding of the patient-healer-disease relationship. It is with this caveat that the study of ancient Near Eastern and Mediterranean medicine proceeds.

## Overview of Chapters

Each chapter typically begins by outlining the location and providing a brief political history of the society. A description of the culture follows with a focus on the main cosmological principles and the supernatural entities such as gods, spirits, and deified personages most important to their medical theories. Each chapter gives an overview of the main sources, both primary and secondary, relating to medicine. This section looks at not only the actual medical texts, but also literature and government documents, as well as artistic representations of the body. In addition, prominent archaeological sites and artifacts are addressed. Once this background is set, each chapter then looks at the dominant ideologies or cultural concepts for the components of the explanatory model of illness: anatomy and physiology, disease etiology, and restoration of health. The types of illness experienced are then discussed using paleopathological research, as well as social behaviors. Finally, the types of healers are analyzed. These sections should not be considered exhaustive or definitive but as highlighting key points for a broad overview. In many cases, more extensive monographic studies exist for each of these topics and should be consulted for a more in-depth and nuanced understanding of individual medical cultures.

11. Georgia Petridou and Chiara Thuminger, eds., *Homo Patiens—Approaches to the Patient in the Ancient World* (Leiden: Brill, 2016).

## Mesopotamia

The chapter on Mesopotamian medicine lays the groundwork for understanding the interplay of communities in a polytheistic society, specifically the relationship between humans, nature, and the supernatural worlds. This idea of community influences their conception of anatomy and physiology as symbiotic, yet another form of community. Focusing on the importance of community captures the Mesopotamian cosmology, because of its hierarchy of wills as well as the need for obedience and consideration for community cohesion. The power of representation in word or image also shows that the Mesopotamian understanding of the body, illness, and healing is communicative. This first chapter addressing a particular culture reinforces the definitions of key anthropological terms. As the study progresses, such repetitions will lessen in favor of highlighting their cultural applications.

## Egypt

The chapter on Egypt is the first encounter with a physiological system that relies upon a concept like irrigation/plumbing and balance as unifying the parts of the body. Egyptian medicine further highlights the idea of community and communication. These ideas incorporate the Egyptian cosmological view of balance, order, and justice (*maat*). This chapter also addresses in more detail the process of accessing supernatural power (*heka*) germane to many ancient medical practices. Access to supernatural power becomes paramount, given the ancient tendency to make the deity that sent an illness the same entity that can cure it, rather than strictly dividing disease etiology and healing between two different gods. A unique feature of Egyptian medicine is the layout for writing some of the medical texts and the formal declaration of one's ability to heal, not heal, or contend with the illness.

## Canaan

Most treatments of medical practices in the Levant completely overlook the Canaanites, focusing instead on the Israelites—a natural tendency since the Hebrew Bible is our most significant textual source for the area during the Late Bronze to Early Iron Age. This chapter tries to address medicine in the Hebrew Bible within its larger Canaanite context. Additionally, the chapter looks exclusively at the Hebrew Bible, leaving talmudic medicine for a later chapter, in its more appropriate Hellenistic world. In order to fully understand healing for the Israelites and other Canaanites, the role of priests and prophets in Levantine medical pluralism is highlighted in the context of a cosmology based on covenants that create and govern the human and supernatural communities. Interestingly, the passages of the Hebrew Bible addressing the priest's role in healing also show a connection between medicine in the Levant and ancient Egypt, indicating the trafficking of medical knowledge apart from the itinerant healer.

## Hittites

The Hittite kingdoms existed at a crossroad between the eastern Mediterranean and the Near East, thus attesting to a blend of cultures. An interesting feature of Hittite cosmology is the claim that gods from other regions willingly joined their pantheon who then met in a council yet retained their native languages. Some of their healing prayers take the form of legal cases, indicating a contractual nature to their idea of community, especially with the gods, much like the cosmology of the Israelites. Their medical culture similarly reflects this syncretizing tendency, demonstrating the fluidity with which healers could move throughout the ancient world without abandoning their original cultural context that informs their explanatory model of illness. The body itself could be just as malleable, particularly with regard to gender; the body functioned as a whole, not according to specific anatomy. This shows a deviation from the beliefs of their Near Eastern counterparts, according to which body parts could have relationships with the supernatural apart from the person as a whole.

## Classical Greece

The previously studied cultures overlapped the categories of disease etiology between natural, individual, social, and supernatural. It is with the Greeks that medical texts begin to focus on the natural etiologies. Certain healers start with the premise that the supernatural links to the natural world in a regular and predictable manner. Therefore, in their view, the natural world should be the primary concern of medicine rather than the gods. Yet Greek medicine still adheres to the common medical principles that the body and illness are communicative and rooted in community cohesion. This chapter explores the coexistence of medical practices of the Asklepiads and the Hippocratics, without falling into the false dichotomy of religious and scientific medicine competing for patients, as the standard history of medicine depicts.

### Hellenism and Hellenistic Medicine: A Brief Introduction

The success of Alexander and his armies changed the political, social, linguistic, and scientific cultures of the ancient world. This brief chapter introduces some key changes in the Hellenistic period, as well as some important figures and texts, aiming to orient readers to the concluding chapters of this volume. As the focus on this book is on the medical culture of Mesopotamia, Egypt, Greece, Rome, the Levant, the Anatolian Peninsula, and the Iranian Plateau, this chapter is necessarily brief. The reader with a focused interest in this period can find helpful resources in the bibliography.

### Ptolemaic Egypt

The chapter on Ptolemaic Egypt marks a shift from a dominant religious culture greatly influencing the prominent medical culture of a society to one in which there may well be a distinction between professional and folk or popular medicine. The professional class of healers tied to the ruling Greek Ptolemies seemed to operate separately from the common Egyptian, who likely held onto his or her indigenous medical culture. The professional healers under the Ptolemies maintained the Greek tradition of writing treatises, arguing with each other in the Hellenistic world rather than trying to win patients away from traditional Egyptian medical practitioners. This focus on philosophical argumentation characterizes Ptolemaic medicine as being far more experimental than its ancient counterparts. Yet this also allowed it to incorporate many ideas from Egyptian medicine, underscoring the lack of competition between Greek and Egyptian medicine.

### Etruscans and Rome

The chapter on Rome starts with the Etruscan and early Roman understanding that supernatural entities exist in the natural realm. This cosmology would allow for Roman adoption of Greek medicine, in which nature obeyed predictable rules laid out by the gods. Roman healers thus engaged in their own epistemological arguments, vying for philosophical if not clinical authority. Yet, like the Greeks, the Romans blended more direct religious practices into their medical culture with the concept of piety as the basis for both disease etiology and healing. Piety or its lack greatly determined the character of Roman relationships with the gods on the personal as well as the state level. This could manifest itself in individual episodes of illness, as well as plagues sweeping the republic or empire. The prominence of blood libations in religious ceremonies also seems to have influenced the role of blood in physiology, as well as in the popular Roman therapeutic technique of bloodletting. The chapter takes as its end point the career of Galen, whose anatomical work on gladiators and championing of bloodletting influenced European medical practices well past the medieval period.

## Second Temple and Early Rabbinic Judaism

The Levant stood within the eastern half of the Roman Empire, but its population did not entirely adopt Greco-Roman medical culture. Various Jewish sects maintained their own medical practices, in keeping with their particular theology of covenantal monotheism, as expressed in the Hebrew Bible. This chapter focuses on the development of medicine in early rabbinic Judaism, insofar as sources are available in the Talmud. This work treats Jewish healers and medicine in a separate chapter on Second Temple Judaism rather than as part of the cultures in the diaspora, such as Alexandria, since there was an attempt to make a community that crossed physical and political boundaries. Here, there is an interesting comparison between the developments in Jerusalem and Babylon, which lay on the fringe of Roman domination. There is a problem of the degree to which Jewish communities interacted with their Hellenistic neighbors. Talmud's prohibition on Greek learning[12] shows that the rabbinic community consciously tried not to blend with them, but apart from that, and even within it, there does seem to be some overlap especially in the realm of medicine.[13] An interesting debate occurs in the talmudic books concerning the efficacy of bloodletting, indicat-

12. Bava Qamma 82b, Sotah 49b, and Menahot 64b.

13. Stephen T. Newmyer, "Talmudic Medicine and Greco-Roman Science: Crosscurrents and Resistance," *ANRW* 37.3:2895–911.

ing an inevitable cultural merge. Additionally, they share the Greco-Roman attention to anatomy in order to better understand and enforce purity laws; this is their own method of establishing epistemological authority. These similarities demonstrate that, as populations adhere to an overarching medical culture for the Mediterranean and Near East, they still negotiate its basic tenets with their particular cosmological beliefs.

### Persia

Closing out this study is the chapter on Persian medicine. Despite the long history of various cultures from the Iranian Plateau, this chapter focuses mostly on the Achaemenid, Parthian, and Sasanian dynasties rather than the earlier Elamites and Medes. This creates a challenge when organizing this study chronologically, since the Achaemenids date to the sixth through the fourth centuries BCE, while the Parthian and Sasanians existed in a more decisively Hellenistic to late antique context. The prominence of Zoroastrianism as a key feature to medicine in these dynasties determines the chapter's position. The Achaemenids gave official weight to Zoroastrianism, but the majority of available sources date to the later Parthian and especially Sasanian periods. This allows the chapter to act as a bridge between the ancient and medieval worlds, much like the analysis of early rabbinic medical culture. Unlike the other cultures of the Mediterranean and Near East, Persian medicine centers on Zoroastrian cosmology and its dualistic struggle between Good and Evil. Rather than the body being a communicative tool indicating a balance of relationships between human and supernatural communities, it is simply a battle ground, with care of the physical body as an act of preserving the greater cosmic Good.

### Absence of Christianity

The absence of a chapter devoted to Christianity might at first be striking in a work collating the medical cultures of the ancient Mediterranean and Near East. For this work, Christianity is not being considered as a subset of Second Temple Judaism, although its formation does occur in the time and place of other sects such as rabbinic Judaism. It is during the late first century CE that Christianity begins the process of seeing itself as something different from Judaism. The development and codification of Christian texts shaping a "Christian cultural approach" to medicine happens with the closing of the Christian canon in the fourth century CE, a point after this study's cut-off at the turn from the second to the third century CE. Although the New Testament texts developed from Hellenism and Israelite religion/Judaism, a separate study would need to be done in order to do justice to the various cultural settings for Christian medicine as they developed from Judaism and Hellenistic practices, especially later Byzantine ones, as well as the infiltration of indigenous medical cultures in areas as far apart as Armenia and Germanic Europe. It is with hope that this study, along with Ferngren's *Medicine and Health Care in Early Christianity*,[14] would work as a foundation for a more in-depth analysis of the development of medical ideas and practices in early Christian culture within the larger context of late antique medicine.

14. Gary B. Ferngren, *Medicine and Health Care in Early Christianity* (Baltimore: Johns Hopkins University Press, 2009).

# 2. Mesopotamian Medicine

## Location and History

Mesopotamia lies between the Tigris and Euphrates Rivers in what is modern-day Iraq. The run-off from the rivers made for a rich soil perfect for farming. Consequently, many textbooks label this area the Fertile Crescent and credit it with the first cities and one of the first civilizations to use writing.

At its most southern point, the two rivers converge into the Persian Gulf, which is the location of the earliest Mesopotamian civilization, called Sumer, with Ur as its most prominent city. The earliest Sumerian cities, though, date to 5400 BCE and flourished until 2234 BCE, when Sargon of Akkad conquered them. A brief renaissance occurred for Sumer in 2047–1750 BCE.

Moving up the rivers north and west from the marshlands of Sumer, Babylonia is the next significant territory within Mesopotamia. The rise of Babylonia is marked by the first law code from Urukagina, the king of Lagash in 2350 BCE. The most notable ruler of Babylonia was Hammurabi (1795–1750 BCE). The fortunes of Babylonia waxed and waned until the Persian king Cyrus conquered Mesopotamia in 539 BCE.

Even farther to the north, approaching the foothills of the Zagros and Taurus mountain chains, lies the region of Assyria, which rose to prominence with the founding of the city of Ashur in 1900 BCE. The Assyrian cities also won and lost control of Mesopotamia, until the Babylonians caused their final collapse in 612 BCE.

It is important to understand that, in this ancient period, there was no nation called Mesopotamia or even ones called Sumer, Babylonia, and Assyria. Each city was its own independent political entity or city-state. Kings or high-priests took charge of the city-state. As cities rose in power, they would control an expanding territory, becoming kingdoms or empires. At times, these would be known by the name of the most powerful city, such as Ur, Akkad, or Babylon. Other times, they are known by the names given to a common culture, linking the cities beyond just political domination. Serving as examples of such cultural links, Assyria and Babylonia both used the Akkadian language and worshiped the same pantheon of gods. The naming of kingdoms/empires by the culture is where we get the names Sumer, Babylonia, and Assyria. In the case of Babylonia, the culture derived its name from the politically powerful city of Babylon. Assyria also derived its name from the city of Ashur, though the capital of its empire moved around to other cities, such as Nineveh.

The proximity of the three regions meant not only did they jockey for political domination, but the oldest of the three, Sumer, influenced the cultural development of the other two. Although Sumer used a different language from Assyria and Babylonia and thus had different names for the gods, they still shared the same ideology of how the gods behaved and how to worship them. It is this common culture that allows us to look at Mesopotamia as a whole when investigating its ancient medical practices.

## Religion and Culture

Ancient Near Eastern cultures did not regularly use a post-Enlightenment scientific method that separates the natural and supernatural worlds. Divine or supernatural entities significantly influenced the human body. To fully understand how the interactions of these realms are significant for health care, we must first take a brief look at the Mesopotamian cosmology.

### Cosmology

All elements of the world, such as trees, rivers, and even the wind, have wills or a type of conscious power.[1] Where modern thought would classify these as natural elements and then explain how the Mesopotamians believed in a supernatural spirit inhabiting the element, the ancient Mesopotamians tended to link the physical entity and the spirit as one. For them, the supernatural meant an entity with greater power than mortals, like ghosts, spirits,[2]

1. A more detailed explanation of the Mesopotamian concept of wills and the interaction of powers can be found in Thorkild Jacobsen, "Mesopotamia," in *The Intellectual Adventure of Ancient Man*, ed. Henri Frankfort et al. (Chicago: University of Chicago Press, 1977), 125–219.

2. The term "spirit" is used in this context to describe supernatural entities not as powerful

and gods. Wind, water, and plants are manifestations and conduits to the greater powers. Sometimes these powerful entities will work with or submit to human actions, such as farming, and other times they will exert their own will and force, as in a storm.

Such a plethora of wills could cause chaos, as each tries to exert its power over another. But the "continual integration of the many cosmic wills"[3] produces a natural social order or hierarchy of wills, such as the family and the state. Just as the king has subjects and some subjects have slaves, the hierarchy is paralleled with gods at the top, spirits in the middle, and humans on the bottom rung. Mesopotamians viewed humans as essentially slaves of the gods. Each of these groups formed communities among themselves, as well as with each other. Humans may form a community with themselves as a city or a larger empire, but they can also form a community with a god, such as the patron deity of a city.

Although an ordered system, it is still fraught with danger for the weakest entities in the hierarchy—humans. One tries to form relationships with the more powerful entities, intercessors, to offset the dangers of life. Sharing the power of gods provides protection from enemies, as well as good health for both the individual and the community. An entity at one level may beseech those higher up on behalf of those lower down. Priests are often thought of in this role, but kings are also important intercessors, as the Code of Hammurabi shows: "When lofty Anum . . . and Enlil . . . established for him in its midst an enduring kingship . . . to promote the welfare of the people."[4] The "welfare of the people" refers to their health, as well as military, economic, and legal protections normally ascribed to the king.

Knowing the character of various spirits and gods allows one to better form these necessary alliances. Within this system, obedience and consideration become important concepts. Lesser entities, humans, must show obedience to the gods, while the gods must listen to the humans. The tale of *Atra-ḫasis* exemplifies this when the god Enlil sent the *šuruppu*-disease:

---

as the gods but usually more powerful than humans. Many texts will designate these beings as "demons," but the English word imparts an inappropriate value judgment of innate evil. Some entities like Lamaštu may always play an evil role, but others, like Pazuzu, can be both harmful and beneficial. These spirits are distinct from the ghosts of deceased humans, although they both occupy the same relative power in comparison to gods and humans.

3. Jacobsen, "Mesopotamia," 127.

4. James B. Pritchard, "The Code of Hammurabi," in *Ancient Near Eastern Texts Relating to the Old Testament* (Princeton: Princeton University Press, 1969), 164.

Because of their uproar sleep cannot seize me
. . . let there be chills.
The pestilence shall promptly put an end to their clamor!
Like a storm it shall blow upon them
Aches, dizziness, chills, and fever.[5]

The hero *Atra-ḫasis* eventually saves the people by imploring the god Enki, who advises him to withhold sacrifices to the gods, with the exception of Namtar, a harbinger of death. Humans then showed obedience to one particular god. Namtar's guilt over receiving the sole sacrifices causes him to revoke the *šuruppu*-disease.[6] His guilt shows his consideration of humans but also his nervousness about now being outside the community of the other gods.

The fundamental principle behind Mesopotamian health care is the relationship between powerful entities. The body becomes a medium by which the various entities communicate their power. Symptoms convey encoded messages to the afflicted and his community. For this reason, explanations of physiological processes such as digestion or circulation have no to little importance in their medical texts. The focus is on reading the symptom and conveying a message of obedience to the natural hierarchy.

Since the natural hierarchy of gods, spirits, and humans is key to understanding Mesopotamian medicine, let us look at a few of the important figures in their pantheon. Ancient Mesopotamians believed not only in multiple gods but also that they often acted as an assembly or divine council. Like the various city-states rising and falling in political importance, so too do the gods. This will have an effect on the character of Mesopotamian medicine over the course of the area's history from 5400 to 539 BCE. In the following descriptions, the Sumerian name of the deity is given first, with the Akkadian following.

5. James B. Pritchard, "Atra-Ḫasis," in *Ancient Near Eastern Texts Relating to the Old Testament* (Princeton: Princeton University Press, 1969), 104–6.

6. Stephanie Dalley, *Myths from Mesopotamia* (New York: Oxford University Press, 2008), 20.

## Mesopotamian Gods and Goddesses of Disease and Healing

### *Marduk*

He began as the patron deity of the city of Babylon. Various localities called him the "bull-calf of the sun," as well as the son Enki. His attributes include wisdom, judgment, magic, water, and vegetation. As Babylonian political power grew, Marduk came to be known as the head of the divine council. This position of supreme power, even within the supernatural realm, made him a natural recourse for alleviating illness. A number of medical incantations refer to him as healer of the gods.

### *Gula*

Although any divine entity can be sought for healing and protection from diseases and injuries, the most consistently prominent one linked to medical practices is the goddess Gula. She is first mentioned during the Early Dynastic period in tablets from the city of Fara (2600–2450 BCE). As the patron deity for the city of Isin, she is called Ninisina or "Lady of Isin." She also becomes a syncretization of healing deities from other cities as well and so takes on the names Ninkarak, Baba, and Nintinuga, which means "Lady who gives life to the dead." Her attributes include healing hands, soothing bandages, and dangerous scalpels, and she is usually depicted accompanied by a dog. She assists in childbirth and takes on some of the characteristics of the divine midwife Ninmah. Her consort is the god Ninurta, a farmer-warrior god noted for defeating the Asag and his stone army, which became the mountains from which the Tigris and Euphrates flow. Gula cures ailments of the skin, abdomen, and the connective tissue of muscles, tendons, ligaments, and blood vessels. Just as Gula may heal, she can also cause diseases. This is a feature common to all deities in the ancient world, in that they control both the negative and positive aspects of their elements.

### *Asalluḫi*

Gula and Asalluḫi are often paired in incantations. He is the son and assistant to Enki, which gives him dominion over the use of magic. Although childbirth usually has divine female attendants, Asalluḫi is the one male deity that assists as a midwife, likely because of his associations with magical incantations.

*Enki/Ea*

He is the god of the fresh waters of the underworld, commonly appearing with water flowing from his arms. He represents wisdom, magic, and generally arts and crafts, and he frequently takes the side of humans in their conflicts with the gods. These attributes often involve him in cases of illness.

*Inana/Ištar*

The name Inana derives from the Sumerian "Lady of Heaven." She embodies love and sexuality (though not marriage), war, and the planet Venus as the morning and evening star, which figured prominently in omens relating to childbirth. She is described as the daughter of An[7] but also of Enlil and Enki. The Akkadian name Ištar may come from the Arabian god Athtar and the Canaanite goddess Astarte. She is usually portrayed as a warrior with wings, as well as being surrounded by stars. In some accounts, Ištar is masculine, particularly when represented by the evening star, the planet Venus visible at night.

*Nergal*

Originally two distinct gods, Nergal and Erra eventually merged over time into just Nergal. A son of An, he was linked to the underworld by his consort, Ereškigal, the queen of the underworld. He ruled over forest fires, fevers, and plagues.

*Ninhursaga*

Originally a Sumerian goddess, she was viewed as the mother of the gods and credited with creating specific deities that favor humans. In this regard, many

7. An is a Sumerian god and the head of the divine council. Similarly, Enlil also has this position in later periods.

rulers claimed descent from Ninhursaga. When the sick sought help from their king, they would also look to Ninhursaga. She becomes syncretized with the goddess Ninmah, the midwife during the creation of humans. The poem *Lugale* explains how her named changed to Ninmah.

### *Utu/Shamash*

The god of the sun, he was fathered by Nanna, the moon. His twin sister is Inana. In other traditions, his father is An or Enlil. He appears at dawn at the doors of heaven, and then he returns to the interior of heaven at dusk through a set of opposite doors. He ruled over truth and justice and thus was viewed as a protector of humans in both legal and medical matters.

### *Lamaštu*

Additionally, spirits may be addressed in an ancient Mesopotamian's quest for medical help. The most significant of these are Lamaštu, Pazuzu, Namtar, and Asag. Lamaštu occupies a position somewhat between a demonic spirit and a goddess in her own right. She is considered a daughter of An and can exercise her own will rather than being confined by the directives of the gods. Depictions of her show the head of a lion, teeth and ears of a donkey or dog, a hairy body with bare breasts, feet as talons, and long, filthy finger nails. She can attack anyone but especially targets babies and pregnant women, as a type of anti-midwife. She is thought to come in on the wind.

### *Pazuzu*

Pazuzu, an underworld spirit, is also associated with wind and becomes the protector against Lamaštu's wind-borne illnesses and attacks on children.[8] Depictions of him show a dog-like face, scaly body, snake-headed penis, talons, and wings. He does not appear in the literature and iconography until the first millennium BCE.

8. Ironically, the image of Pazuzu was used to illustrate the demon possessing the teenage girl in *The Exorcist* (1973).

*Namtar*

He is a son of Enlil and serves as a minister for the underworld queen, Ereškigal. His name means "fate" or "destiny." As a spirit sending disease, he is confined to illnesses that are part of a rightful destiny ordered by the gods. He is often paired with Asag, showing a contrast in their natures.

*Asag/Asakku*

The name Asag means "smashing force," and Asakku translates as "disorder." These indicate his nature as being more capricious; his diseases are not sent by the gods but originate from his own ill-will. He generally attacks the musculoskeletal system and the skin, which puts him in direct confrontation with the goddess Gula.

## Sources

There are two broad categories of sources; one is archaeological, and the other is textual. The textual category can further subdivide into primary and secondary sources. Primary sources are texts written in the ancient world, while secondary sources are modern, scholastic texts pertaining to the topic. Böck estimates that only about 15 percent of ancient Mesopotamian medical texts, the primary sources, have been published.[9]

### Texts

Mesopotamian texts recognized as medical in nature are usually divided into two main groups: therapeutic and diagnostic. The therapeutic texts follow a standard format of symptom description, instructions for preparing and administering a remedy, and occasionally a prognosis.

> If a man gets a pulsating of the temple and has numbness, you grind dried *e'ru*-tree leaves, mix it with wheat flour, *saḫlû* and *ḫašû*-plant and with

9. Barbara Böck, *The Healing Goddess Gula: Towards an Understanding of Ancient Babylonian Medicine* (Boston: Brill, 2014), 2.

beer of a tavern keeper into a paste, you bandage him continually with them and he will recover.[10]

As the above example shows, not all the ingredients can be translated. Numerous types of trees and plants are native to Mesopotamia, so any one of them can be the *e'ru*-tree. Without knowing the exact ingredient or the exact illness, it is difficult to assess the effectiveness of the remedies. We must assume that, since they used these treatments for centuries, they had to have a fair degree of success with them.

Some therapeutic recipes call for unpleasant ingredients or *dreckapotheke*, as this poultice for a headache demonstrates, "ox-dung, gazelle-dung thou shalt pound together, [sift], in Ú.SA-beer [knead] . . . 'shell' of human skull."[11] Originally, scholars thought these prescriptions to be a form of like canceling like by fighting dreadful spirits with dreadful ingredients. More recently, researchers understand *dreckapotheke* as a type of code for various plants, used to fool imposters. A fake healer not knowing the truth would include real feces in his remedies. This would, one hopes, tip off the patient that the healer was a fake.[12] Literacy was a fairly rare skill, so it is not likely that just anyone could read the recipe. But hiring a scribe to read to you was not unusual. Also, a scribe not trained as an *asû* or *āšipu* healer could try to pick up a healing job "on the side," which could pose a threat to the professional healers.

Frequently, the remedies include incantations and rituals alongside these more natural *materia medica*.

> Ea, king who created mankind,
> Šamaš, judge who makes the teeming people go aright,
> Marduk, *āšipu* of the gods, noble god,
> Those[13] who have been angry with me for some time,

10. BAM 11; translation from Nils P. Heeßel, "The Babylonian Physician Rabâ-Ša-Marduk: Another Look at Physicians and Exorcists in the Ancient Near East," in *Advances in Mesopotamian Medicine from Hammurabi to Hippocrates*, ed. Annie Attia, Gilles Buisson, and Markham J. Geller (Boston: Brill, 2009), 27.

11. R. Campbell Thompson, "Assyrian Prescriptions for the Head," *American Journal of Semitic Languages and Literatures* 54 (1937): 21.

12. Markham J. Geller, *Ancient Babylonian Medicine Theory and Practice* (Oxford: Wiley-Blackwell, 2010), 53.

13. Unlike in English, the demonstrative article does not refer to the previously named gods Ea, Šamaš, and Marduk; instead, the construction refers to an unnamed entity that sent the demon.

Wind from an evil mouth has been blown into me; an evil
*rabiṣu*-demon,
Which has been set on me so that it continually pursues me,
Struck the top of my head (so hard that) I bit my tongue;
He struck my legs; my arms were (magically) bound;
He has fallen on me so that he has knocked me over.
That unknown ghost
I have made a figurine of him. I have cried out to you, great gods
. . . .
(Ea), warrior, by your august command, (and)
Šamaš, judge, remove him from my body so that
He may not return to cause me confusional states.
May he swear by your oath to cross over (and be gone).[14]

Many cases will simply state "charm" after the list of ingredients, while the incantation to be recited is placed before or after a set of cases. These will typically call upon the god(s) associated with the disease or body part or just hold a high place in the pantheon.

The diagnostic texts take the form of standard omen literature, with an "if . . . then" construction. Some cases readily appear medical, in terms of looking at the patient's physiology as the omen, but their ultimate diagnosis sounds less scientific. "When a man is heavily feverish and he finds no relief, he burps and coughs and his stomach always turns to vomit, he is sick due to an oath."[15] Other omens are easily mistaken for a pure magic-religious text, with very little connection to the patient's physical condition (e.g., "If a hawk crosses the sky to the left, the sick one will die").[16] Some omens actually combine the medical prognosis and a military outcome (e.g., "If [I throw oil into water and] the oil divides itself into two—the sick person will die; for the campaign: the army will not return.").[17] This type of omen indicates that the pattern of a division equating to a negative outcome has greater value in Mesopotamian culture than investigating each case with a scientific method. It is important to remember that these diagnoses and therapies developed

14. Scurlock, *Magico-Medical Means*, 347.

15. Nils P. Heeßel, *Babylonisch-assyrische Diagnostik*, Alter Orient und Altes Testament (Münster: Ugarit-Verlag, 2000), 253–54, 259.

16. René Labat, *Traité akkadien de diagnostics et prognostics médicaux* (Paris: Académie internationale d'histoire de sciences, 1951), 6–7.

17. William W. Hallo and K. Lawson Younger Jr., eds., *The Context of Scripture: Canonical Compositions* (Boston: Brill, 2003), 423.

from clinical experience rather than an independent process of laboratory testing. Rather than looking at patterns within a case, Mesopotamians apply a culturally acceptable pattern to the cases.

Because divination patterns apply to medical cases, as well as any other situation, many of the Mesopotamian medical texts have been frequently grouped with omen or other religious ritual texts rather than identified and compiled as medical texts *per se*. Consequently, they tend to be widely scattered throughout the literature and create a false dichotomy between "scientific" and "magic-religious" medicine. More recently, scholarship is moving away from the division of diagnostic and therapeutic texts, showing how the different types of texts are integrated in Mesopotamian health care.[18]

A majority of primary sources now commonly used in the history of Mesopotamian medicine were not grouped together until the nineteenth and twentieth centuries. The SA.GIG series of tablets compiled in the ancient period is an exception to this. Yet the modern grouping of texts now reveals other ancient tablet series, such as *utukki limnūti* (ghost trouble) and *šumma amēlu muḫḫašu umma ukāl*[19] (if a man's head holds fever), which were likely subsets of larger collections. These modern compilations contain some overlap, due to the fact that duplicates of ancient texts were found at different archaeological sites throughout Mesopotamia. This attests to their widespread use but also shows that Mesopotamian healers did not strictly adhere to a single canon of medical texts. Variations can be found according to region, with certain texts gaining prominence, while others may have fallen out of favor over time. The following is a brief survey of the most frequently cited collections of Mesopotamian medical texts.

SA.GIG is a Sumerian logogram,[20] originally meaning "sick cords," and was used synonymously with Akkadian *sakikkû*, translated as "symptom."[21] It refers to a collection of tablets that list symptoms and omens by which the *āšipu* may make a diagnosis and prognosis. Different recensions of the catalog were compiled in the ancient world. The earliest datable tablets making up the collection come from the reign of Adad-apla-iddina (1067–1046 BCE), a Babylonian king from the Second Dynasty of Isin. But there is speculation that some may be as early as the Middle Babylonian period (1595–1000 BCE).[22]

18. Geller, *Ancient Babylonian Medicine Theory and Practice*, 89.

19. Tablets from this series are commonly referenced with the simple abbreviation UGU.

20. It is convention to transliterate Sumerian using all capital letters.

21. J. V. Kinnier Wilson, "Two Medical Texts from Nimrud," *Iraq* 18 (1956): 130–46.

22. Martin Stol, *Epilepsy in Babylon* (Groningen: Styx, 1993).

Several tablets preserve the names of two ancient scribes who compiled the SA.GIG series. The first is Ešguziš, whose name means "toward Ešguzi," a reference to the Esagil or "Lofty House," a temple to Marduk in Babylon. Ešguziš claimed to be revising an older collection of the SA.GIG and dated his new version of the tablets to the reign of the Babylonian king Marduk-apli-iddina II (721–710 BCE). The second scribe was Esagil-kin-apli, who worked during the reign of the Assyrian king Assurbanipal (668–627 BCE). The tablets of Esagil-kin-apli comprise the majority of tablets used in Labat's modern translation *Traité akkadien de diagnostics et prognostics médicaux* (TDP).[23] More recently, Heeßel's *Babylonisch-assyrische Diagnostik* updates the translation in German.[24]

Although the rulers of Assyria and Babylonia frequently fought for control over the region of Mesopotamia, the use of the SA.GIG/*sakikkû* series attests to the strong cultural continuity among healers that lasted down to the Persian period (525–404 BCE), at which point the tablet series fell out of use.

A large body of anti-witchcraft texts can be found as early as the second millennium and appear to have been used almost to the end of the first millennium BCE. These contain a blend of magical and medical practices, showing there was no clear distinction between the two. *Maqlû* (burning), dated to the early first millennium, is one of the more important tablet series. Abusch has published extensively on the format, content, and significance of the *maqlû* series, summarizing it as a description of the necessary elements for one long, complex ceremony performed through the night and into the early morning hours at the end of July/beginning of August, a time of year when entities could move more easily between the natural and supernatural realms. The participants are the *āšipu* and the patient.

By the beginning of the twentieth century, modern scholars began to systematize and analyze the varied medical tablets. Published in 1904, Küchler's *Beitrage zur Kenntnis der assyrisch-babylonischen Medizin* is an attempt to compile three texts based on ten tablet fragments from the Kuyunjik collection in the British Museum.[25] The fact that the tablets needed to be joined by modern scholars indicates the problematic nature of reconstructing a corpus of medical texts for ancient Mesopotamia. This work helped

23. Labat, *Traité akkadien de diagnostics et prognostics médicaux.*

24. Heeßel, *Babylonisch-assyrische Diagnostik.*

25. Friedrich Küchler, *Beitrage zur Kenntnis der assyrisch-babylonischen Medizin* (Leipzig: J. C. Hinrichs, 1904).

scholars recognize that the tablets were part of a larger series, now referred to as *utukki limnūti* (ghost trouble).

Similarly, from 1916 to 1923, Ebeling published the four-volume work *Keilschrifttexte medizinischen Inhalts* (KMI),[26] which transliterated and translated into German a number of tablets from the British Kuyunjik collection and the Vorderasiatisches Museum, a part of the Pergamon in Berlin.[27]

The Assyrian Medical Texts (AMT), published between 1907 and 1937, is an attempt to compile the 660 medical tablets from the Kuyunjik collection[28] in the British Museum. These tablets came from the library of Assurbanipal at his capital in Nineveh, which contained roughly five thousand literary and scholarly texts. The scribes at Nineveh copied these from sources gathered mostly from the temples and priests in Babylonia. Because of this scribal activity, the tablets used for AMT date to the seventh century BCE. Yet these are likely copies of much older texts. Each case may be older than the composition of the text in which we find them. A scribe writing in the seventh century may be using a contemporary case, but then the next case was actually written earlier in the 22nd century. The scribe included it without change. So scholars date a tablet to the seventh century, but parts of it may be older. One tablet, K. 4023 in the AMT collection, mentions "the ancient rulers before the flood that was in Shurippak," with a date for the second year of Enlil-bani, king of Isin (2201–2177 BCE). Further complicating the question about the original date of composition for the cases in the texts is the fact that scribes would often claim an older source in order to justify the authority of the text. The regnal date in K. 4023 may be an ancient fiction.

*Babylonisch-assyrische Medizin* (BAM) originally was a six-volume series edited by Franz Köcher from 1963 to 1980.[29] These collect therapeutic tablets from Assur, Nineveh, Nippur, and Babylon. Each volume is based on tablets from a particular city, but often the fragments that make up a single text are spread across different museum collections, in London, Berlin, Istanbul, Paris, and Brussels. A seventh volume, focusing on renal and rectal diseases, was published in 2005.[30] With this new volume, the series will now focus on compiling texts thematically rather than by location.

26. Erich Ebeling, *Keilschrifttexte medizinischen Inhalts* (Berlin: Selbstverlag, 1916–23).

27. Tablets in this collection are designated by VAT, followed by a catalog number.

28. These tablets are typically referred to as K., followed by their catalog number.

29. Franz Köcher, *Babylonisch-assyrische Medizin in Texten und Untersuchungen* (Berlin: de Gruyter, 1963–1980).

30. Markham J. Geller, *Babylonisch-assyrische Medizin: Renal and Rectal Disease Texts* (Berlin: de Gruyter, 2005).

A comparison of SA.GIG and BAM shows a difference between the writing of omens for therapeutic and diagnostic texts, which Geller interprets as a difference in "workshops" that produced the two types of texts.[31] Similarly, he divides the libraries at Nineveh and Assur. He considers texts from Nineveh as reference works for a major compendium on medicine, while the tablets from Assur were for lecturers or practical applications, in essence a textbook. Problematically, though, there is an overlap of recipes in SA.GIG and BAM, which calls into question such a clear distinction between the uses of the original tablets. Complicating the matter is the fact that so many of the surviving texts come from large collections made by kings or priests, who engage in such an intellectual "arms race" as a display of power.

The Harran Plain in southeastern Anatolia linked the cultures of Mesopotamia with the Levant and Mediterranean. The site of Sultantepe on the plain's western edge flourished in the Neo-Assyrian period of the eighth and seventh centuries BCE. Excavations revealed nearly six hundred tablets associated with a priestly family. Gurney published the Sultantepe Tablets (STT) in two volumes, with about fifty-one identified as medical texts.[32] Additionally, these tablets contain other texts pertaining to health care in Mesopotamia, such as the *namburbi* ritual, which attempts to thwart bad omens. *Namburbi* rituals, typically performed by an *āšipu*, involve the smashing of clay vessels inscribed with the name of the misfortune, such as a disease. STT also includes the ghost series *utukki limnūti*.

The study of health care and medicine in ancient Mesopotamia lacks a concise, collated body of all primary texts. Scurlock's recent work on ancient Mesopotamian medicine comes closest, compiling the diagnostic, prognostic, and therapeutic series of tablets.[33] These are grouped according to anatomical and physiological ailments. We have yet to find any theoretical discourse from the ancient Mesopotamians on physiology and likely will not. Mesopotamian literature did not focus on philosophical discussions. This makes it difficult but not impossible to deduce an overall picture of how they understood certain concepts such as physiology or the role of the *asû* and *āšipu* healers. Worthington, adopting categories of patient-healer

31. Geller, *Ancient Babylonian Medicine Theory and Practice*, 91.

32. O. R. Gurney and J. J. Finkelstein, eds., *The Sultantepe Tablets I* (London: British Institute of Archaeology at Ankara, 1957); O. R. Gurney and J. J. Finkelstein, eds., *Sultantepe Tablets II* (London: British Institute of Archaeology at Ankara, 1964).

33. Scurlock, *Sourcebook*.

interaction,[34] tries to address how nonmedical texts like letters can be used to fill these gaps.[35]

The archives of the Assyrian kings Esarhaddon (680–669 BCE) and Assurbanipal (668–627 BCE) contain letters to and from the court healers, both *asû* and *āšipu*.[36] These give us a better understanding of the working conditions of healers, as well as the concerns of the patients. Similarly, letters from Tell al-Rimah and the kingdom of Mari give us an indication of health care during the reigns of the Assyrian Šamši-Adad (1808–1776 BCE), the Babylonian Hammurabi (1792–1750 BCE), and Zimri-Lim of Mari (1775–1762 BCE).[37] It should be kept in mind that these letters reveal life only among the elite classes associated with the court of the king. How healers and patients interacted for the peasant class is, for the most part, unattested.

Governmental texts, such as the Code of Hammurabi, can reveal information on healers in terms of payment or restitution for malpractice. Yet the propaganda function of these law codes should be considered when used to reconstruct the life and social role of healers. Quite often such law codes contain much harsher penalties than what records of actual legal cases indicate. Additionally, the law codes mention the *asû*'s use of a lancet for incisions and the reduction of fractures. Neither surgery nor fractures appear in the medical texts.

The literature of a culture can also indicate the character of health care and healers. But, just like the pitfalls of the law codes, literary depictions cannot be taken at face value. They may represent an ideal form or an exaggeration of problems. Two tactics used by ancient writers to make their points are mediation of tales/reports and acceptable embellishments. An author/scribe can choose what symptoms or contextual elements to include and which ones are unimportant to the overall message of the text. This mediation effects symptoms in the therapeutic texts as much as it colors

34. Laura M. Zucconi, "Can No Physician Be Found?" (PhD diss., University of California San Diego, 2005); Arthur Kleinman, *Patients and Healers in the Context of Culture* (Berkeley: University of California Press, 1980).

35. Martin Worthington, "Some Notes on Medical Information outside the Medical Corpora," in *Advances in Mesopotamian Medicine from Hammurabi to Hippocrates* (Boston: Brill, 2009), 47–77.

36. Steven W. Cole, Peter Machinist, and Simo Parpola, eds., *Letters from Priests to the Kings Esarhaddon and Assurbanipal*, State Archives of Assyria (Helsinki: Helsinki University Press, 1999); Simo Parpola, *Letters from Assyrian Scholars to the Kings Esarhaddon and Assurbanipal* (Winona Lake, IN: Eisenbrauns, 2007).

37. S. Dalley, C. B. F. Walker, and J. D. Hawkins, eds., *The Old Babylonian Tablets from Tell al Rimah* (London: British School of Archaeology in Iraq, 1976).

the mythic stories. Knowing the literature beyond the immediate medically oriented passage in question can help discern patterns to the style of mediation in Mesopotamian texts. Similarly, for authors/scribes to make a point stand out, they can alter or embellish "historical facts." This is most obvious in reported speeches and battle accounts, but patterns of embellishment appear in all types of writing.

Yet one should not discount these literary texts. Because ancient writers did not distinguish between scientific and theological, nor even fiction and nonfiction, as precise categories, any text with reference to sickness, healing, and healers can supply valuable information. Although scribes use mediation and embellishment, they cannot write something too wildly different from the cultural norm, or the audience will not accept the authenticity of the text. The key for medical historians is to develop a sense of the cultural norm.

Obvious examples of informative theological texts come from the many hymns to Gula, a healing goddess. The *Gula Hymn of Bullutsa-rabi*, likely composed between 1400 and 700 BCE, theologically defines and organizes the pantheon relative to Gula and her consort Ninurta.[38] It did not serve any purpose in an exorcism or state ritual. A few lines of a hymn, spoken from the point of view of the goddess, demonstrates their usefulness:

> I am a physician (*asû*), I am able to heal.
> I carry around all kinds of plants, I drive away illness.
> I gird myself with a leather bag with curative incantations.
> I carry around written texts which can restore good health.
> I give cures to mankind.
> My pure bandage soothes a sore.
> My soft bandage brings relief to the sick.[39]

The depiction of Gula, although on a grander scale, has many commonalities with the human *asû*, such as the use of plants, incantations, and bandages, as well as carrying a leather bag and texts. In another passage of the *Gula Hymn*, Gula describes herself as an *asû*, *bārû*, and *āšipu*, which has implications about how the different types of healers may have related to one another.

38. W. G. Lambert, "The Gula Hymn of Bullutsa-Rabi," *Orientalia* 36 (1967): 105–32.

39. Robert D. Biggs, "The Human Body and Sexuality in the Babylonian Medical Texts," in *Médecine et médecins au Proche-Orient ancien* (Oxford: British Archaeological Reports, 2006), 39.

Within the larger corpus of theological literature, one category of texts deals with the problem of theodicy. Much like the biblical story of Job, these involve a suffering man who pleads his case to a god, which often includes descriptions of illness and occasionally their treatments. These are different from incantations in which the supplicant, suffering from the hand of a ghost or spirit, simply apologizes for an unknown or unspecified transgression. Poems such as *Ludlul bel Nemeqi*[40] come closest to a philosophical exposition as to why illness and other misfortunes occur even for those who have committed no wrong. The god to whom the poem is directed acts as the ultimate cause of illness, as well as the underlying source of healing. "He [Marduk] is the one who afflicts with demons of shaking-disease / Through his sacral spell chills and shivering are driven away."[41] If one looks only at the medical texts, it would be easy to mistake the demon as the sole cause of disease, but an analysis of the theological texts reveals another layer to the etiology and can explain why some incantations appeal to gods rather than just commanding the demon to leave.

A popular story found at Nineveh and Sultantepe, *The Poor Man of Nippur*,[42] serves as an example of a nonmedical text that can help us understand healers in Mesopotamia. This comedic tale relates the fictional account of a peasant, Gimil-Ninurta, who exacts revenge on a city official for mistreating him. One of Gimil-Ninurta's schemes involves being disguised as an *asû* from Isin in order to gain entry into the official's house. Although the passage has comedic embellishments that move the plot along, such as driving pegs into the ground to tie up the mayor, the physical appearance of the *asû* and the fact that his remedies are mysterious to the patients must have some credibility to remain in the story. The story also plays up the unpleasantness of many healing tactics, which is why the mayor regards Gimil-Ninurta as a fine *asû*, but it also calls into question whether a patient would recognize the use of real excrement as the sign of a quack, which the coded *dreckapotheke* assumes. Such situations, both real and comedic, rely on the patient's intelligence, or lack thereof, regardless of social class. These details contribute valuable information for the modern analysis of Mesopotamian health care.

40. This title comes from the first line of the poem, "I will praise the lord of wisdom," but translations often give it the title *The Poem of the Righteous Sufferer*.

41. Hallo and Younger, *Context of Scripture: Canonical Compositions*, 487.

42. O. R. Gurney, "The Sultantepe Tablets V: The Tale of the Poor Man of Nippur," *Anatolian Studies* 6 (1956): 145–64.

Later texts, post-dating the heyday of the Assyrian and Babylonian Empires, as well as those from outside observers, can also be informative. Herodotus's *Histories* provides an example of both of these. Written between 450 and 425 BCE, it acts as a vehicle for Herodotus's ideals, especially reciprocity as the foundation of the world's social structure. His account of the common person's access to health care may give us a clue about the practices under Persian domination, but the description of free consultation among the townspeople, essentially crowd-sourcing for diagnosis and treatments, may not be entirely accurate.[43]

## Archaeology

Archaeological finds can often complement textual sources. Several texts reference an *asû*'s bronze lancet or Gula's obsidian blades, while some art depicts Gula holding a stick or sickle-shaped blade.[44] From the city of Babylon, sixteen surgical instruments were found dating to the first millennium BCE, while an earlier text from Ebla is a receipt for bronze instruments made for an *asû* in the mid-third millennium.[45] Much like written letters, seals from different individuals can tell us about the use of titles or iconography for healers and associated gods such as Gula.

Similarly, amulets provide ample sources of information. Archaeology has revealed amulets for Lamaštu and Pazuzu, not only in Mesopotamia proper but throughout the ancient Near East. The Lamaštu amulets contain an image of the demon/goddess on one side and a prophylactic incantation on the other. These would typically be worn by pregnant women or newborns, her favorite targets. But some amulets show a man in bed, which attests to Lamaštu as a carrier of disease in general and not just causing obstetric and pediatric problems. The idea that she can send disease on the winds gave rise to the amulets of Pazuzu, a god of the underworld who protects against wind-borne illness. These amulets took the shape of Pazuzu's head, which could be worn, usually by women, or hung by doorways.

43. Herodotus, *Histories* 1.197.

44. Dominique Collon, "Neo-Assyrian Gula in the British Museum," in *Beschreiben und Deuten in der Archäologie des Alten Orients: Feschrift für Ruth Mayer-Opificius*, ed. M. Dietrich and O. Loretz (Münster: Ugarit, 1994), 43–48.

45. Böck, *Healing Goddess Gula*, 20.

Numerous votive statues from places such as Tell Asmar, Nippur, and Mari provide other sources of information. Worshipers dedicated statues of themselves or others to specific gods in order to plead their cases or give thanks for the gods' beneficence. The votives carry an inscription giving thanks and briefly describing the situation prompting the offering, which sometimes includes a sickness.

Contrary to what one might expect, the numerous liver models that aid in interpreting divinations from animal entrails (haruspication) do not address medical issues, nor do they look like a human liver. Anatomical knowledge gained during animal sacrifices did not, for the most part, inform Mesopotamian concepts of the human body. The culture essentially forbade dissection of humans, thus limiting any type of comparative anatomy.

Even with an underrepresentation of medical tools as artifacts, archaeology can still help develop an overall picture of health care by investigating cities, temples, and priestly houses closely tied to healers and medical practices. Isin and Nippur are two such prominent archaeological sites.

From the late third millennium onward, Isin was an important city for Mesopotamia and enjoyed the reputation of being a center for learning and knowledge. The patron goddess of the city was Gula, who during the Ur III period (2112–2004 BCE) gained the title Ninisina (Mistress of Isin), as well as the epithet "great *asû* of the black-headed."[46] Her temple, Egalmah, became the location for the sacred marriage ceremony for the city's political leader. Additionally, the city had a temple to Nintinuga (a manifestation of Gula) and the Eurgira, or "dog house," a temple to Ninisina. Although this last temple is known only through an inscription from the king, Enlil-bāni (1860–1837 BCE), it served as a main cultic center from about 2000–1800 BCE. Excavations by Hrouda found a cemetery containing thirty-three dog skeletons. Associated votive figurines indicate the "dog house" likely served as a cultic site for Ninisina/Gula rather than simply a kennel.[47]

At the start of the Early Dynastic period (2900–2350 BCE), the originally Sumerian city of Nippur rose to prominence in Babylonia as the center of a fairly unified religious practice, a position that lasted until ca. 1700 BCE. For Mesopotamians, the god Enlil, head of the Mesopotamian pantheon, resided at the Ekur temple in the city, giving its priesthood considerable power. Enlil's temple, though, contained an altar, as well as a storehouse for

46. Black-headed is the phrase Sumerians used to refer to themselves.

47. A. Livingstone, "The Isin 'Dog House' Revisited," *Journal of Cuneiform Studies* 40 (1988): 54–60.

the healing goddess Nin-gagia, a manifestation of Gula. This indicates Nin-gagia/Gula held a prominent position within the pantheon and received a considerable amount of offerings to warrant a storehouse.

Nippur also had a temple complex for the goddess Nintinugga, another manifestation of Gula. This complex was large enough to have stables housing cattle offerings. Inside the temple itself, one could find a cleansing basin, or *apsû*,[48] and an altar to Lama-lugal, the king's protective deity. Additionally, Nintinugga would receive offerings at the city's temple to Ninlil, the wife/consort of Enlil. A later map of the city (ca. sixteenth or fifteenth century) indicates that one of the city gates was called Gula, attesting to her continued prominence within the city.

## Cultural Concepts

Since the hierarchy of wills in the Mesopotamian pantheon can directly affect human health, let us now examine more closely how Mesopotamians understood the causes of disease in relation to deities and their wills. It would seem obvious to a modern person what counts as an illness, but "illness" is a culturally constructed term. A simple definition for disease etiology is the causative agent, such as bacteria or a genetic mutation. But even in modern medicine, an explanation for an illness involves more than just etiology. It includes the patient and healer negotiating their understanding of physiology and treatment along with the etiology. This is what medical anthropologists term an "explanatory model of illness." It determines when someone needs treatment, who will treat the illness, and how it will be treated. Let us first look at the Mesopotamian understanding of anatomy and physiology, before addressing disease etiology and treatment.

### Anatomy and Physiology

Physiology can be defined as a "theory of the normal functioning of living organisms."[49] This brings up the question of what is normal. Normalcy is

48. The *apsû* basin derives its name from the Apsû, or primordial waters of the underworld.

49. Manfred Horstmanshoff, Helen King, and Claus Zittel, eds., *Blood, Sweat, and Tears: Changing Concepts of Physiology* (Leiden: Brill, 2012), 1.

determined according to culture, in this case Mesopotamian culture and not modern medical standards. These standards must be reconstructed from available sources, since Sumerians, Assyrians, and Babylonians did not write out any physiological explanations. Furthermore, Mesopotamians did not make a distinction between the study of anatomy (the structures/organs) and physiology (the function of structures/organs) as in modern medicine. Structures/organs and their functions were intimately linked. Quite often, their physiological concepts find expression in similes and metaphors that fall into three basic categories: object, animal, and person. In some cases, the person is named, but frequently the body part is asked a question about why it does or does not do a common human action. This is the first indication that one's anatomy is a distinct entity with a will or power of its own and that its function or physiology is communicative.

Artistic representations are the best place to start an investigation of Mesopotamian anatomy and physiology. Although the Uruk Vase (ca. 3100 BCE) shows the human body, most early artistic representations of people did not even attempt a realistic portrayal of the body. Geometric forms that suggest a human shape had nearly exclusive use during the Early Dynastic period (2900–2300 BCE). By the reign of Sargon and domination of the region by the city of Akkad (2300–2230 BCE), a more naturalistic depiction of gods and kings came to the fore, but they were still stylized, being idealized physical types rather than the realism of exact portraiture. Whether a commemorative building stela or a votive statue, this ritual iconography tended to show people well-muscled, with thick, curly hair. Texts that named the person always accompanied these images, making individual realism unnecessary, though the images were a necessary component of the rituals.[50] A stock "healthy looking" figure was not only sufficient but a key to the ritual's efficacy. The office of the king is, in essence, a religious one, being a mediator between the people and the divine. So, in the case of royal depictions, "the king's physical representation had to demonstrate that he does not possess any culturally suspect physical features if he is to be considered a legitimate candidate for the throne."[51] Similarly, a votive figure for the commoner must also indicate that the petitioner is of a sound enough body

50. Zainab Bahrani, *The Graven Image: Representation in Babylon and Assyria* (Philadelphia: University of Pennsylvania Press, 2003), 1; Zainab Bahrani, "The Babylonian Visual Image," in *The Babylonian World*, ed. Gwendolyn Leick (New York: Routledge, 2009), 155–70.

51. Jeremy Schipper, *Disability Studies and the Hebrew Bible: Figuring Mephibosheth in the David Story* (New York: T&T Clark, 2006), 74.

to be in the presence of the divine. This is true even if the petitioner is asking for a medical cure.

Art, whether symbolic or representational, embodies and represents a truth for the ancient Mesopotamians.[52] This is an important point for how they understood their world and the interactions between humans, spirits, and gods. Signifiers, word and image, become their own entities. To write a name or to make an image, even an idealized one, calls it into existence in that depicted form.

The votive statue of Lu-Nanna (1792–1750 BCE) shows a healthy body and standard male face with a short, curly beard. There are no distinguishing characteristics of the figure that would indicate the individual as Lu-Nanna. The text on the statue labels the figure Lu-Nanna. Text and figure work together, thus creating a Lu-Nanna[53] that has a healthy body, an acceptable form to appear before a god, regardless of the actual physical state of the human Lu-Nanna.

According to statuary and reliefs, the normal or cultically acceptable body of a male has well-developed upper body musculature, especially the biceps and extensors of the lower arm in profile view and the brachioradialis in frontal view; lower body musculature highlights the calves; hair is thick and curly but limited to the head and face; skin appears smooth, with the exception of occasional wrinkles on the forehead and under the eyes, perhaps denoting age;[54] and the eyes are large and symmetrical.

Females have the same features of clear skin; large, symmetrical eyes; and long, thick, curly hair. Additionally, there are representations of pubic hair, a prominent navel, wide hips, and full breasts, but these tend to be prevalent in works associated with fertility. Reliefs showing women as part of a royal court scene are clothed, thus omitting the pubic hair, navel, and dramatically wide hips. Underlying musculature is minimal—just enough to give shape to the limbs, but it does not show any sense of vigor and strength in comparison to the men.

It should be noted that the intensity of muscular depiction does carry cultural significance, much like the overall size of figures. Women are not as muscular as men, and, among men, muscular definition increases relative

52. Bahrani, *Graven Image*, 74–77.

53. Bahrani, "Babylonian Visual Image," 160.

54. Most figures appear youthful, with a few exceptions, such as the head of a king (ca. 1750 BCE) housed in the Louvre and thought to be Hammurabi. See Bahrani, *Graven Image*, 159.

to social status. The king has more definition than courtiers, soldiers, and slaves in the same scene, while a god displays larger muscles than the king. Creatures in hunt scenes, such as lions and bulls, will also have prominent musculature in their limbs, roughly on par with the kingly hero, indicating an equal and worthy opponent. The use of musculature demonstrates their anatomical knowledge but also highlights its communicative importance in the culture.

Cylinder seals, though, lack these anatomical details for both genders, with the exception of breasts for the women and beards for the men.[55] Limbs of both are devoid of clear muscle definition but tend to use more gentle sloping lines for the shoulders of women, but not exclusively so. The more geometric human form dominates seal imagery, but this is likely due to the small scale of the images, as well as a long-standing tradition of how seals should look.

Not all artistic depictions fall into clear masculine and feminine categories. The Ur-Nanshe statue from Mari and tile fragments from the Ištar Temple in Nineveh serve as examples of ambiguous gender.[56] The Ur-Nanshe statue (ca. 2400 BCE) consists of feminine features such as a clean-shaven face, wide hips, and breasts. Although the breasts are smaller than those of standard female figures, they are more prominent than the pectoral muscles of male statuary. Complicating the matter are the masculine clothing for the figure and the masculine name, Ur-Nanshe. Scholars are divided on whether this represents cross-dressing or a physical condition such as hermaphroditism. The Nineveh tile fragments (ca. 900–800 BCE) show a queen sporting a beard, as well as wearing a dagger, signs of masculinity. Like the Ur-Nanshe figure, debate surrounds the Nineveh fragments, questioning the accuracy of anatomical representation in contrast to blended cultural conventions that show unique behavior rather than physiology. Even if these are cases of the social behavior of cross-dressing, their depiction in physical form does create gender-blended entities acceptable to both the human and divine communities. In these cases, the body type is made to look like the ideal physiology of the preferred gender for that social role. Ultimately, the social role is more important than the original biological sex of a person. A woman filling the role of a king must look like a king, the more important social status.

55. Clothing and posturing also act as gender indicators in seals.

56. Kathleen McCaffrey, "Reconsidering Gender Ambiguity in Mesopotamia: Is a Beard Just a Beard?" in *Sex and Gender in the Ancient Near East*, ed. Simo Parpola and R. M. Whiting (Helsinki: The Neo-Assyrian Text Corpus Project, 2002), 379–91.

Literary representations give us another view on Mesopotamian conceptions of anatomy and physiology. The introduction of commoners in the *Epic of Gilgamesh* tends to focus on their occupations, such as a hunter, with the story quickly moving on to recounting their actions. There are a few minimal physical descriptions that reflect a social status, like the shaved head of the *asû* (a healer) in the *Poor Man of Nippur*, but a commoner's anatomy or physiology is rarely mentioned. Exceptions are descriptions of old age or the effects of famine.

The ideal body appears in literature most obviously with Gilgamesh, who is "perfect in strength."

> The Lady of Birth drew his body's image,
> The God of Wisdom brought his stature to perfection
> . . . his cheeks had a beard like . . .
> The locks of his hair grew thick as a grain field.
> He was perfection in height,
> Ideally handsome.[57]

This description reinforces the same physical characteristics found in reliefs and statues. Also, as Foster notes, the two-fold reference to "The Lady of Birth" (Ninmah) and "The God of Wisdom" (Enki) in the birth of Gilgamesh likens his form to the perfection embodied by the first created humans.[58]

The creation of Enkidu also holds significant clues for Assyrian and Babylonian physiology.

> Aruru wet her hands,
> She pinched off clay, she tossed it upon the steppe,
> . . . Shaggy with hair was his whole body,
> He was made lush with head hair, like a woman,
> The locks of his hair grew thick as a grain field.[59]

This parallel of Gilgamesh and Enkidu illustrates how the defective is defined in relation to the idealized form. The line "the locks of his hair grew thick as a grain field" is used for both characters. But Enkidu is not perfection in the same way as Gilgamesh. Enkidu has too much hair, covering his

57. Benjamin Foster, *The Epic of Gilgamesh* (New York: W. W. Norton, 2001), 4–5.
58. Foster, *Epic of Gilgamesh*, 5n2.
59. Foster, *Epic of Gilgamesh*, 6.

whole body, as well as an inappropriate gender type, "like a woman." This defectiveness does not mark Enkidu as something evil to be destroyed but ultimately as Gilgamesh's partner as the epic bears out. Once again, the image fulfills the important social role. Enkidu may be male, but his social role is in being a companion or consort to Gilgamesh.

The creation of Gilgamesh and Enkidu did not happen by the chance of natural birth, but rather was intentionally crafted. The epic plays up the uniqueness of the characters by the role of the divine in their creation, but this relationship to the gods is not completely lacking for the common person. According to the creation story of *Enuma Elish*, as well as the tale *Atraḫasis*, a god was sacrificed in order to use his body/blood to create humans. This means that all humans share a part of the divine. Let us remember that the divine have greater power than humans and exercise it through their distinct wills. Consequently, humans have a part of themselves that has its own will and power. It is not one particular body part that is so intimately connected to the gods. Rather, the distinct, willful divine element is diffused throughout the human body. Essentially, this is a symbiotic anatomy rather than a symbolic one.

A human's body in itself forms communities. It is a community of the anatomical parts with the human, and it forms a community with the gods as well. To see whether this type of symbiotic anatomy holds true for the ancient Mesopotamians, we must look at their use of similes and metaphors, as well as the symbolic anatomy, in their medical texts.

Traditional symbolic anatomy links body parts to specific gods, usually as protective entities. Bottéro noted that divination from animal entrails worked because the gods inscribed future events on the animal's anatomy.[60] This is no different for humans. The principle of symbolic anatomy functions in both the case of reading animal entrails and the physical symptoms of a human patient. Symptoms such as fever, sweating, and diarrhea allow the message to be read without opening up the patient and looking at his or her liver.

The most obvious link between a body part and a particular deity occurs in the texts focused on diagnoses. For example, one diagnosis, "if his head on the right side is struck, the hand of the god Adad,"[61] associates part of the head with a specific deity rather than just naming a disease. The more

60. Jean Bottéro, *Mesopotamia: Writing, Reasoning, and the Gods* (Chicago: University of Chicago Press, 1992), 125–37.

61. Labat, *Traité akkadien de diagnostics et prognostics médicaux*, 26–27.

frequent phrases used in diagnoses are: hand of, staff of, smite, seize, bruise, touch, and conquer, followed by the name of a deity or attributed to ghosts and other spirits. Interestingly, these phrases diagnose diseases more so than trauma cases, as one would expect with words like "hand," "staff," or "smite."

The texts focusing on therapeutics show an approach to anatomy akin to modern medicine, in their application of medicines through the urethra or nostrils, observations on the pulse, and use of the term *šer'ānu*, which translates to vein, muscle, or tendon, depending on the context; it is anything that has a cord-like structure. But even these texts omit an explanation of how the different anatomical parts function, making the application of medicines effective. In keeping with this absence of physiological explanations, their anatomical terms lack the precision of our modern counterparts, such as *šer'ānu*, meaning widely different organs. Similarly, the Akkadian term *libbu* can mean either heart or stomach, depending on context. This reinforces the fact that Mesopotamians focused on the body's communicative function and its links to the supernatural realm.

Because parts of the body have relationships with the gods, independent of a human, the symbolic anatomy is also a symbiotic anatomy. Descriptions of various anatomical structures and their symptoms in the incantations accompanying the *materia medica* illustrate the idea that body parts exercise their own power while also being subject to greater powers.

The stomach or belly is likened to a lion, in terms of its fearsomeness; it can gore like an ox, and it is a wolf ranging free. Much like the ancient Greek conception of the uterus being able to wander, the stomach for the Mesopotamians could also move. Ancients did not think of organs as being permanently anchored to a specific location within the body. The belly is also anthropomorphized, in that it has eyes that can be discolored yellow, and it is a fisherman with its contents being fish. It is linked to the gods, with Enki as its lord. The daughters of Anu look after its maintenance by "clearing out the canals." And the gods Sîn, Šamaš, and Gula also play a role.

The eyes are personified as two sisters, the daughters of Anu,[62] separated by a barrier such as a mountain, ridge, or wall, representing the nose. This personification means that healthy eyes work together as in a familial association. When Nergal, the god of fevers and plagues, sets up a chair between them, making the eyes unable to relax, it is a sign of illness. As a result, they cannot work together, causing the sisters to weep, which manifests as the

62. Timothy Collins, "Natural Illness in Babylonian Medical Incantations" (PhD diss., University of Chicago, 1999), 212.

symptom of watery eyes. Incantations threaten the eyes to get better.[63] This indicates that the eyes have volition apart from the person. They can obey or not, which means they have a will or power separate from their human host. A person does not have power over his or her own senses; it is not ultimately the person, though he may typically control where the eyes look. The gods usually associated with the eyes are Anu, Nergal, Ea, Asalluḫi, and Gula.

An incantation against a toothache shows how one's flesh and bones are subject to relationships apart from the human. A worm asks Šamaš, "Lift me up and among the teeth / And the gums cause me to dwell! / The blood of the tooth I will suck, / And of the gum I will gnaw / Its roots!"[64] Other gods paired with the teeth are Asalluḫi, Enlil, and Gula.

Although the Mesopotamians never outlined an exact physiology, one can be reconstructed from the description of symptoms, as well as the therapeutic incantations. The body consists of a net of cords (veins, muscles, and tendons) stretched over a skeletal frame and filled in with soft organ tissue.[65] Blood and wind must move through the body. It seems a reasonable observation for them to assume this. Even the simplest scratch would show that blood infuses all body parts. They do not concern themselves with how substances like blood move through the body. It is not clear, like in Greek or Egyptian physiology, whether blood and wind being held within an organ is the cause of a disease or whether the disease causes the retention of the substances. There is also no sense of blood and wind needing to be held in a relative balance or absolute amounts.

Each body part is its own distinct entity, but they do work in conjunction. This is true of obviously paired organs like the eyes. If other organs are near one another, they can have an influence, such as the muscles of the temple causing the eye to hold onto water or to weep. But less obvious associations are also apparent in the medical texts. A blow to the mid-section can cause immobility in the legs. Similarly, a cranial injury can cause disruption with movement of the hands and feet. Modern medicine explains this as a brain and spinal injury that causes impairment of the neural pathways. For the Mesopotamians, a direct mechanical relationship was of little concern. The *šer'anu* (vein, muscle, or tendon) serves as a rudimentary explanation

63. Collins, "Natural Illness in Babylonian Medical Incantations," 91–95.

64. James B. Pritchard, "A Cosmological World Incantation: The Worm and the Toothache," in *Ancient Near Eastern Texts Relating to the Old Testament* (Princeton: Princeton University Press, 1969), 100–101.

65. Adapted from Böck's physiological theory; see Böck, *Healing Goddess Gula*, 27.

of connective tissue. But the healers would need to understand only that these parts have a relationship with each other and not exactly how they communicate with one another across the body.

Little in the texts gives clues about how the body interacted physiologically with the environment, such as how food is digested or why breathing air is necessary. There is an understanding that the stomach acts as a fermentation vat but nothing beyond that to indicate that nutrients are absorbed into the blood from digestion. The point of breathing is omitted, beyond the basic idea of needing to breathe to stay alive. They do have an understanding that the body can function as a barrier protecting it from the outside world. Flesh is taken as anything from the epidermis to deep muscle tissue and is likened to a door. The bone structure upon which the flesh lies is the bar for the door, strengthening it against intrusion.

The Mesopotamians understood time itself as an outside influence on physiology. Some diagnostic texts advise healers that injuries can turn into other types of illness because malignant forces have time to exert their influence. This explains why ancient scribes compiling series of medical cases made time one of the organizing principles for grouping various ailments. The component of time means that physiology for them was not static but changed according to variations in relationships.

Since physiology ultimately is a collection of symbiotic entities who balance relationships with each other—making up their human host, the gods, and other entities—the body acts a communicative object. This communicative ability of the body explains the ubiquitous use of votive statues, as well as the overlap between the medical texts and omen literature. We will return to this point about the medical texts.

## Disease Etiology

Now that we understand how Mesopotamians see the body, let us look at their explanation for what causes disease. Medical anthropology uses four categories for etiology: natural, individual, social, and supernatural. Mesopotamian etiology attributes illness to outside forces, whether it is a god, ghost, human using magic (*kišpu*), or even an animal. For them, the four named etiological categories essentially collapse into just the supernatural.

Since the body functioned as a vehicle for messages from more powerful entities, a diagnosis that identifies the powerful entity functions also as an etiology. By knowing the disease-causing entity, whether ghost or god, the healer may tailor the cure toward it. Yet some diagnoses omit naming the powerful entity, and many of the texts lack a diagnosis altogether. The symptom description itself provides enough information for the healer to find the appropriate remedy. The physical examination essentially acts as a form of divination.

Scholars originally understood the phrase "hand of DN," found frequently in the medical texts, to indicate illness as a form of divine punishment. This may be true in some cases of illness, but not all. It is better to think of illness as a message that prods humans to behave in a particular way.[66] Van der Toorn interprets the phrase "hand of DN" as identifying the god who has ultimate control over the disease, but not necessarily the one who sent it.[67] As the tale *Atra-ḫasis* illustrates, Enlil ultimately controls the *šuruppu*-disease, but it was the god Namtar that sent and eventually revoked it.

This also indicates that one need not have committed a sin to suffer a disease; Enlil ordered up the *šuruppu*-disease because humans made noise, not because they were wicked. *Atra-ḫasis* also sheds light on the ease with which etiological categories can overlap for the Mesopotamians. If one acts unneighborly, such as making a lot of noise (social), a god may warn him with an illness (supernatural). Similarly, an actual transgression (individual) may cause the god to send illness (supernatural) as a punishment. Animal attacks are linked to the supernatural, as seen in the previously stated incantation against a toothache.[68] The worm (natural) requests the human mouth as a place to dwell from the gods (supernatural).

The accessing of power through magic or sorcery (*kišpu*) to cause disease also falls into the supernatural category of etiology. This manipulation of power may stem from someone's attempt to reinforce cultural behavioral norms or from exact retribution for a personal affront. Again, the categories of social, individual, or natural may overlap.

The patient and healer may have to navigate different levels within the power hierarchy in order to account for all the beings involved in the illness. A human may use magic to cause a spirit to attack someone with an illness, or to convince a god that a transgression has occurred, with the god

66. Hector Avalos, *Illness and Health Care in the Ancient Near East: The Role of the Temple in Greece, Mesopotamia and Israel* (Atlanta: Scholars Press, 1995), 134.

67. K. van der Toorn, *Sin and Sanction in Israel and Mesopotamia* (Maastrich: Van Gorcum, 1985), 199.

68. Pritchard, "A Cosmological World Incantation: The Worm and the Toothache."

in turn sending a demon. Ghosts, demons, or other spirits may also act independently from gods and magicians. Some ghosts may cause illness as a punishment or at least a deterrent, but other times they will use a disease simply to capriciously demonstrate their own power.

One would expect workplace accidents and animal bites to fall solely under the natural-world etiology. Animals may attack of their own volition, but even these cases may have connections to the supernatural and other categories. Amulets to prevent snakebites and scorpion stings attest to their connection to the supernatural hierarchy of power. Even the weather can cause disease. As one letter to the Assyrian king Esarhaddon explains, northern winds carried an epidemic from Nergal.[69]

## Restoration of Health

Since illness ultimately stems from an outside source, this essentially leaves two types of remedies for it. The cause of a disease can be either appeased or overpowered. These options appear most readily in the medical incantations. But even in the texts that simply list symptoms and *materia medica* without an incantation (instrumental healing), one can discern the principles of appeasing and overpowering. In fact, these texts, which at first glance lack any type of "magic," most likely have their basis in ritual practices.

Appeasing works when a god sent the illness. At the heart of the appeasing tactic, the patient must show deference or obedience, which can take the form of offerings, sacrifices, and ritual practices. These may include also an incantation containing an apology, even if the patient is oblivious to the exact transgression. "My god, . . . after you will have my eyes recognize my sins."[70] In some cases, appeasing takes the form of the patient proclaiming innocence, explaining that sorcery made him unacceptable and tricked the god(s). "Because a sorceress has bewitched me / They have driven away from me my (personal) god and my (personal) goddess / I have become obnoxious to whoever sees me."[71] While the human shows obedience, the god must consider the appeasing ritual acts and may remove the disease. Consideration by the gods must be a part of the relationship for Mesopotamians, or

69. Robert Pfeiffer, *State Letters of Assyria* (New Haven: American Oriental Society, 1935).

70. Hallo and Younger, *Context of Scripture: Canonical Compositions*, 574.

71. Benjamin Foster, *Before the Muses: An Anthology of Akkadian Literature* (Bethesda: CDL, 2005), 666.

else such medical advice would not work. That is, it would not appear in the texts with such regularity.

The appeasing tactic does not work, and therefore does not appear in the texts, when an illness is caused by a spirit or a ghost. These entities normally do not form a community with humans and would not be moved by any show of obedience; they have no reason to reconsider their actions and to dispense mercy. If the spirit or other entity acts on behalf of a god, then the patient may directly appeal to that god, effectively bypassing the middle-man entity.

For dealing with spirits and ghosts who have sent a disease of their volition, overpowering them becomes the more common healing tactic. But in this action, there may still be an appeal to the gods. The patient asks the gods to use their power, a greater power, against the spirit.

> Let him be put under your oath
> Let him be put under the oath of Ea and Asalluḫi
> Let him be put under the oath of the gods of heaven and earth
> Let him not come near me; let him not come close to me.[72]

Spirits do have a community with the gods and therefore must obey any oath imposed by the gods.

Some healers, though, by acting on behalf of a god, have enough power to directly command the spirit/disease to leave. An incantation for a gastrointestinal illness, followed by an explanation, indicates this:

> May his excrement escape and come out
> May the whirlwind inside him come out and see the sun!
> The incantation is not mine, it is the incantation of Asalluḫi, exorcist of the gods, he cast it and I took it up.[73]

The acknowledgment that the power ultimately rests with the gods is important. Although the healer has specialized knowledge that can access godly power, he must not attribute it to himself, lest he expose himself to the gods' wrath for such pride.

Similar tactics of overpowering were used when sorcery caused the illness. Although human, the sorcerer sending the disease acts outside the

72. Scurlock, *Magico-Medical Means*, 363.

73. Collins, "Natural Illness in Babylonian Medical Incantations," 136.

bounds of the human community, therefore necessitating the same healing strategies as a spirit or ghost attack. The sorcerer may have felt that his actions corrected a wrong, even when contracted by an accusing third party, but such retribution is ultimately decided by the gods. When the patient complains to the gods, they consider his plea. If he is innocent, the sorcery-induced illness may be removed. But if he is not so innocent or not properly contrite, they may allow the illness to continue.

The ideas of obedience, consideration, and maintaining community cohesion, still find expression in the instrumental healing practices in the texts. The traditional assumption of dividing Mesopotamian medicine into symbolic and instrumental healing, more commonly labeled magical and scientific, caused many to overlook the ritualistic nature of the *materia medica*. Rituals typically have three components: the oral rite, the physical rite, and charged substances. The most obvious example is saying a prayer or incantation (oral rite) while sacrificing (physical rite) an animal (charged substance). What appears to be instrumental healing techniques in creating and applying poultices or fumigations are actually the use of charged substances in a physical rite. The medical texts contain abundant cases of ritual in which incantations charge the *materia medica*.

> Before the foremost star . . . lay down a *mersu*-cake of honey and butter . . . mix "wood of release," rosemary, bat dung, *imḫur-ešrā* plant, and "sailor's dung" with oil. Lay it before the star, recite three times the incantation: You, O star, that gives light to . . . may these plants destroy my complaint.[74]

An incantation is not always needed to charge the substances or attract the consideration of the gods.

> If a man's head burns with *sētu*-fever and his skin hurts him, his head being swollen, dry, crush, sieve, branches of *magan*-tree, knead flour of chick peas, flour of lentils, *tappinnu*-flour, *ennenu*-cereal together in beer dregs, shave, ditto.[75]

Some substances naturally have their own charge and can attract the gods and spirits. The patient's act of submitting to the therapeutic treatments

74. R. Campbell Thompson, "Assyrian Prescriptions for the Head," *AJSL* 53, no. 4 (1937): 217–38; Martin Worthington, "Edition of UGU 1 (=BAM 480 Etc.)," *JMC* 5 (2005): 6–43.

75. Worthington, "Edition of UGU 1 (=BAM 480 Etc.)."

(patient compliance) demonstrates his obedience to the hierarchy of power, with the gods at its pinnacle.

As we saw when looking at the archaeological evidence of Mesopotamian medicine, healing could take place in the temples and other sacred sites associated with the gods. Yet healers did not need specialized settings but often worked at the home of the patient. The archive of King Esarhaddon of Assyria attests to the fact that healers, at times, did not need to be near the patient. They could diagnose and advise treatment solely through correspondence. Avalos claims that the social stigma attached to being ill necessitated house calls rather than having the patient appear in public at a temple or other place of healing.[76] Although illness would bar someone from entering parts of a temple, it is not so shameful a state that it would warrant extreme isolation or quarantine, even though there is a natural tendency to avoid people who are obviously sick.

Some treatment rituals required patients to immerse themselves in a river; the Tigris and Euphrates were particularly important ones, as their water was a naturally charged substance. Debate surrounds the ritual hut of Gula as a specialized place for healing or simply as a sacred site.[77]

Most people can recognize when their health has changed for the worse. But having the community recognize it is another thing. Medical anthropology refers to the hierarchy of resort, with recognition of an illness and treatment occurring within the family located at the lowest level of the hierarchy. The highest level would be consultation with a healer sanctioned by the state, religion, or other authoritarian structure.

In Mesopotamia, the complex relationship between the human and supernatural communities made it necessary to seek recognition of illness and treatment from a culturally approved authority such as the *asû* or *āšipu*. Once someone is recognized as being ill, he adopts the sick role, which allows him temporary release from certain obligations but may also suspend certain rights. Various texts attest to workers and bureaucrats who, because of illness, were excused from duties. For example, a letter from the *asû* Ikkaru, on behalf of Iratti, states, "He has not gone in front, the king, my lord let it be known on account of he is sick."[78] Removal of the sick role is not automatic when the symptoms disappear but seems related to the final act of thanking the gods, such as in a libation ritual, for their granting a recovery.

76. Avalos, *Illness and Health Care in the Ancient Near East*, 177–80.

77. Avalos, *Illness and Health Care in the Ancient Near East*, 205; Livingstone, "Isin 'Dog House' Revisited," 54–60.

78. Pfeiffer, *State Letters of Assyria*, 282.

## Illnesses

More often than not, we cannot definitively claim, by their modern names, which diseases were present in ancient Mesopotamia. It is difficult to reconstruct which illnesses were present based solely on symptom descriptions in the medical texts. Quite often these are incomplete and subject to literary conventions that may obscure important factors used in modern clinical diagnoses. We can discern broad categories of ailments that frequently concerned Mesopotamian healers, which in turn can help us understand cultural values for issues about body image, gender, and social roles. To better understand the actual diseases present in ancient Mesopotamia and their effect on demographics, we must rely on the work of paleo-osteologists and paleopathologists who can analyze the biological record from skeletal and other remains.[79]

### Disease

Although the medical texts frequently cite skin disorders as a complaint, no evidence exists discerning between ailments such as eczema, psoriasis, melanomas, or the like. Paleopathologists find no evidence of Hansen's disease, popularly referred to as leprosy, until the Hellenistic period, starting in the late fourth century BCE. The focus on skin conditions should not seem unusual, given the communicative function of the body. The complexion acts as an immediate indicator of whether there is a disruption with the divine community.

Fevers and gastrointestinal upset are other common issues, but again there is no way of pinning down specific diseases by the symptoms of cramping, bloating, vomiting, diarrhea, and constipation, as listed in the medical texts. A variety of parasites like helminths show up in some human remains and other finds in excavations. Even though we know they suffered from parasitic infections, we cannot always link exact cases in the medical texts to the known parasites. The problem is that the symptom descriptions in the cases are not clear enough, due to their brevity or difficulty in translating unusual terms.

Many modern scholars try to ascertain the presence of diseases like tuberculosis, typhus, smallpox, and bubonic plague, but they tend to be

79. Laura Battini and Pierre Villard, eds., *Médecine et médicins au Proche-Orient ancien* (Oxford: British Archaeological Reports, 2006).

limited to the human remains from Egypt and the Levant. They extrapolate their findings to Mesopotamia on the basis of environmental factors and highly interpretive readings of symptom descriptions in the medical texts.[80]

This is not to say that all reconstructions formed on the basis of symptom descriptions are false. The disease *bennu* has such frequent references and sufficient symptom descriptions in the medical texts to translate it as epilepsy.[81] They recognized it as a disease that causes falling, tremors of varying degrees, and at times foaming at the mouth, essentially distinctions between petit and grand mal seizures. But not all references to *bennu* mean epilepsy exclusively. Mesopotamian medical texts actually have three groups of diseases that cause types of "falling." All of them derive from either a malicious demon or a functionary of the moon god Sîn. This cluster of "falling diseases" includes also what are likely forms of mental illness. Direct references to madness or insanity are rare in the medical texts but do appear in texts relating to the sale and activity of slaves. Interestingly, terms for madness are used for female slaves almost exclusively, whereas males tend to have the diagnosis of epilepsy. Within the medical texts themselves, the occurrence of *bennu* as epilepsy is distributed evenly between men and women.

## Trauma

The medical texts do not give lists of how specific injuries were acquired, though it is not hard to imagine that most trauma cases would be related to farming or construction accidents, as well as war wounds. On the basis of skeletal evidence of healed injuries, it is obvious the ancient Mesopotamians could set broken bones. Yet instructions for the reduction of fractures is missing from the medical texts. As noted earlier, they observed traumatic nerve damage, though they did not bother to explain it. Prognoses for trauma cases can be found frequently in the medical texts focused on diagnostics. Injury and poisoning from animal bites and stings do appear in the texts, with dogs, snakes, and scorpions being the more frequent ones.

80. Don R. Brothwell and A. T. Sandison, eds., *Diseases in Antiquity: A Survey of Disease, Injuries, and Surgeries of Early Populations* (Springfield: C. C. Thomas, 1967); P. B. Adamson, "Human Diseases and Deaths in the Ancient Near East," *Die Welt Des Orients* 13 (1982): 5–14; Donald J. Ortner and Bruno Frohlich, *The Early Bronze Age I Tombs and Burials of Bâb-Edh-Drhâ', Jordan* (Lanham, MD: AltaMira, 2008).

81. Stol, *Epilepsy in Babylon.*

They treat the bites and stings with salves, but the texts for these types of cases also show that they practiced preventative medicine. Frequently, people would wear amulets to ward off such animal bites.

## Disability

The ancient Mesopotamians did not medically distinguish between disabilities caused by congenital birth defects or ones acquired over time, such as a grievous injury. Rather, they focused on the inability to perform certain tasks instead of why the disability existed. Like diseases and trauma, a permanent impairment is a message from the gods, but it cannot be assuaged with responses of obedience. They accepted that the gods essentially decreed a unique social role for a person. Sometimes this unique (or new) role could be a positive one, a sign of a special relationship with a god. Other times, it meant that a god has permanently rejected a relationship with a person, which may be a fate worse than death. For children born with certain deformities, the god's rejection is aimed at the parents and not just the child.

Other deformities have nothing to do with the gods' relationships with humans but with each other. The Sumerian tale *Enki and Ninmah* relates how, during a feast celebrating the creation of humans, the gods have a contest. Ninmah creates disabled humans, for whom Enki finds a function and place in society. They then reverse roles, and Enki creates a human that is simultaneously a fetus and an old man, for whom Ninmah cannot find a function and therefore a place in society.[82]

Ultimately, the culture focused on the gods finding a place for the disabled, but this does not mean everyone with a disability was treated equally or even allowed to survive. They did not think that every life was sacred from the moment of birth (or conception) and therefore must be saved. Nor was it a brutal world in which the "weakest" were simply allowed to die. How well a disabled person fared depended greatly on one's social status, as well as the beneficence of individuals in one's immediate community. Someone from an elite family, such as royalty or the priesthood, may have stood a better chance than a peasant in being cared for and in finding a workable place in society. Yet this high social status could also easily mean ostracism for a defect, while a similarly disabled peasant would not suffer from such social demands.

82. Hallo and Younger, *Context of Scripture: Canonical Compositions*, 516–18.

## Conditional States

Ancient Mesopotamians recognized various stages of life, like infancy and old age, as well as conditions such as pregnancy, but they did not necessarily understand or classify them in the same way that modern medicine does.

The Mesopotamian medical texts do not address infancy in terms of growth or developmental benchmarks, such as being able to roll over or speak at certain ages. The cases for infants usually focus on attacks from Lamaštu and other malevolent spirits. The most common advice has parents placing amulets on the newborn to prevent an attack. When a baby becomes ill, it typically signals a disruption to community cohesion on the part of the parents, not the infant. Like most medical cases, the exact offense that warrants the illness is not mentioned. But for these particular pediatric ones, it seems that the parents' neglect in properly protecting the child from spirits is the default explanation. Deformities that the Mesopotamians referred to as monstrous births were attributed to the sinful actions of one or more of the parents.

Whereas modern medicine subdivides childhood and puberty into distinct neurological and biological phases, ancient Mesopotamians had no such conception of human development. There are cultural distinctions between an infant and a child, with infancy lasting until the child is weaned, roughly at the age of two or three. At this point, children are treated as working members of the household. A Sumerian list of food rations divides childhood into the age ranges of one to five, five to ten, and ten to thirteen years of age. This list speaks only to the need for an increasing amount of food as a child grows. Nothing in the written materials indicates other biological or neurological changes at these stages. It is likely though that the type of work given to children would reflect an awareness of increasing maturity and responsibility at different stages.

It is not clear exactly when a child reached an "age of majority" and was recognized as an adult, but most likely it was around the onset of puberty, which seems to have occurred around thirteen to fourteen years of age. The availability of proper nutrition could slightly shift this age range. Mesopotamians based their distinctions between child and adult on cultural behaviors, and therefore when to assume the role of an adult was subject to the maturity of the individual. Social status also played a great part in the exact responsibilities of an adult and when someone was deemed ready to fulfill them.

Modern obstetrics and gynecology view pregnancy as an aberration in the normal, nonparturient state of women. For both men and women in Mesopotamia, having children was an important part of adult life and being a part of a thriving community. For this reason, the medical literature does not treat pregnancy itself as a special medical state needing help from a healer. The medical texts do focus on miscarriages, complications with birth, and postpartum women. When assessing patients with fever, vomiting, or other symptoms, they almost never address whether the patient is pregnant. There is one exception where the line "if a woman is pregnant . . ." appears to be a later insertion into a list of cases for postpartum women. We can only assume that most treatments for women were the same, regardless of their pregnancy status. A Sumerian proverb does express sympathy for ill pregnant women: "To be sick is good, to be pregnant is bad, to be pregnant and sick is too much."[83]

Although the medical texts contain cases of complications during birth, the term for "midwife" never appears in the introductions that list the titles of healers, for whom the writings were meant. Yet as far as the evidence attests, from both literature and legal documents, a midwife was always present at the birth, but not necessarily any of the other healers. Midwives were connected with the mother goddesses in the pantheon. But the second millennium BCE marks a shift in the literature, showing only male gods attending the births of heroes and acting as midwives. During birth, women would sit on bricks, and amulets could be draped across the hips. Midwives were said to "untie the knot" that allows delivery of the child; this is likely a reference to the physiological concept that a net of cords made up the body. The midwife used a sharpened reed to cut the umbilical cord and placed the afterbirth in a special jar. She would then bathe the newborn with salts.

Many texts discuss the favorable conditions for conception, especially for bearing a son, and the omens surrounding childbirth. The fetus is imagined as a boat floating in dark waters, which is consistent with other descriptions of the stomach or belly as a place of dark water. Miscarriages are a concern of the medical texts, which refer to "what has been thrown from the belly," and often they are attributed to an act of sorcery. Temples for Ninisina have a room that is associated with childbirth and may have acted as a cemetery for stillborn babies, as well as a repository for the ritual preservation of the afterbirth. Infertility is another concern in the medical texts, but responsibility lies mostly with the woman in terms of taking prescriptive herbs to "open her womb." Although Mesopotamians understood that both

83. Martin Stol, *Birth in Babylonia and the Bible: Its Mediterranean Setting* (Groningen: Styx, 2000), 203.

parents contribute to the creation of the fetus, male infertility simply did not exist in their concept of the world. For them, semen in itself had potency; so as long as there was an ejaculation, the man was fertile. Men may aid in conception by prayers to the gods or by taking care to have proper positioning during intercourse.

A common misconception about the ancient world is the average life span. Frequently, one hears that it was twenty-five or thirty years, giving the false impression that most people did not live past this approximate age. This is simply not true. Ample records exist indicating that people lived well into their sixties, seventies, and eighties. Some texts refer to a man in his forties as "prime," and sixty as "manlihood." Designations of old age begin in one's seventies. When calculating the average, demographers include all those who died in infancy. The ancient world's high infant-mortality rate skews the final outcome.

Because many lived well past the age of sixty, various illnesses that tend to present themselves as a person ages, such as cataracts or dementia, could then be found among the ancient Mesopotamians. But the treatment of geriatric issues as a distinct category did not exist in their medical texts. Instead, we can find cases for treating hair loss, eye ailments, and other illnesses, which may be age related, but age is not a significant factor in their symptom descriptions or diagnoses.

The issue of menopause is also absent from the medical texts; it was a natural stage of a woman's life and, therefore, not in need of healing. To alleviate its more annoying symptoms, women likely used family or community traditions. In the hierarchy of resort, medical anthropologists would classify these as popular or folk remedies.

## Healers

Typically, the Akkadian term *asû* is translated as "physician," and *āšipu* as "exorcist" or "magician."[84] This creates a false dichotomy of science and magic within Mesopotamian medicine.[85] Coupled with the fact that the *āšipu* gained prominence in the later texts, it appears as if the Mesopota-

84. The Assyrian Dictionary of the Oriental Institute of Chicago (CAD) still uses these translations.

85. Jean Bottéro, "Magic and Medicine," in *Everyday Life in Ancient Mesopotamia*, ed. Jean Bottéro (Baltimore: Johns Hopkins University Press, 1992), 162–82.

mians became more superstitious as time passed. It also raised the question why the culture would increasing rely on magic; there was no satisfactory answer to this.

Texts show that both the *asû* and *āšipu* used instrumental healing as well as the symbolic technique of incantations. The titles could not be differentiated on the basis of science for one and magic for the other. Recently, the *asû* has been described as a pharmacist, and the *āšipu* as a diagnostician.[86] Although more reflective of the ancient medical texts, using these translations obscures the fact that the *asû* could also make diagnoses,[87] as well as unintentionally impart an anachronistic hierarchy, since the modern medical system places a pharmacist in a less privileged position than a diagnosing physician.

It is best to understand the roles of the *asû* and *āšipu* without directly translating the terms. The Hymn to Gula addresses her as an *āsâtu* and *āšipaku*,[88] while Maqlû (an anti-witchcraft text) uses *āsâtu* and *bārâtu* (diviner). This indicates that all healers ultimately owe their skills and powers to Gula. The difference between the titles for healers lies in their focus of communication between the communities of humans and the gods.[89]

### *Asû*

The Akkadian word *asû* derived from the Sumerian A.ZU and appeared as early as 2500 BCE in Old Akkadian. A related term appears in some texts, the *azugallu* and its feminine form *azugallūtu*, which traditionally has been translated as "chief physician," but it is best regarded as "chief *asû*."

The *asû* assesses the physical symptoms of the patient, quite often the signs of communication from the gods most obvious to the human community. Although nonhealers may not know the exact message encoded in the symptoms, they can tell something is wrong. In turn, the instrumental healing techniques frequently employed by the *asû* communicate a ritualistic obedience not only to the gods but also to the human community. Healing

86. Scurlock, "Physician, Exorcist, Conjurer, Magician," 69–79.

87. The diagnostic series SA.GIG in tablet 18 lists the *asû* and *barû* as practitioners alongside the *āšipu*.

88. The feminine forms of *asû* and *āšipu*.

89. Laura M. Zucconi, *Can No Physician Be Found? The Influence of Religion on Medical Pluralism in Ancient Egypt, Mesopotamia, and Israel* (Piscataway: Gorgias, 2013).

practices act as an assurance that the patient is addressing what has gone wrong with the relationships.

### *Ašipu*

The Akkadian word *āšipu* first appears in the Middle Assyrian/Middle Babylonian period (ca. 1500–1000 BCE). The *āšipu* looks at signs from the gods, ones that are not readily apparent to the human community. The focus is on communication from the community of gods. Once a correct reading is given, that is to say, the diagnosis, the *āšipu* may use instrumental or symbolic healing, or the patient can consult another healer for treatment. The upsurge of *āšipu* in later medical texts can be explained by the development in the medical literature itself. As descriptions of symptoms/signs and diagnoses gained prominence in the writing of the texts during the Middle Assyrian and Middle Babylonian periods, the *āšipu*, as the one qualified to read them, also grew in importance. Further investigation is needed about why this section of the medical literature became more developed over time. This literary development does not mean Mesopotamian culture underwent a dramatic shift from scientific to magical. The belief in the gods' role in human activity remained fairly constant.

No information has come to light that indicates a formal education for the *asû* and *āšipu* apart from basic scribal skills. Both types of healers most likely received training through an apprenticeship rather than formal schools. Healers from Isin have the strongest reputations, most likely due to the prominent temple of Gula in that city, which may have been a center for some apprenticeships. Textually and archaeologically, nothing at Isin demonstrates the existence of a formal school, as suggested by Bottéro.[90] Often, priests from the Gula temple are noted for healing, but neither title of *asû* or *āšipu* is used for them.

Other types of healers in Mesopotamia include the king himself (technically a priest *ex officio*) as well as diviners such as the *bārû* and *mašmaššu*. Since kings function as an intermediary between the gods and the people, this places them in a position to heal, but there is little evidence of this being done in practice apart from petitions to the king, asking for his help in matters of health. The *bārû* engages in mediumistic divination, such as reading animal entrails or the shape of oil in water. The *mašmaššu*, commonly

90. Bottéro, "Magic and Medicine."

translated as "exorcist," is another type of healer akin to the *āšipu*, but we lack evidence to distinguish the precise difference, if any, between the two. It is important to keep in mind that these various types of healers were not in competition with one another. A letter from the *asû* Arad-Nana to his patient even suggests seeking a second opinion from a *bārû*.[91]

91. Pfeiffer, *State Letters of Assyria*, 286.

# 3. Egyptian Medicine

## Location and History

Ancient Egypt lies along the Nile River in North Africa, bounded on the north by the Mediterranean coast and on the south by a series of cataracts. At various times in Egypt's political history, the first, second, and third cataracts served as the southernmost boundary. Longitudinally, Egypt can be divided between the Western Desert, the Nile Valley, and the Eastern Desert. Egyptian terms characterized these regions by referring to the deserts as "red lands" or *dšrt*, while the fertile Nile Valley was called the "black land" or *kmt*. The Egyptians also used *kmt* in reference to their political territory, whether it was the river valley or the desert regions.[1] Egyptians additionally distinguished between the territories of Upper and Lower Egypt. Upper Egypt lies between Aswan in the south, at the first cataract, and Asyut toward the north. Lower Egypt covers the delta region from Asyut to the Mediterranean coast. The terms "Upper" for south and "Lower" for north use, as a reference, the Nile's south-to-north direction of flow. At various historical points, the Sinai Peninsula further to the east was also incorporated into the Egyptian kingdoms. Administratively, Egypt was divided into nomes, which varied in number in different periods. As Egyptian pharaohs expanded territory southward into Nubia and Kush, more nomes were created.

Commonly, histories divide roughly three thousand years of Egyptian civilization into the distinct phases of the Old, Middle, and New Kingdoms, punctuated by intermediate periods, incorporating the twenty-two dynasties listed by the Ptolemaic priest Manetho (third century BCE). Modern scholars using both textual and archaeological evidence have fine-tuned and expanded the chronology of ancient Egypt.[2] The Predynastic period

1. The name "Egypt" comes from the Greeks.

2. Dates in Egyptian history are debated between high, middle, and low chronologies

(ca. 5000–2950 BCE) includes the cultures of Taso-Badarian and Naqada. The end of Naqada III saw the rise of a more centralized authority over various cities in Upper Egypt, under King Scorpion in Dynasty 0. The Early Dynastic period followed with the creation of the First Dynasty (2950–2775 BCE), attributed to Narmer,[3] unifying Upper and Lower Egypt. The Old Kingdom begins with the Fourth Dynasty (2575–2450 BCE), lasting until the dissolution of the competing Seventh and Eighth Dynasties[4] (2175–2125 BCE). The First Intermediate period sees the rise of various political centers, until unification and centralization under the Eleventh Dynasty ushered in the Middle Kingdom period (2010–1630 BCE). Again, centralized governance breaks down when the Twelfth Dynasty ends, starting the Second Intermediate period (1630–1539 BCE). During this time, a Canaanite group called the Hyksos came to prominence as the Fifteenth Dynasty (1630–1520 BCE) in the Delta region of Lower Egypt. Their eventual defeat by Kamose (1541–1539 BCE), the last ruler of the Seventeenth Dynasty, paved the way for his brother Ahmose I (1539–1514 BCE) to once again centrally rule Upper and Lower Egypt, as the Eighteenth Dynasty, creating the New Kingdom period (1539–1292 BCE). Under the New Kingdom pharaohs,[5] notably Ramesses II (1279–1213 BCE), Egypt expanded its interests and sphere of influence into the Levant, bringing it into direct conflict with powers such as the Hittite Empire. The Third Intermediate (1069–664 BCE) is another period of decentralization, with certain dynasties trying to assert universal authority by military conquest of resource networks from the Levant. The Late or Saite-Persian period (664–332 BCE) is a time of centralized rule but usually by foreign powers who mostly kept the indigenous religious culture intact. This continued under Greek (332–331 BCE) and Roman domination (31 BCE–330 CE) until the Arab conquest brought in Islam in 641 CE.

Studies on ancient Egyptian medicine, including this one, tend to treat the time span between the Old Kingdom and the New Kingdom as one cul-

---

somewhat reliant on ancient astronomical observations, which can have a plus or minus of several years. This work roughly follows the chronology of Toby Wilkinson; see Toby Wilkinson, ed., *The Egyptian World* (New York: Routledge, 2010).

3. Often referred to by the Greek rendition Menes. The name Narmer translates to "Catfish."

4. Throughout Egyptian history, many dynasties overlap rather than having direct succession.

5. Use of the term pharaoh, *per-aa* in Egyptian, meaning "Great House," did not really take hold until the New Kingdom period. It signifies the separation of the king from the population, just as the gods are hidden within their temples.

tural whole. Others extend this to the Ptolemaic period. This grouping of Old to New Kingdoms is only partially true. Medical practices, as found in the papyri, were fairly constant for thousands of years, but changing political fortunes and the impact of various priesthoods would naturally cause shifts within the medical culture. This is somewhat evident in the ancient glosses for Egyptian medical papyri, indicating scribes trying to update traditional texts. As we shall see in this study, medicine in Ptolemaic Egypt is quite distinct from these predecessors. It is hoped that some of the information in this chapter will highlight areas needing further investigation into the practices of a more specific time and place within Egyptian history.

## Religion and Culture

Through the various dynasties and their favoring of priesthoods for different gods, such as Re and Amun, two basic principles of ancient Egyptian religion remain constant, holding great importance for the study of their medical culture: *maat* and *heka*. The word *maat* means "order, justice, or balance," often personified as the goddess Maat, while *heka* is access to power but commonly and inappropriately translated as simply "magic."

### Cosmology

Many cities and nomes had their own creation myths, with the three most prominent being Memphis, Hermopolis, and Heliopolis. In each of these, a god created himself before making the cosmos, earth, plants, animals, and humans in a balanced world (*maat*). According to the creation myth from Heliopolis, it was the god Atum who made the orderly world with the rising and setting sun, as well as with the regular inundation from the Nile. The gods, in particular the sun god Re, chose the kings to maintain this balance, order, and justice. Iconography of kingship in the "smiting pose," with his right arm raised holding a mace and his left hand grasping the enemy, dates as early as the Narmer Palette (ca. 2950 BCE). Over time, depictions of the smiting pose, as well as of Egyptian military victories, decorated the exterior walls of the temples, reinforcing the link between kingship and the maintaining of *maat*. Other images of the king show him lifting up Maat as an offering to the gods during religious rituals, symbolizing his ability to rule with *maat*.

The mythological struggles for kingship between the gods Horus and his uncle Seth represent the constant battle between order and chaos played out among the living kings. Meanwhile, the deceased kings include the god Osiris, who rules over the underworld. He merges with Re, thus entering the underworld with every sunset and being reborn with the dawn. Sunrise and sunset, as well as life and death, represent *maat* at work in and between the natural and supernatural worlds. But this also brings up the important point that Egyptians do not think of time in only a linear progression. Time is cyclical, and all events are recast in one fashion or another. As we shall see, the ability for things to reoccur impacts the ancient Egyptian concepts of diagnosis and treatment.

*Maat* was important not only for the natural world and politics but also for any social relationship, which included interactions with the natural and supernatural worlds. According to Egyptian cosmology, then, health and illness were manifestations of one's relationship with the communities of gods, spirits, and other people. If the proper balance is lacking in one or more of your relationships, then you will become ill. Yet *maat* works within the body itself, too. The system of bones, muscles, vessels, and fluids that make up the body functions by *maat*; they must have balanced relationships with each other, as well as with the natural and supernatural worlds. Disruption of the physical body's *maat* results in sickness.

Creation stories and other forms of Egyptian literature highlight not only the necessity of *maat*, but also the importance of accessing power (*heka*). The Memphite creation story tells of the god Ptah, who used divine power (*heka*), knowledge/creative thought (*sia*), and command/utterance (*hu*) to create the cosmos. These principles of power, creativity, and utterances underlie the concept of magic itself. Typically, magic has three parts to it: a physical rite, an oral rite, and the charging of a substance. Yet not all three parts need to be present in every instance of magic. The tale of the chief lector priest Webaoner, from *King Cheops and the Magicians*, illustrates how this system works.[6] When the priest Webaoner hears about his wife's infidelity, he fashions a crocodile from wax, awakens its spirit by reading aloud a specific text, and then deposits it in a lake near the greenhouse that his wife uses for her liaisons. After one of her trysts, the lover jumps into the lake to wash, only to be promptly eaten by the crocodile. It is not a coincidence either that the crocodile killing the lover restores *maat*. Webaoner's actions,

6. William Kelly Simpson, ed., *The Literature of Ancient Egypt: An Anthology of Stories, Instructions, Stelae, Autobiographies, and Poetry* (New Haven: Yale University Press, 2003), 14–16.

though, fulfilled the three components of magic by fashioning a wax crocodile and putting it into the water (physical rite), by the reading of a passage (oral rite), which then allowed for the spirit to be awakened (charging a substance), bringing it to life. The entire process is, essentially, Webaoner using *heka*, that is to say, accessing power bridging the natural and supernatural worlds. As we shall see, Egyptian healers similarly harnessed *heka* in their therapies, even for those without obvious incantations.

Theologically, the king naturally imbued with *heka* acted as the mediator between gods and man; therefore, only the king could perform rituals. This is especially important for rituals that maintained *maat* for all Egypt, but it also holds true for smaller issues, such as the health of an individual subject. In reality, priests undertook the rituals on behalf of the king. An important point is that cultic activity drawing upon *heka* can be delegated and carried out by substitutes. Priests had the ability to perform healing rituals, as did other people who had access to power (*heka*), often by having the ability to read the appropriate texts. The act of delegation has divine precedent in stories such as *The Adoration of Re*, in which Re quells a human rebellion by sending out the goddess Sekhmet to destroy them.[7] In this situation, the role of Sekhmet is very telling, in that she is not just acting on behalf of Re but that she is particularly linked with plagues and healing.

Many Egyptian deities play an important role in medicine, quite often based on the principle that whoever causes an illness or trauma can also heal it. The following is a brief description of those deities linked to illness and healing, as known from the papyri, inscriptions, and artifacts.

## Egyptian Gods and Goddesses of Disease and Healing

### *Sekhmet*

Ancient Egyptian iconography frequently represented the goddess Sekhmet with a lioness's head; lions both have an apotropaic function and represent pure fury in Egyptian religion and art. Often referred to as the Fiery Eye of Re, thus his daughter, she stands as the opposite of the more loving daughter, Hathor. As part of Sekhmet's destructive nature, she generates plagues; therefore, she is the deity who could best effect healing from disease. The *wab* (pure) priests of Sekhmet are often noted in the medical texts specifically as

7. Stephen Quirke, *Ancient Egyptian Religion* (New York: Dover, 1997), 32.

healers and are called even "messengers of Sekhmet," while their rituals are referred to as "appeasing Sekhmet." These phrases underscore the communicative nature of illness and the healer's role in facilitating communication between the gods and the human community.

### *Serket*

Similar to Sekhmet, the goddess Serket (Selket under Greek domination) personifies the dangers of the scorpion, particularly the ability to interfere with breathing; thus, she could inflict as well as heal the scorpion sting. She is attested as early as the Old Kingdom. The *sau* (protector) of Serket appears as a frequent title for healers.

### *Maat*

As we have seen, the goddess Maat personifies balance, order, and justice and keeps chaos at bay, with references to her dating back to the Old Kingdom. She is pictured wearing a single ostrich-feather headdress, known as the Feather of Truth. An important ritual involved the king presenting her to the other gods, showing the intimate link between kinship and the natural order of the universe. The public spaces of temples always depicted this ritual, yet no temples were dedicated to her until the New Kingdom period. She is associated with the Opening of the Mouth ceremony, used on mummies to effect a rebirth into the afterlife for the deceased; thus, she is viewed as a protector guaranteeing an afterlife. Scenes depicting judgment of the dead show their heart weighed against the symbolic feather of Maat. She is the daughter and eye of the sun god, often represented as the disc of the sun. As the eye of Re-Atum, she was sent out to find the divine children Shu and Tefnut,[8] and upon her return, Maat finds Re-Atum had grown a new eye. The tears of her weeping become the first humans. This creation story plays on the similarity of the Egyptian words for tear and people, and it underscores a connection between the human body and the divine.

8. Twins of Re-Atum. The masculine Shu personifies air, while the feminine Tefnut is moisture.

### *Heka*

Heka, the personification of power, animates, compels, and protects both the gods and all that they created.[9] Depicted as the son of a universal creator god and Lord of the *ka*-spirits (souls), he has a dual nature. As a protector, he accompanies Re on his daily voyage, but he also embodies destruction that even the gods fear. Heka is morally neutral; the one accessing such power imparts to it a good or bad character, depending on his or her intentions in accordance with *maat*. He appears in the triads at Heliopolis as early as the Old Kingdom, with his worship lasting into the Roman period.

### *Isis*

Attestations of Isis appear as early as Unas's Pyramid Texts from the Fifth Dynasty and depict her with a throne upon her head; thus, she is commonly thought to personify regal power. She is the sister/consort of Osiris and mother of Horus and features prominently in the mythic cycle *The Contendings of Horus and Seth*. Her piecing together the dismembered body of Osiris and then conceiving Horus cast her in the role of protector and healer for the Egyptians. Accordingly, in the role of protector, many incantations for snake and scorpion bites appeal to her powers. Stories of her attending to the birth of Re's sons also made her ideal for invoking during childbirth. Her cult lasted into the sixth century CE, making her one of the longer lasting ancient deities in the face of a rising Christianity.

### *Thoth*

The god Thoth appears frequently in two forms, one as a dog-headed baboon and the other as an ibis or ibis-headed man. His worship extended from the Early Dynastic into the Ptolemaic period. Considered a scribal god or god of knowledge, he oversees not just writing but science, such as astronomy, math, and medicine, whose practices are strongly dependent on written traditions. In this, Thoth is connected to the *per ankh* (House of Life), a scriptorium-type area within temple complexes. Scholars debate its function claiming it was a place of learning specifically for healers akin to a

9. Coffin Text Spell 261.

modern medical school. Thoth is the one who teaches Isis the spells to revive Osiris and who heals Horus of a scorpion sting. He brings back the Eye of Re (the goddess Tefnut)[10] from Nubia; thus, he is seen as healing creation itself. Additionally, he is seen as a fellow deity of Maat, overseeing wisdom, justice, and subsequently world order. This balanced nature of Thoth meant that, by the Middle Kingdom, funerary texts characterized his actions as the intermediary between violence and peace.[11] In essence, this reinforces Thoth's medical aspect, balancing the violence of illness and the peace of health.

### *Taweret*

Two deities intrinsic to the health and well-being of humans are Taweret and Bes. The mother goddess Taweret appears often as a pregnant hippopotamus with pendulous breasts, the arms and legs of a lion, and the tail of a crocodile, accompanied by the *sa* symbol, meaning protection. Her image was used on amulets to protect pregnant and nursing women. Her likeness can be found in domestic shrines and on "magic wands," along with Bes. The worship of Taweret lasted through the Ptolemaic period and into the Roman era.

### *Bes*

Bes is a lion-faced god who often sticks out his tongue and whose body has dwarf-like proportions and bowlegs. He was invoked for protection during childbirth, childhood itself, sleep, and even eroticism. Ultimately, he protects the child Horus. His likeness adorns "magic wands" dating as early as the Middle Kingdom, as well as the walls of Amenhotep III's palace. His imagery is linked to an older deity called Aha (The Fighter). The name Bes could be related to the Egyptian word *besa*, meaning either "to protect" or "a premature child." The latter may explain the odd form of the deity. Like Taweret, the grotesque or "unnatural" physical composition may aid in protection by scaring away the more malevolent forces.

10. The phrase "Eye of Re" denotes children or emanations of the god; thus, both Maat and Tefnut carry this title.

11. Quirke, *Ancient Egyptian Religion*, 32.

### *Neith*

The goddess Neith is attested as early as the First Dynasty in Abydos, with considerable popularity in royal names. She rose to prominence again in the Late period, especially favored by the Twenty-sixth Dynasty. She is depicted both as a deity of war with shield and arrows and as a domestic goddess with a loom. It was during the New Kingdom that Neith took on the role of creator, producing the world and specifically the seed of gods and men, thus making her the inventor of birth and procreation. In this act, she had the role of both male and female, bringing up the issue of her as a bisexual or androgynous figure, something that is not typically debated for male creator gods, such as Atum.[12] This possible androgyny makes her akin to the Mesopotamian war/love deity Ištar.

### *Khnum*

A male creator god often cited as overseeing birth or conception is Khnum, typically depicted with a ram's head. He fashioned newborn babies and infused them with a breath of life. This act is described in a stela, "I am Khnum, your fashioner. My arms are behind you to shelter your body, to make healthy your limbs."[13] Interestingly, this protective stance is seen also in royal statuary, with Horus's wings coming from behind, outstretched around the seated king.

### *Imhotep*

Unlike the other Egyptian gods described in this study, Imhotep is a deified architect from the reign of Djoser in the Old Kingdom; he created the first step-pyramid. Later Greeks syncretized him with Asklepios, a similar deified human noted for healing. The deification of a historical person is quite rare in ancient Egyptian religion, unlike Greek and especially Roman religious culture, which would use this process often to honor military-political fig-

12. Wolfhardt Westendorf, "Götter, androgyne," in *Lexikon der Ägyptologie*, ed. Wolfgang Helck and Wolfhardt Westendorf (Wiesbaden: Otto Harrassowitz, 1977), 634–35.

13. Robert Ritner, "The Famine Stela," in *The Literature of Ancient Egypt*, ed. William Kelly Simpson (New Haven: Yale University, 2003), 386–91.

ures. Although the tomb of Imhotep has never been found, it is likely that he did not carry the title of a healer during his lifetime. But his reputation for skill and intelligence eventually led to his deification in the Nineteenth Dynasty and then linked him to healing by the Thirtieth Dynasty.

## Sources

### Texts

Unlike the Mesopotamian sources, there is not a significant problem with ancient Egyptian medical texts being misidentified as magical texts, because scholars early on recognized a significant medical culture for ancient Egypt. Yet certain texts with a prominent use of incantations were certainly dismissed as important for studying Egyptian medicine well into the twentieth century.

At present, eleven different papyri are classified as medical texts. They are: Kahun, Ramesseum, Ebers, Edwin Smith, Berlin, Hearst, London, Chester-Beatty, Carlsberg VIII, Brooklyn Snake, and London-Leiden. Grapow's series in German, *Grundiss der Medizin der alten Ägypter*, is the most comprehensive translation of all the Egyptian medical papyri. Although particular papyri can be dated to certain centuries or even reigns on the basis of linguistic evidence, some passages claim greater antiquity by noting specific kings, such as "found in a writing under Anubis' feet in Letopolis; it was brought to his majesty of Upper and Lower Egypt Usaphais [Den (2950–2775 BCE)]."[14] Although the prescriptions to which these are attached may have originated during the Old Kingdom, more likely a later scribe simply inserted the names to lend an air of authority. Ancient scribes from around the Mediterranean and eastward into Mesopotamia commonly attached the names of notable figures from the past to create a sense of importance for the texts. Other times, scribes would copy passages from a variety of older texts. Therefore, many papyri end up with considerable overlap, which helps scholars determine the age of medical practices, by tracing them back to their earliest occurrence in the texts.

Early Egyptologists divided medical techniques between scientific or rational somatic medicine and simply magical practices. Those texts lacking a significant amount of incantations fell into the scientific/rational category,

14. Ebers 103.01.

such as the Edwin Smith Papyrus. Oddly, though, other texts without much in the way of incantations suffered from the label magical, such as the Kahun Papyrus. Other texts, like the London-Leiden Papyrus, originally were not even counted as medical texts, since they contain incantations in every prescription, despite their obvious aim at treating medical conditions such as dog bites and fevers. This problem in classification highlights how modern researchers can manipulate the definitions of medicine by focusing on and judging therapeutic measures by modern standards. An alternative approach would have scholars looking at the problems requiring therapeutic intervention, which subsequently allows for an analysis more in keeping with the cultural standards of the society under study.

The medical cases presented in the papyri tend to follow a layout of title, examination, diagnosis, verdict, and therapeutics. This may seem unremarkable at first. But in comparison to other ancient medical cultures, this feature of the Egyptian medical texts begins to stand out. The examination process often requires the healer to physically manipulate the patient's body in order to render a diagnosis and prognosis. Contrast this to Greco-Roman medicine, which eschews physical examinations or otherwise direct communications with the patient. Also, the therapeutic sections often include several treatment measures presented as alternatives, written as recipes "A or B or C." The complexity of the Egyptian cases, again, can contrast with Mesopotamian medicine's simple construction of if/then statements in its medical texts. Variations across cultures, in their writing of medical cases, may be taken as a field of study for understanding the differing values in each medical system. There is more than one way to present a medical case.

An interesting gap exists in the medical texts between the Late period and the latter portion of the Roman Empire. For this study, medical texts produced with a more Greco-Roman approach, especially those originating in Alexandria, will be considered under Greek medicine. This would include not just the treatises arguing points of view from different *iatroi*[15] but also inscriptions relating to practices at the temple for Asklepios. The fact that a late text such as the London-Leiden Papyrus is included in studies on Egyptian medicine speaks more to how modern scholars understand cultural differences, especially since the London-Leiden is noted as containing a considerable amount of magic.

The following is a brief overview of the texts to help identify pertinent ones for particular areas of study. The eclectic nature of some of them indi-

15. Greek for "physicians."

cates that the practices of healing and even of disseminating knowledge were not based upon the division of discrete systems. Ancient Egyptian healing often had a general, interconnected approach.

Kahun is the earliest known papyrus, dating to the Twelfth Dynasty during the reign of Amenemhat III. It contains prescriptions focusing on obstetrics and gynecology. Yet the cases are not restricted to issues with the reproductive tract or pregnancy itself but include other problems a pregnant woman may have, such as a toothache.

The Ramesseum Papyrus focuses on gynecology, as well as gastroenterology, pediatrics, and ophthalmology. It includes also treatment for ailments affecting the *mtw*.[16] Excavators found the papyrus in a storeroom, in a chest belonging to a priest, which included magic wands and amulets. Likely, the priest functioned as a healer, but there was no indication that he officially carried the title of a healer, such as *swnw*.

The Berlin or Brugsch Papyrus dates to the Nineteenth Dynasty and treats issues with the *mtw*, breasts, contraception, and tests for fertility. It has considerable parallels with the Ebers, Hearst, Kahun, and Carlsberg papyri and thus is interesting for comparative work. Unfortunately, no one knows exactly where the papyrus originated, making it difficult to use when determining a more local character for Egyptian medical practices.

The Hearst Papyrus dates to the reign of Thutmosis III (1482–1450 BCE), covering cases for digestion, dentistry, orthopedics, animal bites, and the *mtw*. Many of its passages parallel ones found in the Berlin and Ramesseum papyri, as well as exact copies of cases in the Ebers Papyrus.

The London Papyrus comes from the Eighteenth Dynasty, perhaps the reign of Tutankhamun. It is given the British Museum (BM) catalog number BM 10059, which may be confused with the later London-Leiden Papyrus carrying catalog number BM 100070, if the popular titles are not used. Its contents cover gynecology plus other ailments, but these non-gynecological ones overlap with cases found in the Ebers Papyrus.

The Carlsberg VIII Papyrus was composed in the Nineteenth or Twentieth Dynasty, but it appears to be based on a document from the Twelfth Dynasty. Gynecological cases are on one side of the document, while the other side is dedicated to eye ailments, copied exactly from the Ebers Papyrus.

The Edwin Smith Papyrus dates to the Middle Kingdom, roughly around the seventeenth century BCE. But some of its vocabulary comes from the Old Kingdom, while glosses in the margins are from the New Kingdom.

16. Tube-like structures found throughout the body.

This type of linguistic blending indicates that prescriptions and healing techniques carried through various political and cultural shifts over a thousand years. The papyrus itself likely lasted for a few hundred years in continuous use. One side of the papyrus addresses cases of trauma, progressing anatomically from the head down through the body, but the papyrus breaks off midtorso when dealing with the spine. This portion has only one incantation, so early scholars labelled it a "surgical papyrus." This text became a popular reference among scholars wishing to highlight the scientific aspects of Egyptian medicine, drawing favorable parallels with modern medical techniques. The reverse side of the papyrus (conveniently ignored) contains several incantations for a "pest of the year," menses, the complexion, the anus, and restoring one's youth.

Two translations are available in English. Still popular are reissues of Breasted's 1930 edition, with an emphasis on philology that handily cross references some passages with other Egyptian medical texts.[17] Yet it suffers from the rather dated perspective that Egyptian healers are divided between scientific "physicians," represented by the *swnw*, and the more magical-based practitioners, the *wab* priest and *sau*. More recently, Sanchez and Meltzer have updated the translation and provide modern medical commentary on the cases, with useful anatomical illustrations.[18] It continues, though, the assumption that a division between scientific and magical medical practices existed in ancient Egypt.

The Ebers Papyrus is one of the more popular texts among modern scholars of Egyptian medicine. It most likely dates to the Eighteenth Dynasty. Its cases cover a wide range of ailments, including gynecology, intestinal worms, skin afflictions, dentistry, disease of the anus and heart, remedies created by the gods for the gods, ophthalmology, bites by dogs and humans, and the *mtw*, which delves into the physiology of them. The order in which the cases appear has no discernible pattern, such as starting at the head and working downward through the body or grouping them according to related symptoms or treatment measures. The therapies are a mixture of incantations and more obviously somatic treatments that modern medicine would classify as minor surgery. An interesting feature of the Ebers Papyrus is the

17. James Henry Breasted, *The Edwin Smith Surgical Papyrus* (Chicago: University of Chicago Press, 1991).

18. Gonzalo M. Sanchez and Edmund S. Meltzer, *The Edwin Smith Papyrus: An Updated Translation of the Trauma Treatise and Modern Medical Commentaries* (Atlanta: Lockwood, 2012).

inclusion of a treatment for an eye ailment, referencing its origins among the Canaanites. This attests to the fluid nature of medicine between ancient Near Eastern and Mediterranean cultures. Some cases may have adapted incantations or *materia medica* to local practices, but others intentionally retain foreign elements, such as the Ebers Papyrus keeping incantations in the Canaanite language.

The Chester-Beatty Papyrus was found at Deir el-Medina, the workers village for the New Kingdom tombs in the Valley of the Kings. It comes from the archive of the Nineteenth-Dynasty scribe Qen-her-Khepeshef. His family had it for over a century, but no one from this family carried any of the titles for healers, such as *swnw*. This may indicate that one could practice healing techniques without benefit of a formal title as long as one was literate enough to read the appropriate texts. The papyrus presents therapeutic recipes differently in some portions, using the format "A then B then C," as if compounding over time, rather than alternatives more commonly written as "A or B or C." The text treats a variety of illnesses, one of which may have been epilepsy, as well as impotency, headaches, and scorpion stings.

The Brooklyn Snake Papyrus directly addresses the priests or *sau* of Serket and deals exclusively with bites from snakes, scorpions, and spiders. Unlike other medical texts treating animal bites, this papyrus contains descriptions of various snakes. The treatments are usually somatic in orientation, with only a few incantations. It dates to the Late period, sixth to fourth century BCE, and possibly the Thirtieth Dynasty. Thus, its description of snakes may be in imitation of Greek scientific treatises.

The Crocodilopolis Papyrus is also known as Papyrus Vindob D. 6257. It dates to the second century CE and likely was written in Memphis, but it was found in the Fayum, an oasis area to the west of the Nile. It has no incantations but interestingly combines traditional Egyptian *materia medica* with newer medicants from the Mediterranean, that is, Greco-Roman. The cases are composed mostly in the traditional format of medical texts like the Ebers Papyrus, but it focuses more on the preparation of remedies than on diagnosing through examination. Crocodilopolis may have possibly influenced the pharmacopeia treatises of Dioscorides and Pliny.

London-Leiden is the latest of the Egyptian medical papyri, dating to second or third century CE. It is a papyrus reconstructed by joining fragments held in two different museums, hence the name London-Leiden. Although composed well beyond the Pharaonic period, its contents rely heavily on ancient Egyptian religious culture, with regard to invoking ancient Egyptian gods and a reliance on healing through incantations, with little obvious corruption from contemporary religions such as Christianity. It may be useful in analyzing how Egyptian religious-medical culture survived beyond the political fortunes of Egyptian kings.

As in all societies, a variety of texts may touch upon medical topics, including letters, royal and legal documents, and literary texts. Of particular note is the plethora of literary texts that involve priests. Since there is overlap between the priesthood and healers, close attention to descriptions of *wab* priests may shed light on medicine in ancient Egyptian culture. Similarly, references to the body in love songs or other writings can indicate cultural values for anatomy and physiology.

The Nineteenth-Dynasty story *The Tale of Two Brothers* illustrates the value of literature in the study of medical culture. It recounts the troubles the brothers Anubis and Bata have with their wives, eventually leading to Bata becoming Pharaoh and making his older brother Anubis the crown prince of Egypt. The wife of Anubis inappropriately propositioned Bata and, to cover her violation of *maat*, pretended to be ill, eventually accusing Bata of assaulting her. In Bata's own defense, he both cuts off his phallus and removes his heart. These organs then survive apart from the body, creating effects in fish, trees, houses, and people. Although at first it appears as nothing more than a fairy tale about kingship rife with magic, a close reading of it reveals cultural values about gender and castration, the power of blood, pregnancy, and the independence of organs, all of which impacts the Egyptian conceptions of medicine, as we shall see. Analysis of similar literary texts will uncover Egyptian attitudes about the body, health, and disease that are not obvious through just studying the medical papyri.

Work records and contracts can also shed light on the daily impact of illness as well as the practical role of healers in society. For example, the texts relating to the workers at Deir el-Medina, spanning the reigns of Ramesses II to Ramesses IX, include *swnw* on the payroll.[19] Ostraca record the absence of workmen due to illness and reveal pressure for them to work through their illnesses.[20] Some scholars use this type of evidence in arguments for Egypt having a form of government-provided health care. Other documents of interest are contracts from Sais during the Late and Ptolemaic periods, which show people selling themselves into slavery[21] but include also an interesting

19. O. Cairo J 51518.

20. Ann E. Austin, "Accounting for Sick Days: A Scalar Approach to Health and Disease at Deir el-Medina," *Journal of Near Eastern Studies* 74 (2015): 75–85.

21. It should be noted that ancient slavery, unlike that of the United States in the nine-

line for the study of medicine: "No male or female spirit, sleeping man, ghost, drowned man, demon, ill-fortune or pestilence will be able to exercise power over me except you from today onward."[22] This clause serves as a guarantee of good health at the time of purchase, so any subsequent illness or injury is the fault and responsibility of the new master. It indicates also that health is governed by relationships that exist not only between humans but also with the supernatural and that it can be contractually bound.

Letters provide another good source for ancient Egyptian medical practices. The most frequent mention of Egyptian healers occurs in the correspondence records kept by Assyrian and Babylonian courts. Only a few letters from Egypt mention healers and sickness, typically asking that medicants or other items be sent to help pass the time while ill. A letter on behalf of Ramesses IX (1126–1108 BCE) complains that a medicant used in eye-paint (*galena*) was of an insufficient amount.[23] Several letters over the years, from a man named Dhutmose, mention his illness, though not in any detail that could be used to clinically diagnose an ailment.[24] Dhutmose's letters do give a picture of the cultural context for experiencing illness in ancient Egyptian society. An interesting letter to a deceased wife asks her to help remove an illness using the imagery of her fighting. In return, the widower promises to make an offering for her, much like the exchange one would have with a god when supplicating for healing.[25] Another letter from a man to his dead wife essentially sues her spirit for not leaving him alone. He makes part of his case by noting that he sent for a healer (*swnw*) when she became ill.[26] This is notable in that a written document can transcend mortal boundaries and have an effect on supernatural relationships, much like the slave contract. Underlying this is the idea that the written word calls things into existence; in this instance, it is a court proceeding.

---

teenth century, looked at slaves as permanent children in need of care rather than as sub- or nonhuman chattel.

22. William W. Hallo and K. Lawson Younger Jr., eds., *The Context of Scripture: Archival Documents* (Boston: Brill, 2003), 23.

23. P. Cairo B; see Edward F. Wente, trans., *Letters from Ancient Egypt* (Atlanta: Scholars Press, 1990), 37.

24. Wente, *Letters from Ancient Egypt.*

25. Wente, *Letters from Ancient Egypt*, 215.

26. P. Leiden I 371; see Wente, *Letters from Ancient Egypt*, 217.

## Archaeology

Besides written documents, archaeology can also help us understand how healing was effected in ancient Egypt and the role of religious culture on those practices. Digs have been done in Egypt essentially since the time of Napoleon, but only in the latter part of the nineteenth century has the modern field of archaeology carried out a more systematic method of excavation with attention to documenting the context of artifacts. Because of the long duration and wide scope of Egyptian archaeology, only a few highlights will be given here, which illustrate the controversial nature of interpreting sites and artifacts.

One frequently debated issue is the function of the House of Life. Inscriptions indicate that it is a building attached to or within a temple complex, reserved for either healing practices, medical education, or more likely just scribal activity. It is problematic in that no House of Life has actually been excavated. References to it appear as part of a title, such as the *swnw* of the House of Life. Given that the education of ancient healers is mostly through an apprenticeship or simply the studying of texts in a scribal school, it is hard to imagine the House of Life as a dedicated space solely for learning medicine, akin to a modern medical school.

Other ubiquitous sources are tomb reliefs, scenes of everyday life and exceptional events either painted or carved into the walls, as well as the biographies of the tomb owners. They can show what might be therapeutic, such as manicures and pedicures, as in the tombs of Khentika and Ankhmahor.[27] The tomb of Ipwy from the workers' village of Deir el-Medina depicts industrial accidents, such as a dislocated shoulder and debris in the eyes.[28] The pyramid of Unas (Fifth Dynasty) depicts adult famine victims with extremely narrow waists and protruding ribs, while children have the characteristic extended bellies.

Although not technically textual sources, many names of healers can be found in these reliefs on tomb walls. These can be either the tomb of the healer, such as the case of Sankhu-Ptah, or mentioned in the tomb of another official, such as the *swnw* Tjau, named in the tomb for Hem-min.[29]

A site commonly referred to as the Physician's Tomb at Saqqara is actually the tomb of Ankhmahor, a priest and vizier of the Sixth-Dynasty king

27. John Nunn, *Ancient Egyptian Medicine* (Norman: University of Oklahoma Press, 2002), 133.

28. Nunn, *Ancient Egyptian Medicine*, 57.

29. Nunn, *Ancient Egyptian Medicine*, 134.

Teti. Its appellation, "Physician's Tomb," comes from a number of scenes depicting circumcision and some type of manipulation of the feet and hands. The circumcision scene is repeated on the wall of the Temple of Mut at Karnak, indicating that the practice went unchanged for much of Egyptian history. The image of treating hands and feet is not as clear. Some argue that it is a form of surgery being carried out, due to the accompanying hieroglyphs' use of the word "pain." More likely, it is a massage reminiscent of ones prescribed for aching muscles, which appear in the Kahun Papyrus.

Karnak started as a shrine in the Middle Kingdom, but it became the main center for Amun worship during the New Kingdom and lasted into the Roman period. The site contains temples to Amun, his consort Mut, their son Khonsu, and the god Montu, as well as festival halls, processional walkways, and a sacred lake. In addition to the scene of circumcision, hieroglyphic inscriptions in the Temple of Mut retell the story of Isis saving Horus from poisonous creatures sent by Seth. Elements of the story were used for healing purposes; the same story is recast on Ptolemaic-period *cippi* statues used in healing rituals.[30] Amenhotep III installed roughly seven hundred statues of Sekhmet near his mortuary temple and the Mut Temple, likely as a response to devastating plagues that swept through the region during his reign.

The graffiti at Deir el-Bahri presents an interesting problem in dating the use of funerary cults[31] in medical therapies. The debate centers on the funerary cult for the architect Amenhotep, the son of Hapu, as a center of healing.[32] The funerary cult dates to the reign of Amenhotep III, yet the use of a funerary cult for healing is a much later practice, usually Ptolemaic. The questions then are, When exactly was the graffiti written, and by how much does the site's association with healing predate the Ptolemaic period? Similarly, a stela for Qen her Khepeshef (1295–1186 BCE) attests to sleeping in a temple for healing, but this stands as an anomaly, with dream therapies not being popular in Egypt until the Coptic period in the third century CE.

Like the House of Life, archaeologists have yet to recover any tools dedicated solely to healing, such as a surgical kit. A chest from the Ramesseum,

30. Philippa Lang, *Medicine and Society in Ptolemaic Egypt* (Boston: Brill, 2013), 95.

31. Funerary cults are designed to maintain the tombs and other monuments associated with the burial of high-level officials and lesser members of the royal family. It provides a financial basis and also supplies personnel such as priests to carry out cultic activities on behalf of the deceased.

32. Serge Sauneron, *The Priests of Ancient Egypt* (Ithaca: Cornell University Press, 2000), 157.

belonging to a priest and with the title "Chief of Secrets," did contain magic wands and amulets along with a medical text. Intact pottery is often tested for residues but usually contains foodstuffs rather than medicants known from the medical texts. This is complicated by the fact that the compounding of the medicines likely occurred at the time they were needed rather than when they were premade or stored. Also, these pots tend to be found in tombs, which obviates the needs for medicine. Once the person is deceased, the soul(s) and the body are not as intimately connected; therefore, messages from the supernatural no longer need to be inscribed on the body, nor would the body serve as a message to the wider human community when locked away in the tomb.

Although the practice of mummification is not the process by which Egyptian healers learned about anatomy and physiology, mummies simply being preserved bodies can provide modern paleopathologists information about prevalent diseases and medical practices in ancient Egypt. The use of salts and bitumen in the mummification process can interfere, though, with certain types of paleopathological analyses that rely on the soft tissue. Mummies do provide a good source for analysis of trauma, congenital defects, and disease processes affecting the skeleton. The skull of the Pharaoh Seqenenra shows fractures. The Pharaoh Saptah has a club foot. And the priest Nesparehan from the Twenty-first Dynasty displays spinal tuberculosis. Interestingly, the edges of the fracture in Seqenenra's skull have slightly healed, indicating he lived for roughly a month after the blow. The mummy of a fifty-year-old woman from the Third Intermediate period had an amputated big toe, plus a working prosthesis.[33]

During the process of mummification, the embalmers removed certain internal organs and placed them in special containers known as canopic jars, although they could just as easily have been chests, miniature coffins, and sometimes even masks. The organs were desiccated, wrapped, and placed in the jars, which could then be put back into the body or given a special niche in a tomb. Each jar had a special pairing between the organs, a son of Horus and a goddess. The liver matched with Imsety and Isis, the lungs with Hapy and Nephthys, the stomach with Duamutef and Neith, and finally the intestines with Kebehsenuef and Serket. Although these practices date back to the Old Kingdom, it was during the First Intermediate that the jars developed human heads, which then evolved to animal and bird heads in

33. Andreas G. Nerlich et al., "Ancient Egyptian Prosthesis for the Big Toe," *Lancet* 356 (2000): 2176–79.

the New Kingdom. The original representations stressed the human aspect of the deceased person, whereas later ones emphasized the protective powers of Horus's four sons. This pairing indicates the link between anatomy and cosmology used in Egyptian physiology. Many scholarly texts describe this as symbolic anatomy, in which a body part represents a particular deity. As we shall see, the ancient Egyptian conception of the body understood various organs to be, in essence, the deity thus functioning as a symbiotic anatomy.

Boomerang shaped "wands" made of hippopotamus ivory have been found in tombs dating to the Middle Kingdom. These depict fearsome looking deities and spirits carrying knives, including Bes and, at times, Taweret. Inscriptions on the wands attest to their apotropaic function of protecting infants. The exact ritual use of the wands is not entirely clear, although some suggest that they were placed in the beds of the children or used to scratch a protective circle on the ground around a bed.

A common artifact dating from the Late period and into the Greco-Roman era are the *cippi* statues. These are stelae with carvings of Horus as a child standing on a crocodile. Often they are called "Cippi of Horus." The term *cippus* is Greek, meaning "grave marker" or "tombstone." But this term was originally applied to the Horus carvings on the basis of appearance and not function, which was either to prevent or help cure bites from animals, particularly reptiles. Someone would pour water over the stela, which charged the water with the power to counter poisonous bites or stings and then collect in a basin at the bottom. Drinking the water could either prevent the animal attack or cure one that had already happened. Most *cippi* are small enough to be placed in a private home, but two seem to have had a public placement. The Metternich Stela is the largest and most well-known of the *cippi*, created during the reign of Nectanebo II (360–342 BCE) by the priest Nesu-Atum only a few years before the dynasty fell to the Persians. They likely developed from small, portable amulets of the god Shed, "the Savior," used during the New Kingdom period.

## Cultural Concepts

As we shall see, ancient Egypt shares a number of cultural similarities with Mesopotamia that affect their explanatory model of illness. There is a belief that parts of the body communicate disruptions in community cohesion. Only perfect or pure bodies should be in the presence of the gods. Although their cosmology lacks a divine council, the gods do act with some level of cooperation. And a hierarchy exists between them and lesser entities such as ghosts and spirits/demons, while the king functions as a bridge between the natural and supernatural worlds. Among humans, social roles carried more value than the reality of physical appearances; thus, gender became a fluid concept in certain situations.

## Anatomy and Physiology

Realism in art as an avenue to understanding Egyptian concepts of anatomy and physiology presents a unique set of issues. In keeping with artistic conventions dominating the ancient Near East, Egyptian statues, reliefs, and wall paintings usually depict gods and kings in their most idealized forms. They all appear youthful, lean, well muscled, and properly proportioned. Women were tall and slender. A fat body meant wealth, but artists never used it for images of the royal family. Similarly, kings never appear with common ailments like hernias, but depictions of workers often showed them. This is in contrast to the reality of pharaohs Merneptah and Ramesses V suffering from hernias.[34] Variable conventions for the ideal body image indicated social position. This is an important point when assessing the body's physiology; depending on someone's place in the social hierarchy, his or her body will have a different ideal form.

Realism, however, also played an important part in Egyptian iconography. *Ka* statues[35] needed realism in order for the deceased's life force to recognize itself. Yet the realism of showing supposed defects in the lower classes cannot be taken at face value. For example, achondroplastic dwarfism seems abnormally ubiquitous for ancient Egypt on the basis of its frequency in art. But coupled with the convention of size denoting social status, it becomes apparent that dwarfism simply serves as a way of rendering someone of short stature (not actually a dwarf) while retaining the relative size of figures of varying social status. Similarly, the presence of a hunchback denotes servant status as an artistic convention rather than accurate clinical depiction of a disease process.

34. J. Thompson Rowling, "Hernia in Egypt," in *Diseases in Antiquity* (Springfield: Bannerstone House, 1967), 446; Nunn, *Ancient Egyptian Medicine*, 92.

35. Egyptians divided the soul into multiple parts; the creative life force, or *ka*, could wander but always returned to the body, even after death. *Ka* statues, like the mummified body, gave it a place to return and rest.

The consistent physical prowess of the king in art symbolizes his ability to keep chaos at bay, especially in the rendering of animal-hunt scenes. The king's physiology, by virtue of being both divine and human, is unique in comparison to other humans. This appears in references to kings having skin of gold.[36] For everyone, the *ka* (soul)[37] and the body are created simultaneously, yet the king's *ka* possesses divinity at this early, pre-birth stage. The act of coronation also deifies the king by joining his *ka* with the *ka* of divine ancestors. Interestingly, the divine powers of kingship must be renewed in the *sed*-festival, when it wanes every thirty years, while documents attest to the ritual occurring every three years. The frequency of these physical rituals designed to reaffirm the strength of a king indicate a need for political stability more than a shift in the ideology of a king's physiology.

Egyptian society definitely functioned with a gendered slant toward male dominance, but it did not operate on a simple binary system of only males and females, with rigid gender roles. At first glance, it would appear that gender was biologically determined for the ancient Egyptians, as found in *The Tale of Two Brothers*, which shows the character Bata cutting off his penis and declaring himself a woman. The presence of a third gender, in the form of eunuchs and others, also existed.[38] Elite women could assume a male role, such as the case of Hatshepsut, because of her position as king. Artists depicted her with a beard, and scribes referenced her with male pronouns. Ancient Egyptian has no word for "queen" as a political category. Similarly, Akhenaten took on an androgynous physique in artistic renderings in order to convey his status as the only human mediator between the divine Aten (the sole god under his reign) and the Egyptian people; he was to be both mother and father of Egypt.

Egyptian art appears to use the same human form, without individuality, in constant repetition, especially in depicting workers in tomb paintings and wall reliefs. Royal images tend to show an idealized physical form, but in sculpture, there is some degree of realism in the king's face. This realism

36. Katja Goebs, "Kingship," in *The Egyptian World*, ed. Toby Wilkinson (New York: Routledge, 2010), 275–95.

37. Egyptians conceived of up to five souls for each person. The *ka* is the life force that animates the body. It exists after the physical body dies, thus necessitating mummification or statuary for it to reside.

38. Mark Depauw, "Notes on Transgressing Gender Boundaries in Ancient Egypt," *Zeitschrift für Ägyptische Sprache und Altertumskunde* 130 (2003): 49–59; T. G. Wilfong, "Gender and Sexuality," in *The Egyptian World*, ed. Toby Wilkinson (New York: Routledge, 2010), 205–17.

carries over into sculptures and reliefs of nonroyal administrators. There is remarkable anatomical realism in Third-Dynasty tomb reliefs of Kha-bau-soker and his wife Hathor-nefer-hotep, from the Old Kingdom, as well as images of Hesi-re, which additionally show him with increased wrinkles at different stages of adulthood.[39] By the later Fourth Dynasty, this anatomical realism for the body begins to fade. In terms of facial features, there are trends toward sternness of countenance in the Third and Fifth Dynasties, while the Fourth Dynasty conveys a more serene disposition. It should be noted that in some cases near Saqqara in Upper Egypt, the lack of detailed modeling for anatomical realism is due to the quality of the stone used rather than any cultural values. The Sixth Dynasty has a mixture of realism and idealization, with a slight favoring of depicting people at older stages of life. This might be fashionable because of the age of King Pepy II and the length of his reign. Variations in artistic renderings of the body between realism and idealization change with almost every dynasty, making it difficult to determine an overarching cultural value regarding anatomy. But this also creates an area of fruitful study regarding more detailed dynasty-by-dynasty analyses.

The Egyptians attributed the specific creation of humans to certain gods—such as Khnum, who fashioned newborn babies and infused them with a breath of life, and the goddess Neith, who invented childbirth itself. The *Instruction of Merikare* (ca. 2125–2010 BCE) describes humans as "god's cattle," saying, "He made breath for their noses to live. They are images who came from his body."[40] The eye of Re-Atum was sent out to find the children Shu and Tefnut and, upon her return, finds that Re-Atum had grown a new eye. The tears of her weeping become the first humans; this story plays on the similarity of the Egyptian words for tear and people. Other versions have humans come from the sweat or laughter of the gods. These stories depict a conception of the human body, in whole or in part, as intimately linked with the gods.

The tongue, too, and its role in speech is an important factor in the creation of humans. According to Egyptian cosmology, speech creates the *ka*, one of the five souls that inhabits a person, which then needs a vessel, such as a body, in which to reside. This explains the ubiquitousness of *ka* statues among funeral goods. In terms of anatomy and physiology, the person is his or her soul (*ka*), which is distinct from the body. It may for a time animate

39. Nadine Cherpion, "The Human Image in Old Kingdom Non-Royal Reliefs," in *Egyptian Art in the Age of the Pyramids* (New York: Metropolitan Museum of Art, 1999), 103–15.

40. Hallo and Younger, *Context of Scripture: Canonical Compositions*, 65.

the body, but they do exist separately and, therefore, can have their own relationships to the supernatural realm. How one, either the body or the *ka*/person, interacts with the god can affect the other for positive or negative results.

Protective spells, as well as the canopic jars, link deities to particular organs, thus depicting what is commonly referred to as a symbolic anatomy, in which the invoked god watches over specific organs. As we read in the Book of the Dead, "My eyes are Hathor, my ears are Wepwawet . . . my lips are Anubis, my molars are Selket."[41] Also, Spell 5 states, "Lick with thy tongue . . . for thy tongue is the tongue of the Agathodaemon, thy tongue is that of Atum."[42] Yet this explanation glosses over the important concept in Egyptian cosmology in which the gods are present within objects, including the body. Note the phrasing "Body Parts are Divine Name." Because of this relationship with the divine, the organs of the human body have an identity distinct from the human. The body parts and the person thus exist in a symbiotic anatomy, working together with the person and exerting nominal control over the body. Leiden Papyrus Spell 2 shows how tenuous this control can be: "Dost thou cause my mouth to speak blasphemy?" Instances of illness show that the body parts can act independently of the human will. Similarly, cures also may require the body part to be independent of the person. A spell for a headache depicts the sufferer swapping heads with Isis or Nephthys.[43] In order for this particular spell to work, the patient is first transformed into Horus, who then asks his mother and aunt for help.

This relationship between body and human mirrors a similar symbiotic anatomy that exists among the gods. By the New Kingdom, the Hermopolitan creation myth gave prominence to Amun, syncretizing him with Re—describing Amun's face as Re, while his body is Ptah. At Memphis, Ptah is the creator god, who first thinks of things with his heart and then creates them through the power of speech. Another creation story from Heliopolis draws upon Ptah as creator but with Atum as his heart and tongue.

Although a vessel for the souls, the body itself is a system or network of interconnected tubes known as *mtw*, forming a type of irrigation system. The term *mtw* is not easily translated, since its use in the medical texts could

41. Raymond O. Faulkner, trans., *The Ancient Egyptian Book of the Dead* (London: British Museum, 2010), 62.

42. F. Ll. Griffith and Herbert Thompson, eds., *The Leyden Papyrus: An Egyptian Magical Book* (New York: Dover, 1985).

43. R. Ritner, Presentation at University of Chicago Oriental Institute's Annual Dinner 1998; see https://oi.uchicago.edu/research/individual-scholarship/practical-egyptian-magical-spells.

mean tendon, nerve, or blood vessel; it essentially describes any long, thin tube-like structure in the body. The Ebers Papyrus has the most detailed outline about how the *mtw* functioned.[44] According to this text, the body contains twenty-two *mtw* that all join together at the heart and the anus. The *mtw* also open to the outside world through the anus, as well as through the mouth, ears, and eyes, which allows for the expulsion of substances from the body but just as easily leaves it vulnerable to toxic substances entering the body. Similarly, wounds create an unnatural opening for the *mtw*.

In addition to the irrigation model of physiology, the Egyptians also worked with a mechanical understanding. This is most evident in the description of spinal-cord and brain injuries correlated with a lack of limb movement.[45] The two concepts of irrigation and mechanics worked together to essentially create a body that runs on hydraulics. This meant that disruptions to the hydraulic system would cause illness, and, conversely, restoration of the hydraulics can bring healing. Preventative medicine called for the regular application of diuretics and emetics to keep the system clear and flowing. Underlying the hydraulics, a properly working physiology is a manifestation of *maat* (balance/order), while an illness indicates that the body in its relation to other elements or forces in the world is out of balance.

No specific elements were outlined as necessary apart from the obviously vital blood and air. Yet the texts do identify specific substances that are harmful, like *weḫedew*, which has various translations, such as "pain matter" or "purulency."[46] The Ebers Papyrus describes *weḫedew* as both moving through the body as a natural substance[47] and being a supernatural agent of the gods or the dead.[48] Once again, this demonstrates that the natural and supernatural worlds were not strictly divided in their medical culture. Hence, physical healing and treatments relying on the access of *heka* (power) also did not fall into opposing magical and rational/scientific somatic therapies.

Contrary to popular assumptions, the practice of mummification was not a significant source of anatomical knowledge for Egyptian healers. They did not engage in dissection as part of the mummification process. During mummification, only the brain, lungs, liver, and intestines were removed, extracted through a small incision on the side of the body between two ribs

44. B. Ebbell, *The Ebers Papyrus* (Copenhagen: Levin and Munksgaard, 1937), 114–18.

45. Breasted, *Edwin Smith Surgical Papyrus*, 324–32.

46. Ebers, Berlin, Hearst, Ramesseum, London, and Chester-Beatty papyri.

47. Ebers 856a.

48. Ebers 131.

rather than a large "Y" incision through the chest, as in a modern autopsy. The goal was to preserve parts of the body in order for the *ka* to use it. Additionally, taboos and rituals surrounding the cutting into the body meant the embalmer spent little time inspecting the body itself, which would undermine any study of it or consequent development of physiological theories. Modern theories abound about why only certain organs were removed. One theory holds that the removal would prevent putrefaction from foodstuffs left in the digestive tract. But this does not account for the removal of the brain, while the kidneys, heart, and spleen left inside the body would just as easily cause rotting. The theory overlooks also that a substance made of wine and vegetables was used to wash out the body cavity.

### Disease Etiology

Descriptions of *weḫedew* demonstrate that even this physical, hydraulic system of the body is subject to illness by actions of the supernatural. Unlike later Greco-Roman medicine, the Egyptians did not espouse different theories about disease etiology or specific treatment measures touted by competing healing practitioners vying for authority. The Egyptians, in keeping with other medical cultures of the ancient Near East, understood disease and trauma as rooted in communication from the divine or supernatural realm. Yet the system of *mtw* made the somatic explanation of disease etiology fairly universal among Egyptian healers, whether it was the *swnw*, *wab* priest, or *sau*.

Modern misperceptions or preconceived notions of ancient Egyptian disease etiology misreads the texts, whether medical or literary. In practice, both natural and supernatural forces created illness and trauma; therefore, both somatic treatments and incantations could just as easily heal them. There was no need to determine a natural or supernatural etiology to match a similar treatment. Nor was there a need to determine the type of healer on the basis of somatic or "magical" treatments. The difference in etiology then lies in the intended audience of the texts describing medical issues. The Edwin Smith Papyrus addresses the healer focusing on the alleviation of specific symptoms. Thus, it is weighted toward somatic treatments, making it appear as if it recognizes only natural-world explanations. Yet the Ebers Papyrus has the same target audience, while liberally using what modern medicine considers "magical" therapeutics. In contrast, a text like *King Cheops and the Magicians*, classified as purely literary by modern scholars, describes the supernatural origins of physical trauma in the story of Reddedet's maidservant.[49] Everything that befalls the woman, from beatings by her brother to an attack by a crocodile, results from her moral transgression of betraying her mistress. This, of course, stands as an extreme case, resulting in death. But even survivable trauma—such as snake and scorpion bites, as well as industrial accidents or injury from warfare—stand as testaments to supernatural forces. As in the case of Reddedet's maidservant, they may be a corrective to behavior, but in other cases it simply is the capriciousness of a supernatural entity and the simple failing of the patient to take normal precautions against such predations.

Where modern medicine draws distinctions between disease etiology, symptoms, and ultimately a diagnosis, the ancient Egyptians often conflated these three categories. *Weḫedew* can serve as both the cause of an illness and the disease itself. Similarly, abdominal distention (what the texts describe as a swollen belly) can be found as both the symptom and the diagnosis, in the same case. Modern bio-medicine defaults to this as well when the reduction/causation model hits a road block—hence, diseases like idiopathic pulmonary fibrosis (unknown scarring of lung tissue). For the ancient Egyptians, the etiology and the diagnosis do not separate the illness from the patient, but rather function to connect the illness and the patient to the larger universe, both the natural and supernatural worlds. So *weḫedew*, as a natural and supernatural substance, links the disease to the body.

## Restoration of Health

In keeping with a medical culture that sees physiology and disease etiology as an intimate connection between the natural and supernatural worlds, the process of restoring health also blends the two realms. It should be kept in mind that the natural world is not limited to the body itself and the disease process, but it includes also the community within which a person lives, whether family, work, or even the temple/shrines.

Illness indicates a disruption in the natural order (*maat*) between the natural and supernatural worlds. This disruption can occur between humans and the gods or spirits but can just as easily arise from discord between humans only, which eventually involves the supernatural realm. Regardless of the etiology of the disease or trauma, the communicative nature of ill-

49. Simpson, *Literature of Ancient Egypt*, 21.

ness demands that the patient at some point display obedience to the gods and maintain the proper relationships between the communities, thus restoring *maat*. Obedience can be demonstrated by submitting to the healing techniques, such as bandaging or purgatives, which are the physical rites in accessing *heka* (power). The gods then consider the demonstration of obedience but do not always respond favorably. The power of the charged substances can hedge one's bets, but it is not a simple mechanistic structure in that the gods must respond one way because of the demonstrated obedience.

An important factor is to whom exactly the act of obedience is demonstrated. The use of *heka* automatically connects the patient to the supernatural realm; thus, communication in a vertical direction to the gods or spirits is easily achieved. But there is a need also, in some cases, to communicate one's obedience to the human community, the horizontal direction. This can be done by having the community know you are under treatment by an accepted healer with *heka*, often by displaying signs such as bandaging.

As seen earlier in the story about the priest Webaoner, *heka*, or accessing of power, has three components: the physical rites, the oral rites, and the charging of substance(s). This aspect of healing is most apparent in prescriptions that make use of incantations (i.e., oral rites) and the obvious physical rituals such as the tying of knots. The *materia medica* then becomes the charged substance. Modern scholarship tends to overlook this same process in somatic therapies. As in the other prescriptions, the ingredients are always the charged substance. The use of bandages, fumigations, or emetics constitutes the physical rite. At the beginning of the medical papyri, such as in Ebers, the oral rites appear as catch-all incantations but also in individual cases.

Four basic devices can make up an incantation: a description, a command, a call for protection, and a recounting of myths, especially those involving Osiris, Horus, Seth, and Isis. In the Leiden Papyrus, spells for a headache, calling on Isis and Nephthys, illustrate the latter grouping of calls for protection, with mythic references. A descriptive spell focusing on the illness itself states, "The burdens are relaxed, and the weakness departs that is located in my belly."[50] An example of a command spell directed at the remedy can be found in Ebers 3: "come remedy, come who removes (bad) things in this my heart and in the parts of my body." The incantations can focus on the illness, the remedy, the patient, or the gods, in a variety of

50. Ebers 61.

combinations. The healer must figure out toward which aspect of the illness to best direct a treatment.

But because illness is ultimately a form of communication between the natural and supernatural realms, the healer must also craft the treatments as a response to one or both of those worlds. A healer focused on the divine aspect of an illness will, then, use treatments that communicate more directly with the divine. This does not limit the healer to incantations. Messages to the gods can just as easily take the form of somatic treatments using charged substances in a physical ritual. Similarly, a healer addressing the natural world can rely on spells. The difference lies in that a natural-world–focused healer will address the human community surrounding the patient.

Certain titles of healers might have indicated to the greater public that they focus on either vertical or horizontal communication. By consulting such a healer, the patient demonstrates obedience and concern for *maat* within the human community, even if the treatment itself is not readily apparent. The *wab* priest's function within the Egyptian religious system indicates an orientation toward vertical communication. The *sau*'s association with Serket and work within the royal court represent a unification of the gods with the ruling order and the ruling order's unification of the human community. This chain indicates that the *sau* has both a vertical and horizontal form of communication. The *swnw*, in contrast, has a stronger focus on just the horizontal form of communication. The exclusive use of *swnw* for healers within the community of gods shows that the vertical form is not really present apart from allying a stronger god to a weaker/suffering god. This connotation is then present in the human *swnw*.

The prognosis section of medical cases illustrates how the healer addresses the human community with the key phrases: "an ailment which I will treat," "an ailment with which I will contend," and finally, "an ailment not to be treated." These phrases indicate the patient's status, with regard to the sick role, as either temporary, possibly permanent, or a definite shift in role to either disabled or deceased. When considering the patient's status, the human community constitutes an important part of the natural world that is integral to the healing process.

Full reintegration with the community, whether human or divine, appears in different contexts. A Nineteenth-Dynasty stela from Thebes describes the recovery of Nakht-Amon after intercessory prayers from his father to Amun. The text explains that the illness came from Amun because of a transgression with cattle, while the healing is reported as, "You have rescued for me . . . so I spoke to you and you did listen to me. Now see, I shall do what I have said."[51] In this case, the exchange of messages occurred between the patient and the divine community. Note also the acknowledgment of obedience and consideration between the human and the divine.

Texts do not directly record the patient's reintegration with the human community, but evidence for it can be found in the documents relating to work sites. Healers such as the *swnw* appear on payrolls for Deir el-Medina, and records show a temporary relief of duties for workers because of illness. Although no texts explicitly mention the restoration of health and their return to the work site, it is reasonable to assume that most workers recovered. This is not far different from the modern situation of an employee calling in sick for a few days without a physician's notice either for the absence or giving permission to return to work. Modern examples of such documents indicate the importance of bureaucratic record keeping, which was not present in the ancient world. Egyptian medicine, even if state sponsored, kept minimal records.

A healing technique not reported in the medical texts, likely because of its late date, is the use of *cippi* statues, which also perfectly illustrates the three parts of accessing *heka*. The statues typically depict the child Horus standing on crocodiles and holding snakes, with passages drawn from the Pyramid Texts, recounting his being stung by a scorpion. Water is poured over the statue (charge of substance) and then drunk (physical rite). Recitation of those passages (oral rite) imparts power to the water (charge of substance), which then prevents or cures a poisonous bite or sting. Interestingly, water running over the text and the recitation of it both impart a charge to the water. The exact practice is not clear on who poured the water or recited the text, whether a healer such as a *wab* priest, *swnw*, simply someone who knew or could read the texts, or even the patient. Spells on the stelae take the form of commands toward the gods and, in some cases, allow a transformation of body parts into the gods.

A common feature cited in early scholarship on Egyptian medicine is "*dreck* apothecary," which works by using noxious substances in medicants in order to drive away the "evil spirits" causing the illness. This system of belief draws upon the concept of treating like with like, or true homeopathy. Similarly, it is thought that the fierce or grotesque appearance of certain deities, such as Bes, would ward off malicious entities, as seen in the Middle Kingdom "wands." As far as can be determined from the textual evidence,

51. Berlin 20377; see James B. Pritchard, *Ancient Near Eastern Texts Relating to the Old Testament* (Princeton: Princeton University Press, 1969), 380–81.

homeopathy constituted only one of the ideologies employed in therapeutic techniques. Overall, Egyptian treatments can be described as pragmatic, in that no one theory predominated in how medicants worked. Rather, treatments became established on the basis of either how they interacted with the hydraulic system of the body or, perhaps more important, whether they evoked a response from the gods. Rather than theoretically arguing for these positions, Egyptian healers relied on their proven efficacy over time, as indicated in some of the medical texts with the gloss "works really well."

## Illness

### Disease

Paleopathological investigations reveal a number of diseases suffered by the ancient Egyptians. Thirty percent of skeletal remains indicate malnutrition at some point in their lives.[52] Although gastrointestinal symptoms occur with many different types of infections, diarrhea in its own right was not considered a problem among the Egyptian population, since their regimen for health included, if not regular purges, then at least an open flow through the *mtw*. In contrast, they considered constipation a more serious concern, needing healing.[53] This becomes evident when looking at the language of the medical texts, which advises examination of stools for the process of diagnosis but does not identify diarrhea as an illness in its own right. Typhoid was a likely candidate for many of the infections suffered, since *Salmonella typhi* is particularly suited to the dry climate.[54] Despite the presence of marshy areas like the Fayum, malaria seems not to have presented a particular problem. The tertiary fevers are not a particularly strong focus of the medical texts, especially in comparison to classical Greece, and human remains do not show a marked increase in sickle-cell anemia, a sign of endemic malaria.[55] Dental caries and other forms of tooth decay occurred with an increasing rate throughout the Pharaonic period and into the Roman era—likely attributed to changes in diet,[56] perhaps

52. Lang, *Medicine and Society in Ptolemaic Egypt*, 10.
53. Lang, *Medicine and Society in Ptolemaic Egypt*, 10–11.
54. Lang, *Medicine and Society in Ptolemaic Egypt*, 10.
55. Lang, *Medicine and Society in Ptolemaic Egypt*, 14.
56. Lang, *Medicine and Society in Ptolemaic Egypt*, 14.

even an increase in grain consumption. Out of all the ancient Near Eastern cultures, the Egyptians had the most sophisticated practice of dentistry, even with evidence of successful root canals.

As radiographical and other scanning techniques develop for modern medical practices, researchers can apply these to Egyptian mummies, better determining the types of illnesses suffered by at least the upper classes of ancient Egyptian society. Halioua and Ziskind[57] provide a basic overview of recent paleopathological studies and brief analysis of certain types of diseases that were likely associated with particular professions, such as urinary tract infections for fishermen.

### Trauma

It is hard to determine the incidents of injuries, but as noted in tomb scenes, workplace trauma was likely common, as well as animal bites and war wounds. Mummies reveal some cases of trauma, such as lost toes or fatal battle wounds, but this would be only among the elite classes. To date, no systematic analysis exists of the rate and types of injuries sustained by the ancient Egyptians, especially among the peasant workers. This paleopathological data would be interesting, considering the frequency with which trauma is referenced in both the medical papyri and literary works. Comparing the types of trauma and their rates in the skeletal record, on the one hand, with their appearance in texts, on the other, can give insight into which particular injuries carried any cultural importance.

### Disability

Studies on disability in the ancient Near East and Mediterranean are limited to the Greco-Roman and biblical worlds, although some in this category do pertain to second- and third-century Egypt.[58] The ancient Egyptians did not conceive of disability in the same way that we do. As

57. Bruno Halioua and Bernard Ziskind, *Medicine in the Days of the Pharaohs* (Cambridge, MA: Belknap, 2005).

58. Jane Draycott, "Reconstructing the Lived Experience of Disability in Antiquity: A Case Study from Roman Egypt," *Greece & Rome* 62 (2015): 189–205.

long as a person was able to carry out his or her social role, the Egyptians did not classify them as disabled. Tomb paintings and physical remains attest to the presence of disabilities, whether from congenital birth defects or trauma. The most common tend to be either dwarfism or leg injuries requiring the permanent use of crutches. Dwarfs did carry special value among the Egyptian royal court not only as a source of entertainment but as a type of person specially marked by the gods. This in itself can carry both positive and negative values, just as a goddess like Sekhmet can bring as well as cure disease.

Very little exists recording the perspective of those not fully able bodied. Yet recognition in the medical texts of a permanent change in one's physical state may be found in the prognosis statement "an ailment not to be treated." More frequently, this likely refers to a terminal diagnosis, but it can indicate also that the condition will persist for the person. As many scholars on disability have shown, ancient societies did not uniformly dismiss those with impairments or routinely expose children with birth defects. It would be reasonable to assume that this integration of different abilities existed in Pharaonic Egypt as well.

**Conditional States**

Similar to the Mesopotamians, the Egyptians did not medicalize various life stages such as infancy, puberty, and old age. *The Maxims of Ptahhotep* open with a description of old age, while Ebers and other papyri mention recipes for grey hair, indicating treatment for signs of old age. But the state itself was not viewed as a medical problem. These types of cases show the Egyptian healer's overlap with other types of professionals dealing with the body, rather than demonstrating a medicalization of geriatrics.

Yet pregnancy did appear in the medical literature. The issue of infertility appears more frequently in Egyptian texts than in those from other ancient Near Eastern and Mediterranean cultures. This does not indicate that Egyptians experienced infertility at a higher rate than other peoples; it shows rather that their cultural value for having children highlights infertility as particularly problematic for them. In contrast, Greek medical texts analyze how children are conceived in terms of the formation of the body, but a concern for infertility does not appear as particularly worrisome. Even though Egyptian society placed great importance on having children, there is ample evidence of contraception, such as the prescription of a linen pessary soaked in honey, found in the Ebers Papyrus. And abortion practices, especially for unmarried women, also existed.[59]

In practical terms, the act of giving birth itself was done on birthing bricks and monitored by midwives rather than titled healers like the *swnw*. The ubiquitousness of obstetrics and gynecology in the medical texts indicates that the care of pregnant women came under the healer's repertoire, but the process of birth itself was not their concern.

## Healers

The three main titles used for professional healers in Egyptian medical texts are the *swnw*, *wab* priest, and *sau*. Most studies on Egyptian medicine translate these as "physician" (*swnw*) and "magician" (for both *wab* priest and *sau*). These modern designations create a false dichotomy between scientific medical practices and purely religious beliefs when, in fact, all of these practitioners used both somatic healing techniques, akin to modern biological practices, and the more obvious religious-based access of cosmological power (*heka*). The idea that one title referred to a physician stems from early scholars assessing the Edwin Smith Papyrus as purely surgical, since it contains only one incantation and addresses the *swnw*. But this determination ignores the first medical case, which clearly states, "Now if *wab* priests of Sekhmet or a *swnw* places his two hands,"[60] indicating that both types of healers use the physical treatments stressed in the papyrus. Similarly, the Ebers Papyrus demonstrates that the *swnw* can just as easily use incantations.[61]

It is best not to translate the terms *swnw* and *sau* directly, but to learn how to use these terms with an understanding about how each title functioned in the overall medical culture of ancient Egypt. Since the variety of terms for healers in ancient Egypt does not indicate a fundamental difference in medical philosophy, this raises the question about why a plethora of terms exists. Although each type of healer uses the same therapeutic techniques and underlying concepts of etiology, the focus of each type differs in the web of interaction between the natural and supernatural worlds.

59. Wilfong, "Gender and Sexuality," 215; John M. Riddle, *Contraception and Abortion from the Ancient World to the Renaissance* (Cambridge, MA: Harvard University Press, 1992).

60. Breasted, *Edwin Smith Surgical Papyrus*, 103–4.

61. Ebers 854a; see Ebbell, *Ebers Papyrus*, 115.

Some healers address primarily the communication necessary between the gods and humans, while others stress the human-to-human component of healing.

Other types of titles appear in a few ancient texts, but they appear too infrequently to deserve a particular focus in this work. Their paucity might indicate a hierarchy of resort in which the ubiquitous *swnw*, *wab* priest, and *sau* can be considered professional healers, while the other types could fall into the category of folk or popular healers. The infrequency of these other titles says less about their exact therapeutic tactics or understanding of physiology and disease etiology and more about their relationship to the power structures of temples and monarchs. Additionally, the surviving texts do not allow for an in-depth study of popular or folk healers such as midwives. Ghalioungui has collated all the ancient Egyptian references to healers, making a handy reference.[62] The key to understanding the difference between the various titles for healers in Egyptian medicine is the communicative function of illness. The illness itself is a message that links the human and supernatural worlds. The problem for Egyptian healers lies in trying to discern who sent the message, why the message was sent, and the best way to communicate a response to that message. The type of healer necessary for each case of illness can change, depending on the answers to each of those questions.

### *Swnw*

Although many earlier studies on Egyptian medicine translate *swnw* as "doctor" or "physician," this is highly problematic. The root itself likely derived from the Egyptian verb meaning "to suffer." Yet there is a similar word meaning "to barter" that works well with tomb scenes showing a *wab swnw* with cattle, doing some type of tax evaluation. The specific translations of physician, doctor, or even surgeon should be avoided so as not to inaccurately impart traits of a modern physician to the ancient Egyptian *swnw*.

Ghalioungui's research shows that the title *swnw* has the most frequency, spanning from the Old Kingdom to the Late period.[63] Often the title is used in connection with a place such as the "*swnw* of the Great House"[64] or "*swnw*

62. Paul Ghalioungui, *The Physicians of Pharaonic Egypt* (Cairo: Al-Ahram Center for Scientific Translations, 1983).

63. Ghalioungui, *Physicians of Pharaonic Egypt*.

64. A palace or other royal residence.

of the House of Ptah."[65] The title appears also on the payroll of a work force found at Deir el-Medina, the workers' village for the Valley of the Kings necropolis. The workers' payroll, however, stands as an exception for the Pharaonic period. This creates doubt about the extent of a state-sponsored health-care system. Their presence in temple and royal structures indicates that their services were available to those elites with access to these places. Most *swnw*, though, worked on a patronage system, lending credence to the idea of the *swnw* as a professional healer.

In addition to the *swnw* being attached to certain government and religious structures, there is evidence also that they made visits to private Egyptian homes and to foreign courts in Mesopotamia. The *swnw* both worked in a stable place and moved around for work as necessary. Yet no facility existed that functioned as a dedicated healing space, akin to the modern hospital, from which the *swnw* carried out his treatments. Debate surrounds the function of places such as the House of Life and the Mansion of Life, with the former being thought of as a medical school and the latter a hospital. But these conjectures stem from assumptions about the *swnw* as physician rather than historical or archaeological records.

In keeping with the association of *swnw* with power holders, this is the title given to various gods when described as healers. For example, Horus carries the title "*swnw* for the House of Re," as other deities also do. These types of references indicate not only that the title is associated with power structures, but also that the *swnw* communicates within a community, god to god, rather than bridging communities, such as gods to humans. From this, it can be concluded that the human *swnw* similarly focuses on communication within a community. A patient seeking healing from a *swnw* wishes not only to understand the message but also to express that message to others in his community, aiming to respond appropriately through the guidance of the *swnw*.

### *Wab* Priest

The term "*wab*" means "purity" and designated the lowest level within the priesthoods for the Egyptian gods. In order for any religious ritual to be effective, it had to be done in a state of physical purity, so as not to offend the gods. Purity could be achieved by at least bathing, while at the higher

65. A temple dedicated to the god Ptah.

levels, such as the lector priest, circumcision was required. The body itself, in this manner, communicated messages to the gods. The *wab* priest's actions appear to focus on vertical communication between the afflicted and the gods in comparison to the horizontal form of communication associated with the other healing titles. The *wab* priest made diagnoses and prognoses after an assessment of physical symptoms. The diagnosis of a disease was not linked to a particular transgression of the patient. Instead, the *wab* priest focused on the patient's willingness to show obedience to the more powerful deities. The patient demonstrated his or her obedience by submitting to the *wab* priest's treatment measures of bandages, laxatives, or other therapies, as determined by specific symptoms.

As indicated in the Edwin Smith and Ebers papyri, the *wab* priests of Sekhmet usually carried out healing, although in theory a *wab* priest of any deity could practice medicine through *heka*. The term *wab* priest in itself indicates temple personnel. Yet their healing practices were not limited to the temple. Texts indicate that the *wab* priest was attached to the *per ankh* (House of Life), but it is not clear to what extent this structure was distinct from the temple or even whether it had exclusively a medical function. Many *wab* priests are noted as attached to work sites as well as to harems. In fact, some *wab* priests practiced exclusively for kings or nomarchs during the Old and Middle Kingdoms rather than rotating through temple service.[66] Only in the New Kingdom do we see the *wab* priest of Sekhmet working more directly with the temple rather than for private families, hinting at the growing power of the temples in contrast to ruling families.

### *Sau*

The term *sau* most likely derived from the word for "amulet" or "protection." This association meant that earlier English translations often referred to the *sau* simply as a "magician" or "exorcist," even though a *sau* could use somatic treatments just as easily as the *swnw* or even the *wab* priest. Within the ancient Egyptian medical texts and inscriptions, the title is always paired with the goddess Serket. The title *sau* can also appear in a military context

66. In ancient Egypt as well as other ancient cultures, priests did not live in the temple exclusively but would serve for several weeks and then rotate home for a few weeks. This would allow them to engage in practices such as medicine or scribal activities on the side as well as in the temple itself.

to designate a troop that protects the king's interests rather than a specific person. These associations throw doubt on the overly simplistic translation "magician," referring to the *sau* as a healer. More recently, scholars[67] favor the translation "protector," which better captures the original meaning of the term and accounts for its presence in military contexts as well as in medical texts using a variety of therapeutic measures. Despite its association with Serket, the *sau* does not seem to have worked within the temple like a *wab* priest, but the title is found for healers in the royal court. This exclusive link between the *sau* and Serket indicates that, like the *wab* priest, the *sau* most likely focused on vertical communication with the divine.

67. J. F. Borghouts, "Witchcraft, Magic, and Divination in Ancient Egypt," in *Civilizations of the Ancient Near East*, ed. Jack Sasson (Peabody: Hendrickson, 2000), 1783–84; Robert Ritner, "Magic," in *The Oxford Encyclopedia of Ancient Egypt* (New York: Oxford University Press, 2001), 326.

# 4. Canaanite Medicine

## Location and History

Ancient Canaan, or the Levant, lies on the far eastern shore of the Mediterranean, incorporating the modern states of Israel, the Palestinian National Authority, Lebanon, and Jordan. The topography and climate vary not only between the north and south, but also from west to east.[1] The north tends to be wet and forested, giving way to desert further to the south through the steppes of the Negev, and finally ending in the arid, rocky landscape of the Sinai Peninsula. The west has a coastline that quickly switches to low coastal mountains, which drop off into a valley consisting of the Sea of Galilee, the Jordan River, the Dead Sea, and the Wadi Arabah.[2] This rises up into a mountain chain made up of the Hauran, the Central Highlands, and the Southern Highlands, all of which are known collectively as the Transjordanian Plateau. Further to the east, the land opens to the Tigris and Euphrates Rivers in the north and the Arabian Peninsula to the south. This west-east division is bisected by other wadis, such as the Jezreel Valley.

Politically, the area was just as fragmented, with various states rising and falling through the centuries. The term "Canaanite" itself does not necessarily denote a specific ethnicity, but the inhabitants shared a common culture and Semitic languages, generally labeled "Canaanite." During the Bronze and Iron Ages, the area came under domination by varying groups, such as the Assyrians, Babylonians, Egyptians, and the Arameans. When the fortunes of these larger empires waned, especially around 1200 BCE, smaller local polities began to assert themselves, such as the Phoenicians, Amorites, Ammonites, Moabites, Edomites, and, most famously, the Israelites. Indo-

1. The topography and climate are reminiscent of California in the United States.

2. Wadis are seasonal riverbeds like an arroyo or gulch. The Arabah itself is part of the Dead Sea Transform that meets the Red Sea Rift and then joins with the East African Rift.

European language groups from the Aegean also settled in the Levant, such as the Philistines and later the Greeks and Romans.

The name Phoenicia comes from the Greek word for purple, but the people referred to themselves as *can'ani*, hence the term "Canaan," used frequently in the Hebrew Bible.[3] This term likely derived from a root meaning "trade" and developed because of the extensive trade networks through the area. The Phoenicians did not possess a central administrative state but functioned as a collection of autonomous city-states along the northern coastline. Sidon, Tyre, Byblos, Dor, and Ashkelon served as major trading ports, with the three most prominent exports being purple dye, cedar wood, and metals. Trade connections with Egypt are attested during the Twentieth Dynasty (1200–1087 BCE) by the *Tale of Wenamun*. Because of their trade routes, the Phoenicians established colonies throughout the Mediterranean, including Carthage in North Africa and Gadir (modern Cádiz) in Iberia. Power shifted from the Levantine coastal cities to Carthage during the sixth and fifth centuries, due to the rise of empires like the Neo-Assyrians and Persians, as well as the Seleucids and Ptolemies. Expansion into the western Mediterranean brought them into conflict with the Greeks, and finally they succumbed to the Romans during the three Punic Wars (264–146 BCE).

The Amorites derive their name from the Old Akkadian word *amurru*, which means "the west" and was used as a geographical and ethnic term for those residing to the northwest of Mesopotamia all the way to the Mediterranean Sea. They were mainly settled, as farmers, between the Euphrates and Anatolia, roughly modern Syria. But the more pastoral elements of Amorite society stretched southward toward the Arabian Desert, therefore occupying parts of the Levant. Expansion of the Amorites started in the late third millennium, continuing into the mid-second millennium, with some Babylonian kings possessing Amorite names such as Hammurabi. This expansion seems to be in response to pressures from the Indo-European Hurrians/Hittites in Anatolia, who reached as far south as the Canaanite area of Hebron. According to the Hebrew Bible, Amorites politically controlled cities such as Jebus (Jerusalem). By the Late Bronze Age, Amorites assimilated into both Mesopotamian and Canaanite cultures but left a significant mark by influencing grammatical changes in Akkadian and Canaanites languages, as well as by introducing gods such as Baal, Yam, and Anat to Canaanite and Babylonian mythic cycles.

3. Antonis Kotsonas, "Phoenicia," in *The Encyclopedia of Ancient History*, ed. Roger S. Bagnall (Oxford: Wiley-Blackwell, 2012).

Similarly, the Kingdom of Aram, centered on Damascus, had significant political and cultural repercussions for the Canaanite states of the Levant. The Hebrew Bible reports that King David occupied Damascus[4] in roughly the late eleventh and early tenth centuries BCE. Yet by the ninth century BCE, Aram became a sizable kingdom, threatening the borders of Israel and creating an alliance with the kingdom of Judah. Additionally, the expansion of the Neo-Assyrian king, Shalmaneser III, was stopped by a twelve-state coalition headed by Aram during the mid-ninth century BCE. By 796, the Assyrians forced tribute from Damascus, making Aram a vassal state. In 735 BCE, Radyan of Aram tried to form another coalition to rebel against Assyria, which included Israel but not Judah. The Arameans then turned on Judah, which allowed Tiglath-Pileser III to quell the rebellion, finally destroying Aram in 732 BCE. The more lasting influence came from the continual use of Aramaic throughout Canaan. The Persians made Aramaic the official language of the region in the sixth century BCE. With dialectical variations, Aramaic, in both written and spoken forms, lasted into the third century CE.

Returning to the Canaanite states proper, little is known of the Ammonites, whose homeland lies in the northern section of the Transjordanian Plateau along the Jabbok River, being a major trade route linking Egypt to Mesopotamia. Their formation as a centralized kingdom occurred in the Iron Age, with the annals of Neo-Assyrian kings[5] mentioning them in the eighth century BCE. We have some evidence of Ammonite kings from the Hebrew Bible and inscriptions ranging from the late eleventh century to the early sixth century BCE, although archaeological evidence shows occupation for the city of Rabbath-Ammon as early as the eighteenth century BCE. This city would later be renamed Philadelphia, under Ptolemy Philadelphius II.[6] The Hebrew Bible claims that the Israelite tribes of Reuben, Gad, and Manasseh settled around Ammon without attacking it by order of God.[7] Yet other references show that Gad, by warring against the Amorites, had expanded to incorporate Ammon.[8] During the Iron Age, the Ammonites were part of an unsuccessful coalition with Moab and Edom, conspiring against the kingdom of Judah in the ninth and seventh centuries BCE.

4. 2 Sam 8:5–6.

5. Tiglath Pileser III, Sennacherib, and Esarhaddon.

6. The city is now called Amman and serves as the capital of Jordan.

7. Deut 2:19 and 37.

8. Num 21:21–31.

Another Transjordanian group are the Moabites, situated immediately east of the Dead Sea, between Wadi el-Mujib and Wadi el-Hesa. Egyptian execration texts and the Megiddo List, from the reign of Thutmosis III (1482–1450 BCE), mention cities and rulers in the area of Moab but do not give an indication of any centralized authority. A campaign list from Ramesses II (1304–1237 BCE) uses the name Moab. The earliest textual reference to them as the kingdom of Moab comes from the Hebrew Bible, mentioning King Mesha and the allotment of the land to the tribe of Gad. This is corroborated by the discovery of the Mesha Stela, dated to the ninth century BCE, in the modern city of Dhiban, which served as the capital of Moab. Ironically, the Mesha Stela claims that the tribe of Gad always resided in the area. The Moabite kingdom likely grew out of the Dibon tribe occupying the area south of the Wadi el-Mujib. The kingdom became a vassal to the Assyrians during Tiglath-Pileser III's campaigns. Culturally, the Moabites focused on Baal and Chemosh worship, having some Egyptian elements mixed in with their religious iconography and geographical names of shrines. Both the Mesha Stela and passages from Jeremiah depict the same type of vassal-state relationship between the Moabites and Chemosh that the Israelites had with Yahweh.

The southernmost of the Transjordanian kingdoms is Edom. The area, rich in copper mines, has been occupied since the late Chalcolithic era. The earliest textual references come from the reign of the Egyptian king Merneptah (1224–1214 BCE) using the names Edom and Seir. Yet earlier inscriptions, from the reign of Amenhotep III, use the word *shasu* to designate the people of Edom, and possibly of Moab. In this case, *shasu* is not an ethnic marker but a term to denote pastoralists. Most likely, the tribes of the area coalesced into a centralized kingdom free from Israelite and Judahite domination during the ninth century BCE. Complete independence was short lived, as the Edomites paid tribute as a vassal state to the Neo-Assyrian king Adad-Nirari III (809–782 BCE). Throughout the eighth century, the Edomites began to make incursions into Judahite territory, capturing the port city of Elath and settling as far west as Beersheba. Early archaeologists thought the Wadi Arabah served as a border[9] between Edom and the later kingdom of Judah, but more recent excavations revealed that Edom stretched westward into the southern Negev.[10] As the Assyrians fell to the Babylonians,

9. Nelson Glueck, *Exploration in Eastern Palestine II* (New Haven: American Schools of Oriental Research, 1935).

10. Laura Zucconi, "From the Wilderness of Zin Alongside Edom: Edomite Territory in

it appears that the Edomites switched vassalage. An unclear population shift occurred, starting in the Persian period and resulting in the Nabateans dominating the area by the Roman period.

During the reigns of Merneptah and Ramesses III (1182–1151 BCE), a coalition of nine tribes from the Aegean, collectively known as the Sea Peoples, encroached upon the eastern and southeastern shores of the Mediterranean. Unable to fully stop their advance, Ramesses III settled them along the Levantine coast as a contingent of mercenaries. Most of the tribes comprising the Sea Peoples had quickly assimilated into the local Canaanite populations. The Peleshet, or Philistines, who migrated both by sea and land (through Anatolia), retained a distinct cultural identity and a loose confederation of city-states; especially notable are Gaza, Ashkelon, Ashdod, Ekron, and Gath.[11] Yet they did adopt the worship of the Canaanite gods Dagon, Baal, and Astarte. And they also generally switched from their original female-centric pantheon to a more male-dominant Canaanite style of pantheon. According to the Hebrew Bible, Israelites demanded a king in the face of Philistine expansion.[12] Philistia came under Assyrian domination during the reign of Tiglath-Pileser III. The city-states of Philistia participated in a series of rebellions fostered by the Egyptians during the late sixth century BCE, but these were put down by the Assyrian kings Sargon and Sennacherib. During the early fifth century BCE, Esarhaddon launched attacks on Egypt, using the Philistines as auxiliary troops or mercenaries. As Assyrian forces gave way to the Babylonians, the Egyptian king Neco II established control over Philistia, inciting them and Judah to fight against Babylon. Upon the capture of Jerusalem in 586 BCE, the Babylonians exiled not only the people of Judah but also the Philistines, settling them around Nippur, near a tributary of the Euphrates.

The most well-known group from Canaan are the Israelites. The earliest mention of Israel comes from the Merneptah Stela (1207 BCE), which ironically claims, "Israel is laid waste, its seed is no more."[13] The hieroglyphs reference a pastoral-nomadic group[14] who likely lived in the central portion

---

the Eastern Negev During the Eighth-Sixth Centuries B.C.E," in *Milk and Honey: Essays on Ancient Israel and the Bible in Appreciation of the Judaic Studies Program at the University of California, San Diego*, ed. Sarah Malena and David Miano (Winona Lake, IN: Eisenbrauns, 2007), 241–56.

11. This city has yet to be accurately identified and excavated.

12. 1 Sam 13.

13. Pritchard, *Ancient Near Eastern Texts*, 378.

14. The name Israel is followed by a hieroglyph of a man walking with a staff. This is in

of Canaan. Although the Hebrew Bible depicts the history of Israel with the patriarch Abraham having come from Ur of the Chaldeans[15] in Mesopotamia and the Israelites later conquering Canaan from Egypt, there is no archaeological evidence that the Israelites originated outside of Canaan or launched a large-scale invasion before creating significant settlements. Ample textual and archaeological evidence attests to the cultural influence of Egypt and Mesopotamia on the Israelites as well as on other Canaanites. Early in the Iron Age, the Israelites began to distinguish themselves as an ethnic and political group distinct from the surrounding Canaanites, as did the Phoenicians and Philistines—a trend that saw the later development of kingdoms for the Ammonites, Moabites, and Edomites. This is not to say that the Hebrew Bible lacks historically reliable information but that one must remember that it, like all ancient documents, is cast in a light to promote the interests of particular power groups at the time of its composition.

The history of Israel as a distinct political entity can be divided into three main periods: (1) the period of the judges (1200–1000 BCE); (2) the united monarchy (1000–922 BCE); and (3) the divided monarchy of the separate kingdoms of Israel/Samaria in the north (922–722 BCE) and Judah in the south (922–586 BCE). During the period of the judges, the Israelites formed a coalition of tribes, without much central authority. The judges acted as military leaders rather than civic ones, organizing the collection and redistribution of resources. The reigns of Saul, David, and Solomon comprise the united monarchy and constituted the typical central authority, overseeing resources from the capital in Jerusalem.[16] Rehoboam, the successor to Solomon, refused to alleviate the taxation policy toward the northern portion of the kingdom, fomenting a rebellion centered at the city of Shechem. A number of different dynasties ruled the northern kingdom, eventually moving its capital to Samaria. The kingdom of Israel would alternately engage in border wars and join forces with Judah, depending on political expediency in the face of the empires of Egypt, Assyria, and Babylonia. In 722 BCE, Samaria ultimately fell to the Assyrians, who exiled the elites of the population. This

---

contrast to the other names in the list, which are followed by a circle with a cross in it, usually denoting a city.

15. Gen 11:31. In this context, the term Chaldeans refers to the Amorite dominance of southern Mesopotamia.

16. The debates concerning the veracity of a truly united monarchy go beyond the scope of this brief history. It is a distinct possibility that David and his heir Solomon ruled two kingdoms and that the biblical image of their unification is propaganda to bolster their position in the northern kingdom.

became known as the ten lost tribes of Israel, while many of the remaining Israelites fled into Judah. The Assyrians brought in a new population for Israel, who quickly adopted the religious practices of worshiping Yahweh Elohim. The southern kingdom of Judah maintained the Davidic line until the destruction of Jerusalem by the Babylonians in 586 BCE. The elite population was also exiled to Babylonia, but once the Persians gained control of the Levant, the exiles were allowed to return in 539 BCE, rebuilding the walls and temple in Jerusalem.

For most of the Persian to the Roman period, Judah existed as an administrative unit with no king. The high priest at the temple in Jerusalem acted as a *de facto* leader of the population until the Hasmonean Revolt in 165 BCE, which allowed for a brief interlude of independence from Seleucid and Ptolemaic control until 63 BCE, when a succession dispute among the Hasmoneans brought in Roman control.

## Religion and Culture

In addition to the Hebrew Bible, the archives from the ancient Syrian cities of Ugarit and Ebla shed light on Canaanite religion. Although the following is a general picture of Canaanite religion, it will highlight the Israelite religion where applicable. This study will focus mostly on the Israelite medical practices up to the Babylonian exile in 586 BCE. After this point in time, the influences of Greco-Roman medicine—a significant shift in religious practices creating Judaism—and the advent of Christianity will all greatly alter the medical culture of the Levant to the extent that it could no longer be termed Canaanite.

### Cosmology

Like the political landscape, the religious practices of Canaan varied depending on the particular region or ethnic group. Overall, the Canaanites were a polytheistic society, with the exception of Israelite monotheism developing in the first millennium. But staying true to their monotheism occasionally even proved to be a struggle.

Unfortunately, no explicit creation stories for the Canaanites still exist, other than the two accounts in the Hebrew Bible. Genesis 1 describes the formation of the cosmos and earth through a series of separations, with the creation of humans on the sixth day: "And God created man in His image, in the image of God He created him; male and female He created them."[17] Other than the vague idea that humans in some way share in the likeness of the deity, there is no explanation about how exactly the human body was formed, making it difficult to discern any links to a concept of physiology. This particular creation account does indicate that there is no fundamental difference between male and female bodies, with regard to their connection to the divine, nor is there a priority between them, asserting that males give rise to females. Their creation on the sixth day once the world was fully formed and dominance of that world show that humans exist both within nature and stand apart from it. These ideas can prove useful in understanding the underlying relationships governing illness and healing.

The order and lack of details in Genesis 1 stand in contrast to Genesis 2, in which male humans are created first: "The Lord God formed man from the dust of the earth. He blew into his nostrils the breath of life, and man became a living being."[18] In this account, humans are very much a part of the natural world, having their physical form come directly from it. Yet they also have an intimate relationship with the divine, since the animating force, life itself, comes from God. Females also have this dual relationship, since "He took one of his [man] ribs and closed up the flesh at that spot. And the Lord God fashioned the rib He had taken from the man into a woman."[19] This story can be read as females occupying a subordinate position due to the fact that they are created from males, as a helper; or it can be seen as females enveloping the whole of creation—positioned, like males, as dominating the natural world and, in that sense, equal to males. It should be noted that this equality is not one of social roles but that the male and female physical body have the same relationship to the divine; thus, treatment measures for illness do not vary by sex. Again, this idea impacts how relationships inform illness and healing. It is interesting to note that between the two accounts, Genesis 2 depicts a human body much more integrated with the natural world. Although coming second in the Bible, the text of Genesis 2 was composed a few centuries earlier than Genesis 1.[20]

Another feature to note about the Hebrew Bible and its place in Canaanite religion is the use of divine names. Where Genesis 1 uses simply the

17. Gen 1:27. All Hebrew Bible translations are from JPS unless otherwise noted.

18. Gen 2:7.

19. Gen 2:21–22.

20. R. E. Friedman, *Who Wrote the Bible?* (New York: Harper Collins, 1997).

translation "God," this stands for the Hebrew text's use of the plural name Elohim, the singular form being El. For the Canaanites, El is the creator and chief god in the pantheon, heading up a divine council; the other gods in the council are often referred to as the "sons of El." This council aspect, similar to Mesopotamian theology, is important to the Canaanite conception of how divine entities and hence humans interact with one another. Although an entity may have extreme power, it does not act unilaterally. Community cohesion is paramount. This ideology finds expression in the Hebrew Bible not only by use of the phrase "divine council" but also with the system of covenants that govern God's relationship to the Israelites through Abraham, Moses, and David, which solidifies the Israelite's identity, using the same expression as the divine council, "sons of El."

Presiding over the divine council with El is his consort Athirat, the mother of the gods. She is often represented by a wooden pole or stylized tree, the Asherah, which appears in the Hebrew Bible in stories about apostasy. An Ugaritic poem presents Athirat as the benevolent personification of El,[21] thus indicating a certain degree of fluidity in the gendering of the divine. Yet this benevolence is balanced out by the violent actions that can be undertaken, such as the sending of plagues.

In Genesis 2, the phrasing rendered "Lord God" is a translation of the two names Yahweh Elohim. The name Yahweh is first mentioned in the Egyptian texts from the reign of Amenhotep III, in which the Canaanites in the region of Edom are referenced with the phrase "the land of the Shasu of Yahweh." It is unclear in the Egyptian texts whether this is simply a place name or the name of a god. It is not uncommon for the names of a god to be grafted on to place names and, in turn, for one term to stand for another. The goddess Athirat began as the name of a place sacred to El. The earliest uses of the name Yahweh in the Hebrew Bible can be found in Judges 5 and Deuteronomy 33, which locate Yahweh in southern Canaan, around Edom, and depict him as a warrior storm god. Eventually, Yahweh is syncretized with El and takes on the consort Asherah, as attested in the Kuntillet Ajrud inscription (late ninth to early eighth century BCE). This inscription denotes Yahweh of Samaria, although it was found in the Sinai.

A more prominent storm god for the Canaanites is Baal, but the name originally served as an epithet meaning "lord" for the god Hadad (thunder). The Baal cycle depicts the struggle of Baal against Yam (the sea)—a demand that El allow Baal his own palace—and then finally Baal's struggle against

21. KTU 1.65.

Mot (death), involving his own death and rebirth. The goddess Anat frequently appears as the consort of Baal, but in Phoenician inscriptions it is the goddess Astarte. The god Dagon is a popular grain god and thought of as the father of Baal. He dwells in Tuttal, mentioned in snake charms from Ugarit. A common phenomenon is the use of Baal in connection to a place or characteristic, so it appears as if there are many gods, such as Baal-Shamem (Baal of the Heavens), Baal-Hammon (Baal of the incense altar), and Baal-Zaphon (Baal of the Mountains). But these are simply variations on the god Baal rather than being completely distinct entities. This practice is common with other gods, such as El-Shaddai (El of the Mountain), in the Hebrew Bible. As different polities developed, certain gods became syncretized, especially Yahweh and El to become Yahweh Elohim, as well as Yahweh and Baal in terms of cultic activity and mythic descriptions (Leviathan, storm god, etc.)

The pantheon of the Canaanites—like many ancient Near Eastern and Mediterranean pantheons—had a loose tripartite ranking of the gods, with deities such as El at the top. Gods associated with natural phenomena and human activities, such as Baal for storms and Kothar-wa-Hasis for craftsmen, occupied a second tier. Wright asserts that the Canaanites understood their gods as being analogous to natural phenomena, the active agent behind storms or the sun rather than actually being the storm or the sun.[22] In this, he emphasizes the human aspect of Canaanite gods, noting that their depiction is always anthropomorphic. Yet texts habitually refer to the gods in animal form, such as the ubiquitous "El the bull from Heaven," or even claim that a goddess is the manifestation of a concept, such as benevolence. This would indicate that the gods are not limited to only a human form, and all their associations are not simply an analogy. Another category of lesser entities, including messengers (angels) and ghosts, ranked third. This essentially mirrors human society, with its class divisions of nobles, peasants/freemen, and slaves.[23]

A more striking parallel between the divine realm and human society is the conception of how the two relate to each other. Just as the human king

22. Wright does acknowledge evidence that some deities are the natural phenomena, especially for celestial bodies, but he is quick to dismiss this. See David P. Wright, "Syro-Canaanite Religions," in *The Cambridge History of Religions in the Ancient World*, ed. Michele Renee Salzman (Cambridge: Cambridge University Press, 2013), 129–50.

23. Some scholars divide Canaanite cosmology into four tiers, with gods of natural elements ranked second and gods representing human activity ranked third, which parallels a human division of kings, nobles, peasants, and slaves; see K. L. Knoll, "Canaanite Religion," *Religion Compass* 1 (2007): 61–92.

acts as patron for nobles and protector of freemen and slaves, the gods are patrons for the kings and protect the lower classes. A king such as Mesha of Moab would single out a particular patron god, such as Chemosh, as his divine patron. At this point, the other gods would fall into a subordinate position, assisting Chemosh in his relationship to Mesha. For this reason, Canaanite gods did not have a static hierarchy but fluctuated over time and place. The Israelite conception of divine patronage expressed in the Hebrew Bible understood the divine patronage of Yahweh Elohim as extending to all the people of Israel. Yet the typical form of divine patronage can still be seen in the selection of men, such as Saul and David, for kingship. The king then stands as an intermediary between the divine realm and the human world, since he both has a god as patron and himself is a patron to the people. Kings may also take on the role of intermediary by simultaneously fulfilling the function of a priest, such as Tabnit, the Phoenician king of Sidon, who also was a priest for Astarte. To this end, kings needed to be ritually pure and of the highest ethical standing, with the duty to protect the poor, widows, and orphans.

Apart from this political system, other intermediaries between gods and humans were prophets. The prophet Balaam son of Beor is found both in Numbers 22 and the Deir Allah inscription (700 BCE). Ancient people could hire such prophets to pronounce curses on their enemies, making the episode in Numbers seem believable to its contemporary audience, especially using the name of a relatively popular prophet-for-hire. The Canaanites stand out as fairly unique[24] in the ancient world in that they had ecstatic prophecy. The ecstatic prophet simply receives messages from a god rather than using divinatory practices, such as reading animal entrails, although this type of prophecy was also common throughout Canaan. Liver models found at Hazor and Meggido indicate such a form of divination, and a text on unnatural births at Ugarit attest to another common form. The Hebrew Bible particularly depicted the ecstatic prophet as a moral check on the political activities of the king of Israel and Judah, ensuring that the king always behaves according to the dictates of his patron Yahweh Elohim.

More often, the priest represented the intermediary between the gods and people that most Canaanites would encounter on a regular basis. The priests' main function was to care for the gods by carrying out the ritual sacrifices and maintaining the temples and shrines. Canaanites frequently placed their sanc-

24. The only other place attesting to ecstatic prophecy in the ancient Near East was the archive at Mari on the Euphrates River.

tuaries on hilltops, the "high places" mentioned in the Hebrew Bible. These sanctuaries consisted of altars and incense stands, wooden poles representing a female deity, such as Asherah, and stone pillars for males, like Baal.

Sacrifices occurred throughout Canaan as a means of feeding the gods, as one ancient story illustrates: "Danel made an offering to the gods, an offering for the gods to eat, an offering for the holy ones to drink."[25] This is not far different from its conception in Mesopotamia when Atra-ḫasis withheld sacrifices to alleviate the plague. Theologically, the blood of the sacrifices ritually purified the altar and the people, as well as bonded the people and the gods in a community. A day of atonement in conjunction with a new year and fall harvest celebration involving such a purifying sacrifice is attested both in the Hebrew Bible and in the archive at Ugarit. The most common forms of sacrifice were peace and thanksgiving. The peace offering gave a portion of meat to the gods, but the majority was consumed by the people as a way of signifying a wholeness of the community, both among humans and between humans and the god. The thanksgiving offering, also referred to as the burnt offering, required the entire animal to be consumed by fire, offered up in this way for the god to eat. No people ate of this offering, yet it still bonded them to their patron god. As states became centralized, the locations for sacrifice became more restricted, with the ultimate case being the temple in Jerusalem as the only proper sacrificial location for the Israelites. Both textual and archaeological evidence, though, argue against the accuracy of this biblical assertion.

Debates surround the issue of human sacrifice in Canaanite religious practices. Its use appears limited only to times of crisis, such as a city under siege. Child sacrifice is even more contentious. Archaeological evidence for it appears mostly from Carthage and other Punic settlements in the western Mediterranean. No such evidence exists in Phoenicia itself or other regions of Canaan. Biblical references, most famously the near sacrifice of Isaac, leave the matter unclear. If such a practice did exist among the Israelites, it is possible that the act of circumcision ritually replaced child sacrifice. This seems most evident in the passage from Exodus in which Moses and his family are fleeing from God, when Zipporah suddenly circumcises their son and flings the foreskin at God, thus satisfying him and stopping the chase. Since the passage begins *in media res*, it is unclear why God is pursuing them or why the foreskin mollifies him.

25. Michael David Coogan, *Stories from Ancient Canaan* (Louisville: Westminster John Knox, 2012), 32.

Some part of the person is thought to live on after death, but this soul does not enjoy any type of significant afterlife. They seem to be simply lurking shades that can positively or negatively affect the living if not properly respected. Some evidence exists that banquets were held for the dead. Such ghosts are referred to as *rephaim*. Linguistically, this term is related to the one for healing; thus, *rephaim* can also mean "healers," as found in literature from Ugarit. Yet, at Ugarit, an afterlife in the form of deification is especially true for the kings. Scholars debate whether the people of Ugarit considered their kings as gods while alive. These beliefs indicate that Canaanites understood a distinction between the physical body and their identity.

An overarching cosmological point of view for the Canaanites can best be described as behaving in the appropriate manner to maintain the patronage between the gods and people, obedience and consideration. Disruptions to this system result in the gods using outside forces, whether armies or illness, to punish those not obeying their patron. To this end, law codes become paramount in order for people to know the proper course of action. Yet these were not limited to regulations on sacrificial matters but stretched well into the social interactions of the human community.

The covenants in the Hebrew Bible best outline the patronage relationship governed by law that existed between the gods and people. The first covenant with Noah guarantees that God, who controls all natural phenomena, will not destroy the earth and that he will pay heed to supplicants.[26] The second covenant with Abraham designates the Israelites as having a unique relationship with Yahweh, forming a congregation (vertical relationship), thus making them a community or camp (horizontal relationship) distinct from the rest of the Canaanites; circumcision stands as the marker of the Abrahamic covenant.[27] The covenant with Moses elucidates the Israelites' obligations to God (within the congregation) and to each other (within the camp) in order to enjoy the protections of God.[28]

This system of covenants impacts Israelite medical practices. All illnesses, whether disease or trauma, stem from God. But if the patient adheres to his obligations to both the congregation and the camp, then God must pay heed and decide whether healing should occur. The role of the healer is to figure out the message God is sending through illness and how best to have the patient demonstrate his or her fulfilling of obligations. But,

26. Gen 8–9.
27. Gen 15 and 18.
28. Exod 19–24.

as the story of Job shows, God has relationships with entities other than the Israelites, and this impacts the sending of illness as well as its possible cure. It is not a simple one-to-one correspondence resulting in the righteous never suffering.

Although the Hebrew Bible's slant toward monotheism means that the Israelites have to concern themselves with their relationship only to Yahweh Elohim, the rest of the Canaanites must navigate their way among the various gods to understand the messages encoded in illness. The following is a list of Canaanite gods with particular connections to disease and healing.

## Canaanite Gods and Goddesses of Disease and Healing

### *Athirat/Asherah*

The goddess Athirat, also called Asherah in Phoenician and Israelite contexts, is the consort of El and mother of the gods. Images from Ugarit show her nursing royalty and holding snakes, which links her to symbols of fertility and healing.[29] Her most notable connection to medical practices comes from the story *Kirta*, in which Asherah sent disease as punishment to Kirta for not fulfilling his vow to her. She appears also in the Hittite myth *Elkunirsha*, which uses Canaanite deities. Again, she sends disease to an unnamed storm god as punishment for his humiliation of her.

### *Astarte and Anat*

Astarte appears frequently throughout the ancient Near East in various parts of Canaan and Egypt, as well as in Mesopotamia as Ištar and among the Greeks as Aphrodite. These cultures linked her with the planet Venus as the evening star, while Venus as the morning star is masculine. Despite this ubiquitousness, scholars have difficulty characterizing Astarte apart from her tendencies to violence and sexuality. The Hebrew Bible refers to her as Ashtart or Ashtaroth. The form Ashtaroth has a feminine plural ending but is frequently used as a singular noun, indicating the Hebrew Bible's tendency to dismissively collapse all the Canaanite goddesses, including Astarte and Anat, into one indiscernible mass.

29. Knoll, "Canaanite Religion," 61–92.

The two goddesses appear together in charms against snakebites, found at Ugarit. In these, the formula always reads in the order of Anat and then Astarte. This combination is found also in New Kingdom Egyptian texts to ward off animal and demon attacks. The goddess Anat is a young huntress and patron of warriors, often depicted as wading knee-high in the blood of the slain, with the hands of her victims dangling from her belt. Despite this ability to wreak havoc, she is not known for the converse of healing, unless linked with Astarte in snake charms. The one exception to this is their healing of a hangover, found in KTU 1.114. This text begins as a story of El becoming dangerously drunk and ends with a recipe for curing a hangover, based on the actions of Astarte and Anat. Interestingly, the order of the goddesses is reversed from the snake charms.

### *Baal*

The word *baal* itself is just a common noun meaning lord or owner, but it becomes cast as the name of the storm god in Ugaritic texts, syncretized with the Canaanite god Hadad, as well as in the Hebrew Bible. The story of Baal's struggle with Death (Mot) and eventual resurrection in essence made him a patron of all those suffering illness and having their own struggles with death. In conjunction with this, some literary fragments give Baal the epithet of healer (*rapi'u*),[30] which connects him to the deceased ancestors, the *rephaim*, who are considered supernatural healers in their own right.

When Baal had temporarily succumbed to Death, the earth became scorched and barren, making him an ideal deity for incantations against infertility, especially among the royal families of Canaan. The ever-present anxiety of kingship is the lack of an heir to the throne. Baal's characteristic of being the ultimate king, in connection to his ability to protect against chaos, renders him perfect for such appeals against barrenness. Similarly, his battle with Sea/River (Yam) makes him the victor against all chaos and thus appropriate for any healing incantations. The dragon-like depiction of Sea/River also makes Baal appropriate for incantations against snakebites.[31]

30. KTU 1.108 and KTU 1.113; see Dietrich and Loretz UF 1980.

31. KTU 1.82.

### *Resheph, Rephaim, and Raphael*

More confusing than the connections between Astarte and Anat are the relationships between the god Resheph, the *rephaim*, and the biblical name Raphael. The name Resheph, as used for a god, is attested as early as the third millennium, but texts that round out his image come from the Late Bronze and into the Iron Age. Resheph functions in the underworld as the gatekeeper and is equated often by the Mesopotamians to their god Nergal. He has a destructive force expressed as arrows that send plagues. This imagery appears also in the Amarna Letters from Egypt, where he was first introduced during the reign of Amenhotep II. Passages in the Hebrew Bible describe Resheph as the arrows of Yahweh.[32] In a marching order, the Canaanite god Deber precedes Yahweh, as plague, and Resheph follows him as pestilence.[33] Resheph appears often with the two companions Deber and Mot. His popularity spread to Cyprus, where he was equated with the Greek Apollo, another healing deity who can send plague by arrows, as evidenced in the *Iliad*. His name, like many other Canaanite deities, appears in snake charms.

The *rephaim* are ghosts of ancestors, under the dominion of Resheph. They enjoy the same power as low-level deities that can affect the living. Like all supernatural entities, their actions can stem from their own volition, as well as from the direction of a more powerful god. To this end, they can both bring healing and inflict illness. This makes one's relationship to dead ancestors an important factor in Canaanite medical culture. The term *rephaim* becomes synonymous with healers, but it is unclear whether this applies equally to human healers or is limited to supernatural entities.

The linguistic root "rph," from which *rephaim* derives, is also the root for the Hebrew term *rophe*, meaning healer and applied to both God and humans. There is a slight difference in the phrase El Rophe, meaning "El, the Healer,"[34] and the name Raphael, "the Healer of El," meaning one who heals by the power of El. No study yet directly connects the term *rephaim* with the name Raphael.[35] Named angels are a late development in Israelite religion, roughly at the end of the first millennium BCE. Raphael, an angel

32. Deut 32:23–24 and Ps 76:4.

33. Exod 9:3 and Jer 21:6.

34. Exod 15:26 and Ps 103:3.

35. K. van der Toorn, Bob Becking, and Pieter Willem van der Horst, eds., "Resheph," in *Dictionary of Deities and Demons in Bible* (Grand Rapids: Eerdmans, 1999).

or messenger of God who is known also as a healer who can bind demons, first appears in the book of Tobit. He heals blindness with parts of a fish—interestingly a somatic treatment that is not unreasonable to find human healers using in their therapeutic repertoire.[36] In 1 Enoch, Raphael heals all the earth from the fallen angels and presides over all diseases and wounds. He later appears in the rabbinic text *b. Yoma* 37a.

Traditionally, there became an ordering of angels with Gabriel, the Warrior of El, marching in front of God, while Raphael, the Healer, follows behind God. It is fairly reasonable and tempting to think that the figure of Resheph and his minions, the *rephaim*, who originally walked behind God, eventually transforms into the angel Raphael by way of the healing abilities of El Rophe himself. A more in-depth study is needed, focusing on the terms in their changing cultural context from the Early Iron Age to the later Roman period with the development of rabbinic Judaism and Christianity.

### *Eshmun*

The chthonic god Eshmun is a healing deity attested throughout Canaan and the ancient Near East as early as the eighth century BCE. The Canaanite pantheon has Eshmun in a triad as the son of Baal and Astarte. By the late sixth century BCE, he became the chief god of the Phoenician city of Sidon, with local kings such as Eshmunazar II, who built the temple to Eshmun in Sidon. Votives of children at the Sidon temple indicate that he is a protector of the young and not necessarily a god of pediatrics, as some would claim.[37] The god's worship spread to Cyprus, Egypt, and the western Mediterranean through Punic settlements. Upon contact with Greek culture, they equated Eshmun to their healing god Asclepius. The Greco-Roman geographer Pausanius (110–180 CE) claims that Apollo was the father of Eshmun, grafting on to him the mythic traditions of Asklepios. The Greek equation of Apollo and Resheph could create a genealogy showing that Eshmun was the son of Resheph, but this is never articulated either by the Phoenicians or even the Greco-Romans. Instead, Eusebius (260–339 CE) preserves a tale of a deity, called the Righteous, who has an eighth son with one of the female titans; this child is Eshmun, which means "eight," according to his etymology.

36. Tobit 6.

37. Contra S. S. Levin, "Eshmun, Healing of God of Sidon," *Adler Museum Bulletin* Special Issue (1983): 39–42.

The name Eshmun likely derived from the same Canaanite word for "oil" or "fat," thus connoting a link between fat and a healthy body. The imagery used in a shrine to Eshmun in Sidon shows a rooster, which is also frequently associated with Asklepios, thus furthering their connection for the Greco-Romans. Eshmun is also depicted as a hunter god who is responsible for feeding men, as well as healing them, an overall protective role much like Baal. For the Greeks visiting Sidon, statuary of Eshmun as a young man created an association between him and Adonis, another Canaanite deity. For the Mesopotamians, Eshmun's ability to heal means also an ability to punish; thus, they employ him in political matters with the Canaanites. A treaty of Ashurnerari V with Mati'ilu of Arpad[38] includes Eshmun in a list of divine witnesses. Another treaty between Esarhaddon and the king of Tyre invokes Eshmun and Melqart in a curse against any possible violator of the treaty. In Cypriote inscriptions, over time, these two gods meld into one entity, Eshmun-Melqart.

### *Kotharat and Bes*

Kotharat is a collective term for seven goddesses, but debate surrounds their actual function. Based on the tale of *Aqhat*, it was thought that the Kotharat functioned as midwives. But others interpret the passage as their power focusing on fertility, since they appear before and not at the birth of Aqhat. A deity similar to the Kotharat is the Egyptian god Bes. Southern Canaanites adopted Bes, likely as a collective term for a group of deities, retaining his general character of protecting women and the household in general.

### *Shataqat*

In the story *Kirta*, the goddess Asherah has stricken the hero Kirta with a plague for not fulfilling his vow to her. El asks among the divine council for one to heal the diseased Kirta, but none respond. This forces El to create the goddess Shataqat out of clay as a manifestation of his healing power. Shataqat's healing ability mirrors the story of Anat rescuing Baal from Death (Mot). Her description in *Kirta* gives her the epithets "expeller" and "ban-

38. A city north of Aleppo in Syria, which served as the capital of the Arameans under King Mati'ilu during the mid-eighth century BCE.

isher," indicating the manner by which she heals. These verbs appear also in the Baal cycle as the names of the clubs Baal uses to slay the Sea/River (Yam). To date, no other texts or inscriptions with her name as a healer have been found.

### *Horon*

The god Horon appears in medical incantations from Ugarit, Arslan Tash, and the Harris Papyrus from Egypt. He is the only one to provide charms to the sun goddess who seeks them.[39] One particular incantation has him accepting myrrh in exchange for healing, which seems to make a pun on the similar words for sickness and myrrh.[40] Like Resheph, Horon is a god of the underworld and rules over harmful creatures. He possesses a neutral character so can be invoked either to send illness and harmful creatures or to heal their effects. His cult spread to Egypt during the reign of Amenhotep II, where he protects against attacks from various animals, including snakes, especially those from the desert. This is in keeping with many Canaanite deities becoming associated with the desert regions in the Egyptian worldview. The Egyptians depicted Horon as a falcon, a natural snake killer, and thus linked him with the god Horus. His knowledge of subterranean passageways connected him also to newborns finding their way to life; thus, Horon oversaw childbirth and protected parturient women from a malevolent entity called the Strangler.

## Sources

Sources for tracing Canaanite medical history are problematic. Archaeological sites have yielded little that can be directly linked to medical practices. The situation for documents is much like the one in Mesopotamia, in that a clear distinction between medical texts and religious ones is not easy to make, since many texts coming from archives like Ugarit are in the form of incantations. Similarly, modern scholars tend to let the religious nature of the Hebrew Bible obscure passages that read like other ancient medical texts. One must look at the genre of "professional instruction literature" or

39. CAT 1.100.
40. CAT 1.124.

"procedural texts" that are directed at specialists, usually religious functionaries carrying out rituals, in order to discover medical-oriented documents. Within this category, only the priestly instructions in Leviticus qualify. The hippiatric texts from the archives at Ugarit also qualify as professional instruction literature for the Canaanites.

## Texts

For the medical culture of the Israelites, one can gain a clearer picture by comparing the Masoretic text of the Hebrew Bible (MT) with the Septuagint texts (LXX). Most people consider the MT the traditional, authoritative text of the Hebrew Bible. The LXX is a Greek translation of the Hebrew Bible made during the Hellenistic period but of a recension different from the MT; thus, it reflects cultural shifts from the biblical to Hellenistic periods. A third set of biblical texts that could be used for comparison are the Dead Sea or Qumran Scrolls. These papyri contain the books of the Hebrew Bible, the Apocrypha, and documents relating to the community that used them. They date from the mid-third century BCE to the first century CE. The Qumran scrolls contain versions of the biblical books that are proto-MT, LXX, as well as Samaritan and more local versions.

The closest parallel to known ancient medical texts appears in Leviticus 12–15. These chapters address the problem of cleanliness connected to childbirth, skin afflictions, fungal growth in houses, and bodily discharges. They follow a similar procedural format to that found in the Egyptian texts, such as the Ebers Papyrus, having a title, examination/symptom description, a diagnosis/prognosis, and treatment measure.

> When a man has on the skin of his flesh a swelling, a rash, or a discoloration, and it develops into a scaly affection on the skin of his flesh (title) . . . the priest shall look at the affection on the skin of his flesh: and the hair in the affected patch has turned white and the affection appears to be deeper than the skin of his flesh (symptom description), it is a skin affliction[41] (diagnosis) and the priest shall look on him, and pronounce him

41. The Hebrew term *tzaraʿat* covers a wide range of ailments for the skin; thus, the translation "skin affliction" is more accurate. The traditional translation "leprosy" is an anachronism, because the disease referred to as leprosy, that is, Hansen's disease, was not known in the Levant until the Hellenistic period.

> unclean (prognosis). . . . And the priest will look at him on the seventh day again and, behold, if the affection has faded and has not spread not in the skin (examination/symptom description), the priest shall pronounce him clean; it is a rash (diagnosis/prognosis) and he shall wash his clothes, and be clean (treatment).[42]

When broken down into the procedural steps, the similarity is striking. This is in contrast to the Mesopotamian medical texts that use an if-then construction, which is common to the genre of omen literature.

The difference between Egyptian and Israelite medical procedural texts is that the therapies in Ebers appear to focus solely on treating the somatic symptom, while those in Leviticus are concerned only with purity. The Egyptian medical texts contain therapies directed at all types of healers, those communicating vertically with the community of the gods, as well as those directing messages horizontally toward the human community. Leviticus, though, directs its therapies only at the priest, who communicates vertically in order to maintain the community/congregation with God. There is an underlying assumption that the somatic symptoms will clear up, but the text never specifies how this is accomplished apart from God allowing it. The practice of isolating the afflicted from the camp or human community does act as a form of communicating with them, demonstrating the patient's obedience to the relationship with the divine. But this is less of a concern for the priest than removing an offensive entity from the presence of God, thus risking the entire congregation's relationship with God.

Apart from the Hebrew Bible, the next closest set of documents akin to medical texts comes from an archive at Ugarit, which lies in the modern coastal city of Ras Shamra in Syria. Ugarit is important for understanding Canaanite society and the historical-literary context for some books of the Hebrew Bible. Scribes from Ugarit wrote in the city's own form of Semitic language (Ugaritic), using cuneiform symbols as an alphabet.[43] All together about five thousand tablets have been found, spanning roughly from 1350 to 1175 BCE, the period when the city was under the domination of the Hittite Empire. Most of the tablets come from the royal district of the city, but the more religiously oriented texts were found near the temples of Baal and Dagon. In addition to the literary tales of *Aqhat* and *Kirta*, this particular archive also contained incantations against evil spirits, scorpions, and

42. Lev 13:2–3, 6.

43. The cuneiform symbols in Akkadian actually represent syllables rather than letters.

snakebites. These are the closest scholars have to Canaanite medical texts concerning human patients, but they do not read as procedural texts like Leviticus or its Egyptian counterparts. The Ugaritic incantations often use a command form with analogies, followed by descriptions of objects and creatures departing, such as smoke and snakes.[44] When the priest speaks, the affliction is to depart like the named objects.

The only professional instruction literature from Ugarit are the hippiatric texts, which are veterinarian cases for horses.[45] Mesopotamian and Hittite archives have revealed texts concerning horses, but they focus on training them, whereas the Ugaritic documents give symptom descriptions and treatment measures for sick horses. The only other known veterinarian documents from the ancient Mediterranean basin and Near East are later Greco-Roman ones. Until the discovery of more Canaanite archives that prove otherwise, it appears that Ugarit valued the health of horses more than other cities in the region did. No titles distinguishing a healer for horses exists, so most likely the healer for humans also treated the horses. In form, the Ugaritic hippiatric texts follow the if-then format common to Mesopotamian medical literature, and some of the therapeutic drugs used in the Ugaritic hippiatric texts match the same medicant found in Mesopotamian drug lists.

The paucity of Canaanite texts that are strictly dedicated to medical issues means that literary texts must be relied upon more to develop a picture of their health practices. One must remember that these are mediated tales and reports intended to promote particular agendas, quite often religious-political ones centered on the issue of legitimate kingship.

A striking feature of ancient literature, but especially so in Canaanite stories, is the appearance of formulaic, repetitive phrases and scenes. Most literary analyses understand these repetitive passages as mnemonic devices helping a storyteller to remember longer sections of the stories. For example, the speech by Asherah in Baal's battle with Yam contains such repetitive phrasing: "May Horan break, my son / May Horan break your head / Asherah name of Baal your skull." This speech has Asherah calling upon the god Horan to use his powers against Yam, which is essentially a curse formula, but it ends with the curious construction of "name of Baal" as a verb. This phrase appears to function as part of the curse by charging the entire speech

44. KTU 1.169.

45. Chaim Cohen and Daniel Sivan, *The Ugaritic Hippiatric Texts: A Critical Edition* (New Haven: American Oriental Society, 1983).

with the power of Baal.[46] There is the possibility that these repetitive curse formulas teach the audience how to use them. This is a dangerous proposition, because the common person having memorized the spell may not use it effectively, since he or she does not have the proper training or purity to access the gods in that manner. At the same time, it reveals the potential for practitioners of folk medicine, among the more daring, to use the same therapies that the official healers use, such as priests connected to the power centers of temples or royal courts.

Besides the Baal cycle, other stories with potential for understanding Canaanite medicine are the *Healers* and *Kirta*. It is not clear whether the characters called "healers" refers to humans with a cultic function tied to healing, divine attendants of El, or minor deities of the underworld, who would actually be deceased ancestors, the *rephaim*, since this is the term used in the text. Coogan agrees with this last explanation as the most likely.[47] If they are underworld deities, then this brings up a curious feature of Canaanite theology and medicine—namely, that healing comes frequently from the underworld/ghosts, as opposed to a celestial deity. This may stem from the idea that the one who causes illness also brings healing. The text itself does not provide information for discerning clinical medical practices, but it illuminates the term *rephaim* as one of healing.

The story *Kirta* has parallels with biblical Job and the Mesopotamian *Ludlul bel nemqi*, in that a man suffers at the hand of the gods with the loss of his family. In his prayers for a family, Kirta makes a vow to Asherah, which he neglects to fulfill. So, unlike the Israelite and Mesopotamian stories, there is a degree of culpability in Kirta's personal illness, although the beginning of the story about why he lost his initial family is not known. His illness prevents him from fulfilling the duties of a king, which can be seen also in the biblical description of King Azariah of Judah, who suffered from a skin affliction that forced him to live in isolation.[48] Yet, in *Kirta*, this situation causes a crisis of succession, with a son trying to usurp the king's power, much like the fulfilling of the curse on David in 2 Samuel 15. It appears that, for the Canaanites, illness signals disruption of the relationship between god and king, which places at risk not only the individual but also the entire human community; illness is a community concern.

46. Theodore J. Lewis, "'Athtartu's Incantations and the Use of Divine Names as Weapons," *Journal of Near Eastern Studies* 70 (2011): 207–27.

47. Coogan, *Stories from Ancient Canaan*.

48. 2 Kgs 15.

A problematic literary source is *Elkurnisha*, a fragment of a Hittite myth using Canaanite gods El, Asherah, and possibly Baal. The god is referenced simply as "storm-god." Asherah tries to seduce the storm god, but he humiliates her. Then, in turn, she injures him. Subsequently, though, the storm god is healed. The content of this particular story does not match any other known Canaanite myth. Quite possibly, it is actually a Hittite myth but, for some reason, cast with Canaanite deities. If it is truly Hittite, then it would not be applicable to understanding Canaanite medical practices. Yet the possibility exists that this could at least shed light on how the Hittites understood and incorporated the Canaanite gods and medical practices, since it would be highly unusual for the Hittites to simply use Canaanite names in a story wholly their own. More comparative work between Hittite and Canaanite religion and medicine is needed to fully appreciate the significance of *Elkurnisha*.

Apart from the mythic tales, official documents, such as treaties and royal correspondence, provide insight into medical issues for the Canaanites. Of particular interest is the Sefire inscriptions from the ninth century BCE, which is a series of treaties between Mati'ilu of Arpad and a king, Bar-Ga'yah, from an unidentified city-state. These Mati'ilu treaties, like all, make use of a curse formula that includes a description of a ritual causing blindness to the violator.[49]

Official documents from outside Canaan are also useful, such as the archive from the Egyptian New Kingdom capital Akhetaten, modern el-Amarna, just south of Cairo. This royal archive contains about thirty years of foreign correspondence to the Eighteenth-Dynasty pharaohs Amenhotep III, Akhenaten, Smenkhkhare, and Tutankhamun; they are sent from Assyria, Babylon, Mittani, and Hatti, as well as Canaanite vassal kings and chieftains. The language of the letters is a blended form of Hurrian and Akkadian, in keeping with the *lingua franca* of the ancient Near East in the mid-second millennium, but simultaneously reflecting a particular west Semitic vocabulary of the Canaanites. The areas of Canaan under Egyptian control reflected in the letters can be divided into three districts: Amurru, the Phoenician coast headquartered at Gaza, and the region between Qadesh and Hazor, including the Transjordan. Most of the letters from Canaanite vassals deal with the political situation, particularly the rising power of the Hittites and Amurru. Of interest to the

49. Joseph A. Fitzmyer, "The Aramaic Inscriptions of Sefire I and II," *Journal of American Oriental Society* 81 (1961): 178–222.

study of medicine are four letters describing a plague sweeping through Canaan.[50]

The most informative collection of texts for medical practices in Canaan is the Hebrew Bible. A number of passages describe different ailments, such as skin afflictions for Miriam in Exodus and for Na'aman in Numbers, as well as the illnesses of various kings in the more historical books. One should note the overlap between these literary accounts of skin affliction and the priestly concern over purity with skin afflictions in Leviticus. In terms of a clinical setting, they do show how prophets function as healers much in the same manner as the priest, but their focus is on horizontal communication, making sure the camp (human community) understands the relationship with God is in jeopardy. It should be noted that, in some cases, a somatic treatment is used, such as eating fig cakes or bathing in the Jordan River. These passages are not only useful for the assessment of a clinical approach to the disease process but also highlight the cultural perception about disease etiology and its overall function in the cosmology of the Israelites.

While using the Hebrew Bible in the study of ancient medicine, one must keep in mind that early rabbis collated the texts into a single work for the MT. The composition of the books occurred over several hundred years, with some passages, such as Exodus 15 and Judges 5, dating to the late thirteenth century BCE, while others, like Daniel, came about in the Hellenistic period. Although this study takes the Hebrew Bible as a whole to understand a general picture of Canaanite medicine over time, a more in-depth study of particularly Israelite or biblical medicine must account for the variations in date and authorship.

## Archaeology

Although archaeological research is extensive throughout Israel and across the Mediterranean basin, including Punic settlements of the Iberian Peninsula, there are few sites and artifacts related to Canaanite medicine. The character of Canaanite medicine meant that healing occurred in a variety of places rather than by pilgrimage to a specifically constructed healing shrine. For the Israelites, going to a temple for healing usually meant the temple in Jerusalem or perhaps a competing site, such as Bethel in the north. Offerings

50. EA 11, 35, 96, and 932; see William L. Moran, ed. and trans., *The Amarna Letters* (Baltimore: Johns Hopkins University Press, 2002).

of thanks for healing at them would normally take the form of animal sacrifices and not material votives, as found in the Greco-Roman world. Other Canaanites, such as the Phoenicians, could have dedicated shrines to healing gods with inscriptions of thanks, such as a fifth-century BCE sanctuary to Rephesh-Melqart in Ibiza. But the eventual conversion of these sites into Greco-Roman shrines to Asclepius or other deities often obliterated the data necessary to reconstruct distinct Canaanite medical practices. An example of this is the temple of Eshmun in Gadir[51] in Iberia. Polybius describes it as a temple to Asclepius, created by Asdrubal. The Roman takeover of Punic-Phoenician territory makes it problematic to tease apart Canaanite from Greco-Roman practices. A few highlights can be gleaned, but each Canaanite site must be closely analyzed for the smallest clues.

Excavations at Ugarit revealed a section of the city now referred to as the Acropolis, since it contained temples to Baal and Dagon. On the south side of the Acropolis, archaeologists found a private residence of a priest, which contained instruction manuals for sacrifices as well as models of sheep livers and lungs inscribed with divinatory interpretations.[52] Although akin to the haruspex models of Mesopotamia, a comparative study of the two in terms of religion or medicine has yet to be carried out. Nearby, texts were found about the Mesopotamian demon Lamaštu, as well as treatments for eye ailments and birth rituals. Original excavators thought a tomb in this south section was a temple to El, calling it the Rhyton on the basis of a Cypriote-made, bull-shaped vessel. Because of this find, early scholarship on Ugarit associated the structure with healing practices using water rituals. Such misidentification highlights the difficulty in interpreting the functionality of material culture without accompanying texts.

In Fluminimaggiore, on the island of Sardinia, archaeologists uncovered an ancient site of the indigenous Nuragic culture, with a healing shrine to the god Sid, dating to about 500 BCE. Phoenician contact with Sardinia started in the ninth century BCE, but colonies that took over Nuragic settlements did not occur until the fifth century BCE. By this point, the shrine to Sid became a temple to the Phoenician god Melqart. Excavations uncovered votive statues dedicated to the healing god Horon, while a nearby burial site of a woman contained a snake ring that could possibly represent Horon. Later Romans who moved into the settlement created an association of Sid-Addir

51. Modern Cadiz in Spain.

52. Marguerite Yon, *The City of Ugarit at Tell Ras Shamra* (Winona Lake, IN: Eisenbrauns, 2006).

and Melqart with Hercules for that temple. Today, on tourist itineraries, the site is referred to as the temple of Antas.

During the 1960s, Dunand excavated the ancient temple to Eshmun, which lies just north of Sidon. Three volumes of excavation reports have been published by Stucky,[53] but they contend with the shoddy documentation by Dunand during the original excavations and the unfortunate looting of 90 percent of the artifacts during the Lebanese Civil War in the late 1970s. For years, locals dismantled the limestone blocks of the structure to repurpose for other buildings. Many interpretations and analyses of the artifacts and buildings have to be done from subpar photographs.

The initial building phase of the sanctuary dates to the late sixth century BCE, during the reign of Eshmunazar II. The shrine had continuous use into the Hellenistic period. Here, statues of Eshmun depict him as a young, handsome hunter with a lion skin, wielding a mace, making the god's association with Adonis easy to see. It is thought that the healing aspect was a later addition to Eshmun at Sidon. The original temple construction stood over a small river that may have been used in rituals. Roughly during 390–370 BCE, the temple was rebuilt in the Ionic Greek style, with a canal connecting it to the nearby Nahr el-Awali, known at that time as the river of Asclepius. Some conjecture that the Phoenicians originally called the river Eshmun, after the god.[54] It appears that during the Hellenistic period, the temple of Eshmun employed incubation or other water-based rituals common to the asklepieia throughout the eastern Mediterranean. Scholars do not know how close this parallels earlier Canaanite healing rituals at the Eshmun temple or whether any were carried out there prior to the influx of Greek culture. No textual sources for Canaanite medical treatments prescribe temple-based water rituals.

Since the Canaanites did not practice any type of surgery, there are no medical kits to be found. The expense of testing residue in jars makes it infrequent, but even then, identifying and matching the substances to known medical recipes is difficult. Votives, such as ones from Sardinia, can transmit significant information but are scant and rarely published. With these problems, two types of artifacts relating to Canaanite medicine do stand out, the Arslan Tash plaques and the copper *nehuštan* from Timna.

At Arslan Tash, a site in northern Syria, archaeologists uncovered a collection of apotropaic plaques written in Phoenician, dating to the sev-

53. Rolf A. Stucky, *Das Eschmun-Heiligtum von Sidon* (Basel: Vereinigung der Freunde antiker Kunst, 2005).

54. Levin, "Eshmun, Healing of God of Sidon," 39–42.

enth century BCE. One depicts a malevolent entity devouring a child on one side, while the other side shows an unnamed deity carrying an axe. The inscription[55] on it relays an incantation against demonic entities, including a group called "the stranglers." Protection comes by invoking a treaty with the Mesopotamian god Ashur and a divine council. The reciter also claims an oath with the wives of the god Horon, reminiscent of similar Akkadian incantations drawing upon Ereškigal, the consort of Nergal. Although no specific medical ailment is mentioned, its use of Horon and "stranglers" can indicate an underlying concept of physiology along with the role of gods in that physiology.

The Hebrew Bible relates a story that God sent serpents to attack the Israelites who complained to Moses during the exodus. God then later instructed Moses to construct a serpent out of bronze, the *nehuštan*, and to have the victims gaze upon it in order to cure those same Israelites.[56] This is in keeping with the common ideology that the cause of an ailment can also cure it. Interestingly, King Hezekiah destroyed the *nehuštan* of Moses when clearing out the symbols of idolatry, such as the *asherah*.[57]

Excavations have discovered a number of small[58] bronze serpents throughout Canaan. The earliest dates to about 1600 BCE from a temple complex in Megiddo. Although one was found in a room associated with a palace, the majority do come from sanctuaries in Hazor, Shechem, and Timna and date to the Late Bronze and Early Iron Ages (ca. 1400–1200 BCE). Snake imagery in the ancient Near East and even in Canaan alone has a variety of meanings, including fertility, wisdom, health, and immortality, apart from the obvious dangers of an actual snakebite and its underlying cultural tradition of punishment from the gods. The context of the various bronze serpents attests to a number of these concepts at work in the cultic centers; thus, it is difficult to characterize one particular snake cult for Canaan or to tie them all to a specific healing deity such as Eshmun or Horon.[59]

55. Kevin J. Cathcart, "The Phoenician Inscriptions from Arslan Tash and Some Old Testament Texts," in *On Stone and Scroll: Essays in Honour of Graham Ivor Davies*, ed. James K. Aitken, Katharine J. Dell, and Brain A. Mastin (Boston: de Gruyter, 2011), 87–99; Theodore H. Gaster, "The Magical Inscription from Arslan Tash," *Journal of Near Eastern Studies* 6 (1947): 186–88.

56. Num 21:5–9.

57. 2 Kgs 18:4.

58. The figures range in size from three to eight inches; one is fashioned in such a way as to be worn as a pendant.

59. Contra Maciej Münnich, "The Cult of Bronze Serpents in Ancient Canaan and Israel,"

## Cultural Concepts

Canaanite artistic representations of the human form make it difficult to estimate their underlying concepts of physiology. No comprehensive or synthesized study of the artistic traditions across Canaan exists. Studies tend to focus on particular ethnicities, such as the Phoenicians, and within that they center on just the Iron Age. A few works that do analyze the development of Canaanite artistic traditions from the Bronze to the Iron Age note that particular regions have heavy influence from politically dominant cultures, such as Egypt, or borrow from areas with consistent exposure, like Cyprus.[60] Other works collate evidence that pertains to a specific research question, such as the development of aniconism among the Israelites.

The aniconism of Israelite religion—or at least a cultural tendency to not represent many humans and anthropomorphized deities—leaves little evidence. The Bronze Age does provide more images from Canaan than the Iron Age, which leads some to argue that the aniconism of Israelite monotheism is a development of the Late Iron Age.[61] Most of the representations are likely of the gods, either in a smiting pose or enthroned. A few humans are shown in the act of presenting offerings to the gods. Females are frequently depicted as holding either their pubis or their breasts. For some of these statues, the nipples do allow for the passage of liquids. The style of these representations reminds one of the early art from Mesopotamia, in that they have a geometric form, although not of the exact same character as to think the Canaanites merely lifted the iconography. The modeling of the arms, legs, and torsos tends to be rather "soft," in that they display no muscular striations. None of them show extreme weight variation, such as emaciation or rolls of fat, denoting social status, although the female figures tend to be more rounded than the males. In a few cases, the absence of genitalia makes it difficult to determine the intended sex, if any, of the figure. From this, it can generally be concluded that the Canaanites did not use art

---

in *IGGUD: Selected Essays in Jewish Studies, Volume 1: The Bible and Its World, Rabbinic Literature and Jewish Thought, and Jewish Law*, ed. Baruch J. Schwartz, Abraham Melamed, and Aharon Shemesh (Jerusalem: World Union of Jewish Studies, 2008), 39–56.

60. Glenn E. Markoe, "The Emergence of Phoenician Art," *Bulletin of the American Schools of Oriental Research* 279 (1990): 13–26.

61. Christoph Uehlinger, "Anthropomorphic Cult Statuary in Iron Age Palestine and the Search for Yahweh's Cult Images," in *The Image and the Book: Iconic Cult, Aniconism, and the Rise of Book Religion in Israel and the Ancient Near East*, ed. Karel van der Toorn (Leuven: Peeters, 1997), 97–155.

to convey specific physiological concepts linked to cultural traditions. The actions of the figures, such as smiting or nursing, were of more importance than the body itself.

## Anatomy and Physiology

The Canaanite understanding of anatomy and physiology must, therefore, stem from the surviving written documents. This does weight the matter toward the Israelite conception as expressed in the Hebrew Bible. Unfortunately, the Bible does not provide a handy outline of the internal system(s) governing the human body, like the Ebers Papyrus does for the *mtw* in Egyptian medicine. When applicable, the incantations and religious texts from Ugarit and Phoenicia will be incorporated to show either continuity or a variation on the Israelite model.

Preuss's seminal work *Biblical and Talmudic Medicine* reconstructs ancient ideas of physiology but focuses on the mechanistic aspects akin to later Hippocratic and Galenic medicine, with attention to rabbinical concerns for precisely identifying anatomical parts.[62] Its references to the Bible support rabbinic interpretations rather than analyzing those passages on their own terms to understand the physiological concepts used by the ancient Israelites. This over-reliance on interpreting the Hebrew Bible through either a talmudic or Greek medical lens obscures the biblical expressions of anatomy and physiology. But even with these limitations, it is not impossible to uncover from Israelite and Canaanite sources a conception of physiology being a three-way relationship between body parts, humans, and god, similar to that held by the Egyptians and Mesopotamians.

To recreate a sense of Israelite anatomy and physiology that underscores their explanatory model of illness, let us start with the creation of humans. The Hebrew term *nefesh* denotes life itself, often translated as "soul," in the texts of Genesis and Deuteronomy. When creating man, Yahweh Elohim "blew into his nostril the breath of life (*nishmat*), and man became a living being (*nefesh*)."[63] The term appears again when Deuteronomy outlines the rules by which the Israelites can consume meat, noting "that you do not partake of the blood; for the blood is the life (*nefesh*), and you must not

62. Julius Preuss, *Biblical and Talmudic Medicine*, ed. and trans. Fred Rosner (Northvale, NJ: Jason Aronson, 1993).

63. Gen 2:7.

consume the life (*nefesh*) with the flesh."[64] From this, we can understand that the Israelites saw breathing and blood as the most vital elements to the body's operation as a living entity. This would seem intuitive, since people die when they either stop breathing or lose too much blood. But Knoll points out that the Israelite value of blood in Deuteronomy is in contrast to the Ugaritic texts, which do not give such priority to blood.[65] Use of the term "stranglers" in the Arslan Tash plaque to highlight the physical dangers of malevolent night entities only reinforces the concept of the breath being the key to life, while making no mention of blood in any parallel context. Although the Hebrew Bible as a whole presents breath and blood as equal, the fact that the passages come from two different authors underscores the idea that physiological ideologies may have shifted over time and across sub-ethnicities of the Canaanites. All Canaanites did not necessarily view blood as a fundamental part of human physiology, but the importance of breath seems universal among them.

Apart from the breath of life, Genesis 2 depicts an important aspect for Israelite physiology: the physical body of humans exists prior to life itself. The idea that God has to form a physical entity and then infuse it with life is not unique to the creation story of humans. God recapitulates this process with every human. "For you created my kidneys; you wove me together in my mother's womb. . . . For I am a wonderful thing, extraordinarily distinct."[66] The Jewish Publication Society uses "consciousness" rather than the literal translation "kidneys," reflecting the ancient belief held by both the Israelites and Mesopotamians that one's thoughts and feelings originate in the kidneys rather than the brain. The Psalmist here gives a further clue about how physiology in the Hebrew Bible works. The uniqueness that makes one a living human, the soul, derives not just from God's breath, but the kidneys channel these divinely inspired thoughts and feelings. Similarly, the blood holds this *nefesh*, the life or soul of the person.[67] Although the life/soul that makes someone a person comes from God, it has a connection also to the body, namely, through the blood and kidneys. Yet the body as depicted in Genesis and the Psalms can exist as a tangible entity without such a soul.

Once made and infused with life, the body parts are not completely at the will of the human host. God can cause them to act a particular way,

64. Deut 12:23.

65. Knoll, "Canaanite Religion," 61–92.

66. Ps 139:13–14. Author translation.

67. Lev 17:11.

as in the famous case of Exodus: "I will harden Pharaoh's heart, that I may multiply My signs and marvels in the land of Egypt."[68] This is repeated when Pharaoh at times agrees to let Moses and the Israelites leave; God, in order to demonstrate his own power, keeps changing Pharaoh's heart.[69] Despite having a soul (*nefesh*), Pharaoh is not in complete control of his heart and its decisions. Organs, whether in an Israelite or an Egyptian, have a symbiotic relationship with the person.

The Bible also depicts organs that act independent of the human, without God directly influencing them: "My kidneys admonish me at night"[70] or "let my right hand forget its cunning."[71] This last phrase may be interpreted as yet another example of God simply controlling the body part. But, in order for God to take the cunning away, it means that the hand possessed cunning in its own right. Although this phrase is normally taken (dismissed even) as simply a description of one's skillfulness as a craftsman, such as carpentry, by the fact that it is written out, it thus creates an entity, a hand, that possesses cunning just as the incantations and votive statues have done for the Mesopotamians. Kotzé establishes that the use of similes and metaphors in the Hebrew Bible does create the depicted entity in the same way that representations call forth entities in Egyptian and Mesopotamian cultures.[72]

For the ancient Israelites, though, the mere existence of body parts like the hands, eyes, and ears do not give them their independence. Psalms 115 and 135 both caution that just because idols have such organs, it does not mean they can see, hear, or touch.

> They have mouths, but cannot speak,
> Eyes, but cannot see;
> They have ears, but cannot hear,
> Noses, but cannot smell;
> They have hands, but cannot touch,
> Feet, but cannot walk;
> They can make no sound in their throats.[73]

68. Exod 7:3.

69. Exod 10:1 and 14:8.

70. Ps 18:7. Author translation.

71. Ps 137:5. Author Translation

72. Zacharias Kotzé, "Humoral Theory as Motivation for Anger Metaphors in the Hebrew Bible," *Southern African Linguistics and Applied Language Studies* 23 (2005): 205–9.

73. Ps 115:5–7. A similar refrain can be found in Ps 135:16–17.

They may have anatomical parts, but they lack a soul and the relationships necessary for a proper physiology. In order for them to work properly, they must have a relationship with God. Conversely, if one is to trust in the idols, the functioning of their own senses, their own physiology, will cease, despite the presence of anatomy. "Those who fashion them, all who trust in them, shall become like them."[74] This underscores the idea that proper physiology is dependent on the body parts, as well as on the human having a relationship with God. In Psalm 137, the hand has cunning, but only because in the writing of the psalm, that hand is supposed to exist in a symbiotic relationship with an Israelite and also to have a relationship with God.

Although the psalmist gives some sense of the internal anatomy and physiology connected to the soul and how a particular body part like the skin may exhibit symptoms, the Hebrew Bible overall portrays the disease process as affecting the entire person. As we shall see, therapeutic measures do not target an isolated body part but treat the whole person, especially as an indication of the relationship between God and humans. The body as a whole undergoing suffering brings up an important point about the Israelite conception of physiology, namely, that the body functions as a messenger between communities.

It is interesting to note that the LXX uses anatomical parts differently than the MT—in particular, books such as Lamentations. Where the MT has "bowels" and "liver," in keeping with a general ancient Near Eastern form of expression for emotions, the LXX changes this to "heart" and "my honor," respectively, indicating a much more Hellenistic sensibility about the organs or lack thereof associated with such feelings.[75] Another common idiom, completely missing from the LXX, is the imagery of a burning nose, associated with anger, or a long nose, meaning slow to anger, as ubiquitously found in the Hebrew Bible and other ancient Near Eastern texts.[76] This variation shows that the LXX does not necessarily provide insight into a pre-Hellenistic Israelite/Canaanite culture but that it can be used to understand the shift into a more hellenized Jewish culture.

74. Pss 115:8 and 135:18.

75. Angela Thomas, *Anatomical Idiom and Emotional Expression: A Comparison of the Hebrew Bible and the Septuagint* (Sheffield: Sheffield Phoenix, 2014), 1.

76. Thomas, *Anatomical Idiom and Emotional Expression*, 308.

## Disease Etiology

If the proper functioning of human physiology rests upon a symbiotic, working relationship with God for both the human and the body part, then it stands to reason that illness stems from a disruption of those relationships. Frequently in literature, disobeying the cosmological order—that is, a lack of piety—is punished with illness or even the threat of death. This stance appears in Canaanite literature apart from the Hebrew Bible. Kirta's illness comes from his lack of piety in not fulfilling a vow to Asherah. Political documents reinforce this disease etiology, such as the Sefire inscriptions, which use a particular curse formula describing various illnesses and trauma for violating the treaty terms.

The Canaanites, and even the Israelites, shared in the ancient Near Eastern conception that disease and trauma represented messages from the gods, indicating problematic relationships on a cosmological level. But these messages are not restricted to just the individual who made a transgression. The intimate relationships within the human community mean that someone can suffer an illness as a result of another person's lack of piety. This is especially true for family members and the king, two categories that are supposed to act as protectors, safeguarding the relationships with community and God. The stories of King Jeroboam of Israel and King Azariah of Judah exemplify the important link between disease etiology and family relationships.

The terminal disease suffered by Jeroboam's son stems from the king worshiping other gods in direct violation of the required relationship with Yahweh Elohim, as stipulated in the Mosaic covenant. The text notes that the son will have a proper burial, because "in him alone . . . has some devotion been found to Yahweh, the God of Israel,"[77] while the rest of the dynasty will fall—a message the human community will surely notice. Similarly, King Azariah must suffer from a skin affliction because he did not remove the shrines to other gods scattered throughout Judah, allowing the Judahites to break the covenantal relationship with God.[78] The fact that he lived many years with this condition, forcing his son to rule in his stead, would indicate to the human community a disruption in the relationship with God. In both of these stories, the body acts as a communicative tool relaying messages to both the individual and the community at large.

77. 1 Kgs 14:13.
78. 2 Kgs 15.

But one does not have to commit a transgression or be in a position to prevent others from doing so in order to suffer from disease and injury. Most famously, the story of Job illustrates the very point that the relationship between God and other entities can result in human suffering. The text characterizes Job as "blameless and upright; he feared God and shunned evil,"[79] and he petitions God based on his keeping of the covenants, denying the accusations of his friends that he had done something wrong to warrant such misfortune. God's answer to Job at first seems to dodge the issue: "Who is this who darkens counsel, speaking without knowledge? . . . I will ask and you will inform Me. Where were you when I laid the earth's foundations? Speak if you have understanding."[80] Yet this is the very crux of the matter in Job's disease etiology, events beyond his knowledge and understanding. The relationship between God and the Adversary,[81] essentially laying a wager, causes the illness.[82]

The idea that disease etiology depends on relationships between God and others also finds expression in other Canaanite cultures. The treaty of the Sefire inscription contains an interesting line in its curse section: "just as a man of wax is blinded, so may Mati'el be blinded."[83] This indicates that someone can fashion a wax figure representing a particular individual who then suffers the same malady as that wax figure. The ritual physically demonstrates the disruption of a human-to-human relationship, causing the illness or trauma. In the case of the treaty, the invoked ritual works because the gods as witnesses can determine whether one of the contractual parties violates the terms. But the possibility exists that someone can carry out such a ritual without the intended victim having done anything wrong within the human community. Although no Canaanite texts directly speak to the gods being fooled in such a way, other ancient Near Eastern cultures, like Egypt and Mesopotamia, with a similar disease etiology provide ample evidence that such situations did exist. But like Job, the innocent victim shows a community disruption that needs to be addressed, such as ferreting out the improper use of such rituals. The process of obedience and consideration is a community affair and not just an individual matter.

79. Job 1:1, 8.

80. Job 38:2–4.

81. The Hebrew *ha-satan* is usually rendered as the proper noun Satan, but this is a later Christian overlay to the text. The literal translation, "the adversary," indicates a particular functionary within the divine council without naming a specific god fulfilling that position.

82. Job 1:6–12.

83. Fitzmyer, "Aramaic Inscriptions of Sefire I and II," 178–222.

It is interesting to note that actually performing rituals, like the creation and the blinding of a wax figure, does not appear necessary for the treaty curse to work. The written description of the act is enough to charge the words with the same power as the act. This brings up the issue of scribes or any literate person having access to the level of power necessary to effect both sickness and healing. Perhaps the literate constitute a class of healers in their own right. This notion would be supported by the occurrence of scribes with the title of healers in other cultures, such as Egypt and Mesopotamia.

Another facet of disease etiology, like the unfounded curse, stems from the malevolent actions of supernatural entities. The disruption of the vertical human-to-god(s) community does not always have to be the fault of the person suffering; it can originate with the gods. The Hebrew Bible demotes the other Canaanite gods to functionaries of Yahweh Elohim, as seen in the imagery of Deuteronomy. "The LORD will make pestilence (*daber*) cling to you until he has put an end to you in the land that you are entering to possess."[84] This passage anthropomorphizes the disease as an entity distinct from humans, as well as God. The term *daber* developed from the god Deber, overseeing pestilence and healing, in the Canaanite pantheon. Yet his name is not as frequently attested as Resheph and Horon. In many cases, Deber appears in a triad with Resheph and Mot (death). Apart from the Hebrew Bible, we can see malevolent entities acting of their own volition in the ancestral ghosts, the *rephaim*, in other Canaanite texts.

**Restoration of Health**

Like disease etiology, the restoration of health depends upon community involvement in the obedience and consideration process. Ultimately, the relationship between the god(s) and humans must be restored, but the process of doing just that also requires the community of gods to be in agreement with each other, especially if the illness stems from a disagreement between supernatural entities. Illness also entails a separation of the afflicted from the human community. While the divine realm coheres to restore the physical health of a person, the afflicted must also find a way to reintegrate with the human community once the illness has departed.

One must be careful not to assume that the physical healing of an ailment is the same as restoration of health. As we see with Egyptian medical

84. Deut 28:21.

documents, the prognostic phrases "with which I will contend" and "not to be treated" acknowledge that the physical state may not change. In modern society, a physical problem that becomes permanent categorizes one as disabled, placing the person in a liminal social state, partially able to fulfill society's expectations while carrying a variety of stigmas. In the ancient world, no such category of disabled existed; the extent to which someone cannot perform social obligations is, especially among the Israelites, indicated in terms of pure and impure. A physical ailment can be categorized as impure, such as a skin condition, thus excluding the afflicted from participating in the human community or camp, as well as the community/congregation with the divine. Yet the physical clearing of the skin, modern healing, does not automatically allow the person to resume community participation. The restoration of health that reintegrates a person with the two communities usually depends upon ritual acts and a new declaration of purity.

The Hebrew Bible stands as our most thorough source on purity in relation to medical practices. Much is made of the issue of purity in Leviticus,[85] with scholars like Milgrom seeing it connected to issues of mortality[86] rather than morbidity; therefore, he divorces Leviticus from any medical practices. Others claim the Levitical laws are the earliest examples of using hygiene as preventative health care, especially citing the prohibition on consuming pork as knowingly avoiding trichinosis. There is no evidence that the Israelites were aware of such infections of pork meat, and more importantly, the dietary restriction on pork appears to be an imitation or emulation of such practices by an elite level of priests in Egypt. It is only coincidental that kosher laws prevent certain infectious diseases.

Not just the Israelites but all the ancient Near Eastern cultures work with a conception of pure and impure that blocks someone from entering holy spaces. For our purposes in this broad study, it is better to work with the general definition of impure, as "that which is not acceptable to be in the presence of the divine" rather than try to puzzle out the precise mechanism by which something is categorized as pure or impure. With this in mind, we can then investigate the involvement of the human community in the restoration of health.

85. Many use the anthropological work of Mary Douglas as the definitive source for understanding the categories of pure and impure; see Mary Douglas, *Purity and Danger: An Analysis of the Concepts of Pollution and Taboo* (London: Routledge, 2005). Lately, Douglas's study is being reevaluated for its applicability to the issue of purity in the Hebrew Bible.

86. Jacob Milgrom, *Leviticus 1–16: A New Translation with Introduction and Commentary* (New York: Doubleday, 1991; repr., New Haven: Yale University Press, 2009).

The more obvious role of the human community in healing comes from Leviticus. Once the priest has declared a woman unclean due to childbirth, she "should not touch any sacred thing and not go into the sanctuary"[87] for a period of days, from fourteen to thirty-three, depending on the gender of the child. This separates her from the community of the divine but also signals to the human community that she is entering the healing process that began with the priest's declaration. A similar process appears in the following chapter regarding skin afflictions, but with a slight change where the "priest should shut up the marked [person] for seven days."[88] This indicates a more severe separation, in which the afflicted must not have contact with the entire human community. Although Leviticus calls for reinspection every seven days, there comes a point when the priest declares a person permanently unclean, who must then "dwell alone outside the camp."[89] Again, the process of healing begins with declaration and separation. The acts of isolating one's self, either from the presence of the divine or the entire community, demonstrates obedience, the functional aspect of the healing process.

In both cases, restoration of health occurs when the person is reintegrated into the community. For the parturient woman, the healing process ends with two acts: her bringing a lamb and a dove to the priest and the priest performing the sacrifice ritual with them. Bringing the animals to the priest who accepts them signals that she has now returned to the presence of both the divine and the human community. Those with a skin affliction have a more complex process.[90] The priest must go outside the camp to the afflicted; perform a sacrifice with a bird, red thread, hyssop, and fresh water; sprinkle a mixture of the blood and water over the afflicted; and set free a live bird. The afflicted must then wash his clothes, shave all his hair, and bathe. This set of rituals allows the person to move back into the camp, but he is not fully integrated into the community, signaled by his staying outside his tent for seven days. A full restoration of health and reintegration occurs when he brings lambs to the priest, who performs a sacrifice with them, rubs oil on the right ear, thumb, and big toe of the afflicted, and pours oil on his or her head. Only at this point is the person declared clean. The declaration of clean indicates that God has considered the plight of the afflicted and acted accordingly.

87. Lev 12:4. Author translation.
88. Lev 13:4. Author translation.
89. Lev 13:46. Author translation.
90. Lev 14.

Apart from Leviticus, the Hebrew Bible has several stories indicating that one is isolated from the camp or human community due to impurity. These usually center on skin afflictions, such as the one that befell Miriam.[91] Miriam is never declared impure but is still excluded from the camp; the skin affliction marked the shame she bore for speaking against Moses. Unlike the instructions in Leviticus, this story does describe how the people of the community help the process of healing the physical ailment. Healing comes in two parts: God answering Moses's prayer of intercession and her exclusion for a prescribed number of days. Living outside the camp shows her renewed obedience to both the divine and human communities, but God's consideration comes from listening to Moses, who directly asks for healing (*repha*). Prayer then plays an important part of the healing process. The intercessional prayer shows the community's obedience apart from the afflicted's act of obedience. It is interesting to note that there is no ritual of reintegration such as bathing or sacrifice. She is simply readmitted after the appointed time.

For other Canaanites, the story *Kirta* exemplifies the involvement of the human community. A banquet is held for Kirta with his nobles, at which they weep for him as mourners. Coogan interprets this fragmented passage as Kirta becoming ill just before an already planned banquet,[92] perhaps to highlight Kirta's impiety. But it could be read that the banquet was undertaken as part of a healing strategy. In a later passage, Kirta sends for one of his daughters to pray for him and host a banquet, demonstrations of community obedience. This brings up the question about the relation between mourning and healing rituals. It is possible that mourning prayers before the actual passing of a person can sway the gods to heal the afflicted. Lewis makes a convincing linguistic argument for the possibility that a healer's weeping and mourning can have therapeutic effects.[93] The mourning prayers in *Kirta* would also parallel the story of Miriam in which Moses's prayer effects healing. The description of Miriam "as a dead one"[94] underscores the relationship of mourning prayers and healing.

Ritual actions for healing, apart from prayer, do appear in the Hebrew Bible, especially in the cases of King Hezekiah of Judah and the Aramean

91. Num 12.

92. Coogan, *Stories from Ancient Canaan*, 53.

93. Theodore J. Lewis, "The Sha'tiqatu Narrative from the Ugaritic Story about the Healing of King Kirta," *Journal of Ancient Near Eastern Religions* 13 (2013): 188–211.

94. Num 12:12.

general Na'aman. The case of King Hezekiah demonstrates that a ritual somatic treatment can act not only as a sign of obedience to God but that God is considering the prayers of the afflicted.[95] The prophet Isaiah declares to Hezekiah that he will die. As expected, Hezekiah immediately turns to prayer. Like the case of Miriam, God considers and responds that Hezekiah will live as well as protect Jerusalem from the invading Assyrians. Although Elisha relays God's message, indicating that the sign of healing will come from a shadow on the steps of the temple, Elisha also orders that a poultice of fig cakes be applied to Hezekiah's rash.[96] Use of the fig cakes demonstrates Hezekiah's obedience, but the resultant clearing of the rash in turn demonstrates that God considered the prayers, essentially to trust Isaiah's pronouncements and healing.

Although not an Israelite who is part of the camp, God favored the Aramean general Na'aman, thus making him part of the congregation. In this regard, Na'aman must be pure, but his skin affliction made him impure. Eventually, he seeks healing from the prophet Elisha, who tells Na'aman that he must bathe in the Jordan River, a somatic treatment with a charged substance. Note that his restoration of health is not as elaborate a ritual as the Israelite wishing to integrate with the human community. At first, Na'aman scoffs at the therapy, stating he thought the prophet would just speak to heal the skin and then asking why the Jordan River is better than ones near Damascus. This story illustrates that despite the similarity of healing tactics among the Canaanites, essentially an ethnic difference still exists rooted in the variation of religious practices between the two groups.

Humans are not the only ones employing ritual actions to fully restore health. The goddess Shataqat effects Kirta's healing by using a staff that forces the disease, personified as dragon-like, to fly not just away from Kirta but beyond civilization. Once she safely removed the illness, she then returns her attention to Kirta to "wash off his sweat"[97] and restore his appetite by opening his throat. This demonstrates that returning to health involves more than just the simple absence of illness. The signs of health, such as an appetite, must be ritually reinstated in their own right.

95. 2 Kgs 20.

96. The text repeats itself, with God speaking to Elisha and Elisha repeating it to Hezekiah, but the part describing the fig cakes is missing from God's speech, as are the precise directions concerning the shadow on the steps. This may be a scribal error due to haplography, a common occurrence with repetitive texts.

97. Coogan, *Stories from Ancient Canaan*, 72.

While the afflicted tries to show obedience and the surrounding human community joins with prayers, the divine community must now work together in considering whether to heal. Since the Hebrew Bible reduces the Canaanite pantheon down to one god, it is difficult to see this among the Israelites. The story *Kirta* provides a clear example in which healing for Kirta can happen only after El consults with the divine council, reinforcing the idea that healing and community cohesion are linked. An interesting aspect of the *Kirta* story is that no god dared try to cure the disease except El.

> Who among the gods can expel the sickness, drive out the disease?
> But none of the gods answered him.
> He spoke a second, then a third time:
> Who among the gods can expel the sickness, drive out the disease?
> . . . .
> He spoke a sixth, then a seventh time:
> Who among the gods can expel the sickness, drive out the disease?
> But none of the gods answered him.
> Then El the Kind, the Compassionate, replied:
> My sons, sit down upon our thrones, upon your princely seats.
> I will work magic, I will bring relief:
> I will expel the sickness, I will drive out the disease.[98]

This indicates that the gods did not wish to cross Asherah, thus leaving it to the superior El, whom Asherah could not counter. Their silence retains cohesion among the divine; to do otherwise would cause strife among the council, possibly leading to more sickness and death within the human realm. Additionally, this represents a conception of disease that some are more difficult to cure than others because of its relationship to the divine. The healer must ultimately try to figure out these relationships to determine the ease with which he can heal each case.

In keeping with most ancient cultures, Canaanites can directly involve the divine in healing by the use of incantations that draw upon the mythic cycles invoking the power of cyclical time. Incantations from Ugarit use analogy with particular mythic scenes to effect the desired outcome.[99] These passages create a parallel between the supernatural and natural worlds that force the gods to act by recreating the events in writing and speech. The

98. Coogan, *Stories from Ancient Canaan*, 72.
99. CAT 1.100, 1.107, 1.114, and 1.124.

incantation creates a specific relationship between the afflicted and a god, such as Baal, so that when Baal is healed in that passage of the story, so too must the patient be healed in that moment of time. The divine realm must reenact the story as written, since time is not linear but circular. If time were linear, then the gods could take a different action, but the circularity of time means that the actions are consistently the same for each occasion that invokes the myth.

A notable feature of these healing stories and rituals is the lack of a specific place dedicated to healing, like the asklepieion in Greco-Roman culture. It seems that, for most Canaanites, any temple could serve the purpose of accepting sacrifices as part of the restoration of health. This might explain the paucity of archaeological evidence for such sites. Under monotheism in the Hebrew Bible, the temple in Jerusalem would be the only appropriate spot for the sacrifices. The priests, whether Levitical or not, do not have to remain at the temples but can go out to the patients. Some scholars take issue with the temple or shrine as a healing location or the thanksgiving sacrifice as part of a ritual reestablishing purity, because the illness and its uncleanliness would prevent someone from going to the temple prior to the required rituals. Restrictions based on purity usually applied to the interior portions housing the statue of the god or, for the Israelites, the ark of the covenant. Outer spaces of the temples could hold those in a state of impurity seeking to do the necessary sacrifices to complete the healing process. The lack of dedicated healing spaces applies also to the prophets. For them, the locus of healing is wherever the patient may be.

## Illness

As with all ancient documents, cultural values imparted to the texts describing various illnesses skew the data for use in clinically assessing the diseases and traumas suffered by the people of ancient Canaan. The curses listed in Deuteronomy 28 stand as a prime example of such problematic texts. For the most part, it gives general symptom descriptions, such as hemorrhoids and fever, but it also designates a specific illness as the "boils of Egypt."[100] One must take care not to mistake this for a particular disease spread from Egypt but to recognize that this phrase draws upon the Exodus narrative in which God sent a plague of boils upon the Egyp-

100. Deut 28:27.

tians.[101] Yet certain documents, such as the Amarna texts, can provide evidence for the presence of an epidemic, even if we cannot discern which specific disease swept through the populations.

A cultural bias, in both texts and material remains relating to medicine, appears in relation to snakebites, but there is no indication that Canaanites suffered a far greater number than in other regions of the ancient Near East, such as Egypt. This is an incomplete picture, since we have no soft-tissue remains by which to test for the presence of snake venom. Additionally, not all snakes are venomous but merely painful, which would necessitate symptom alleviation at the time but leave no record on a body discovered thousands of years later. Nor have studies been conducted on the snake population in the Levant, either for the modern era or the Late Bronze and Iron Age, to determine whether there was truly a higher frequency of contact with snakes. Interestingly, when doing cross-cultural comparisons, the Canaanites make little mention of eye ailments, while the Egyptians, who have a clear obsession for ophthalmological matters, note a number of their medical treatments originated with the Canaanites. These variations indicate cultural values at work.

Ideally, bioarchaeological finds could supplement the unclear textual descriptions, but unfortunately, not many human remains in sufficient condition for testing have been found in the Levant prior to the Hellenistic period. Of those found, there is no soft tissue left to carry out paleopathological analysis for diseases, such as malaria or other infections. Based on the dry environmental conditions, we can rule out the presence of diseases like malaria, which plagued Mesopotamia, but this leaves still a number of other diseases as distinct possibilities.

## Disease

For many, the first illness that springs to mind when discussing biblical Israel is leprosy. The Hebrew term *zara'at* is a catch-all for a variety of skin afflictions, such as eczema and psoriasis, rather than meaning a specific disease. The modern conception of leprosy as a disease that causes necrosis and loss of extremities is anachronistic. This type of leprosy is actually the ancient Greek term for what is today called Hansen's disease, which did not appear in the Levant until the Hellenistic period, well after the texts of Leviticus,

101. Exod 9:9–11.

Numbers, and Kings were written with passages focusing on skin afflictions. The spread of Hansen's disease by Alexander the Great's troops, from the Indus River toward the Levant, is attested in documents referring to necrosis and extremity loss, symptoms absent from the biblical descriptions of skin afflictions. Corroborating this later date for the appearance of Hansen's disease is the osteoarchaeological record. Hansen's disease leaves traces in the skeleton; none of the tested human remains prior to the Hellenistic period shows these traces, whereas a number of Hellenistic skeletons do.

Several of the Amarna Letters attest to a plague that swept through Canaan in the mid-fourteenth century BCE. King Alishiya, in explaining why his gift of copper to the pharaoh is rather small, claims that the "hand of Nergal is now in my country; he has slain all the men of my country and there is not a single copper worker."[102] This letter brings up several points of interest for investigating Canaanite medicine. First, it opens with the standard greeting saying all is well in the land and listing the required gifts sent with it, but it then immediately describes a devastating plague. The close of the letter mentions a death even within the king's own household but assures the pharaoh that the Egyptian envoy, living in the plague-stricken land, has nothing to worry about concerning his health. This demonstrates the cognitive dissonance between reporting events of the plague to excuse certain behaviors while keeping to socio-cultural traditions. Not only must the standard letter formats be adhered to, but it must also be stressed that the powerful king of Egypt and his associates are immune to such misfortune by the virtue of their superior position relative to King Alishiya. In reality, such people are just as easily victims of an epidemic, but this cannot be acknowledged in official correspondence. Second, the letter ascribes the plague to Nergal, since that is the Mesopotamian god, and Akkadian is the diplomatic language used in official correspondence even with the Egyptian king. Yet the Canaanite equivalent is Resheph, and perhaps the Egyptians reading the letter understood the plague to be the work of Sekhmet. This indicates a fluidity across cultures with regard to the names of the deities involved in causing illness and restoring health, while also maintaining continuity in the idea that a divine entity lies at the heart of illness.

102. Moran, *Amarna Letters*, 107.

## Trauma

One would expect more certainty when looking at incidences of trauma for the Canaanites, since the osteoarchaeological record could provide more solid evidence, but this area, too, has its problems. Many studies for Canaan focus on the early Neolithic period to understand the impact of the shift to a farming economy. The exceptions are the Punic-Phoenician *tophet* from Carthage, as well as the sites of Jericho northwest of the Dead Sea in Israel and Bab edh-Dhra' along the southeastern shore of the Dead Sea in Jordan. Since the remains in the *tophet* are children frequently less than a year old, their bodies simply lack the wear and tear indicative of the living conditions in ancient Canaan.

From Bab edh-Dhra', thousands of shaft graves dating to the Early Bronze Age (3150–2300 BCE) give ample samples for paleo-osteological studies. The earliest graves (3150–2950 BCE) are not associated with a settlement and so most likely served as a burial site for a pastoral-nomadic population. By 2550 BCE, the site had a sizable urban settlement with irrigation canals and a town wall. The number of bodies over this period during a shift in settlement patterns and subsistence strategies allows researchers to study how the social organization affected the skeleton, especially joint damage.[103] The problem with using bodies from Bab edh-Dhra' is that no soft tissue was recovered, and the skeletons were not complete. Upper limbs could not be matched to lower limbs. Variations, though, could be found based on time period, as urbanization increased due to different repetitive tasks, like grinding of grain. According to analysis of cranial and forelimb fractures, there was also an increase in interpersonal violence as urbanization progressed.[104]

## Disability

As noted previously, the ancient Canaanites did not have a medical or legal classification of disability. Yet the Hebrew Bible uses precise vocabulary to

103. Jamie M. Ullinger, Susan G. Sheridan, and Donald J. Ortner, "Daily Activity and Lower Limb Modification at Bab Edh-Dhra', Jordan, in the Early Bronze Age," in *Bioarchaeology and Behavior: The People of the Ancient Near East*, ed. Megan A. Perry (Gainesville, FL: University Press of Florida, 2012), 180–201; Jane Peterson, *Sexual Revolutions: Gender and Labor at the Dawn of Agriculture* (Walnut Creek, CA: AltaMira, 2002).

104. Matthew Alexander Gasperetti and Susan G. Sheridan, "Cry Havoc: Interpersonal Violence at Early Bronze Age Bab Edh-Dhra," *American Anthropologist* 115 (2013): 388–410.

make distinctions between different categories of ailments that may or may not preclude one from being in the presence of the divine. One can then think of disability, for the Israelites, as a nuanced form of community created between the body parts, humans, and god(s). This understanding of a symbiotic physiology may clarify issues regarding an apparent disability, such as deafness and muteness, being classified as stigmatizing defects in association with the cursed, weak, and vulnerable[105] but not legally defined as blemishes (*mumim*) prohibiting sacrifice at the temple.[106] This gives us some indication as to how people carrying some impairment were treated among the Israelites, especially with regard to the relationships governing the communities between humans and the divine.

Interestingly, in the position of custodian of the body, as warranted by a symbiotic physiology, an Israelite may intentionally take on a defect, purposefully creating a physical aspect that makes him or her socially marginalized, and potentially ineligible to be in the presence of the divine, for the exact purpose of regaining favor with God. "But I am like a deaf man, unhearing, like a dumb man who cannot speak up; I am like one who does not hear, who has no retort on his lips. But I wait for You oh LORD; You will answer, O LORD, my God."[107] Since writing something brings it into existence, the author of the psalm has created a version of himself that has a series of defects. Rather than waiting for his physical body to exhibit the signs excluding him from God, he has fashioned a disabled version in the prayer/text, thus preempting God's action. He may now continue (he hopes) to be acceptable to the divine, which would allow God to hear his pleas.

It seems ironic that one would create a defective form in order to be acceptable in the presence of the divine. The difference between the broad category of defects and the highly particular legal category of blemishes (*mumim*) becomes the key to understand how this preemptive move works. The defects are deafness and muteness, which do not fall under the legal classification of blemish that excludes a person from temple activity or, essentially, from being in the presence of the divine. Yet deafness and muteness as defects can still demonstrate a problem with the relationships between body parts, human, and God. By assuming a lesser problem, the human host uses the symbiotic physiology to begin the process of healing his relation-

105. Saul M. Olyan, *Disability in the Hebrew Bible* (Cambridge: Cambridge University Press, 2011).

106. Lev 21:17–23.

107. Ps 38:14–16.

ship with God before God uses that symbiotic physiology to exact a greater punishment. If Olyan's reading of these two categories is accurate,[108] then slotting apparent disabilities into either broad or narrowly defined classes of defects and blemishes allowed ancient Israelites to navigate the mosaic of relationships needed for a properly functioning physiology.

## Conditional States

Apart from pregnancy, conditional states as treated by physicians in the modern world tend not to be a prominent concern for Canaanite healers. Menopause and general geriatric issues were likely treated at the level of folk medicine, for particular symptoms, thus not normally making their way into the few pieces of extant medical literature. As in most ancient societies, Canaanites viewed puberty as a social concern, in terms of investing one with obligations.

On the issue of pregnancy, there is not much clinical information for most of Canaan beyond the general use of midwives, since pregnancy also was not medicalized, unlike infertility. Literary sources give ample information though. The prevalent thought about childlessness in ancient Canaan and Israel depicts the barren woman in a socially precarious situation, on the verge of becoming a pariah. Yet a more nuanced study shows that in certain contexts infertility has a valuable religious function. The question whether a woman's normal state is the ability to conceive underlies the significance of fertility/infertility. Moss and Baden make a convincing case that, according to the Hebrew Bible, a woman's natural state is infertility, and only through an act of God can she conceive.[109] The lack of curses for infertility underscores this position, especially in contrast to the surrounding cultures of Mesopotamia and Egypt, in which curses for infertility abound.[110] This perspective, however, assumes that infertility is a problem with conception and not necessarily gestation, since there are curses directly invoking miscarriage, such as in Hosea 9:14.

Two exceptions to the dearth of information on pregnancy itself and infancy come from the Hebrew Bible's determination in Leviticus that child-

108. Olyan, *Disability in the Hebrew Bible.*

109. Candida R. Moss and Joel S. Baden, *Reconceiving Infertility* (Princeton: Princeton University Press, 2015), 55–59.

110. Moss and Baden, *Reconceiving Infertility*, 84–97.

birth places a woman in a state of impurity, and the other is the alleged Punic-Phoenician practice of child sacrifice. An analysis of the *tophet* in Carthage indicates that the number of bodies roughly corresponds to standard infant mortality rates. Some scholars, however, have noted that about 60 percent are stillborns or newborns and so hypothesize that the Carthaginians practiced infanticide as a form of population control.[111] They assert that the festivals for Melqart-Adonis included sexual licentiousness resulting in pregnancies and that these children, essentially, were culled, which may also explain the mixing of lamb remains in the graves. The theory is highly dependent on the reconstruction of a ritual calendar to time the death of the children with the birth of the lambs. The presence of lambs in the graves of infants can indicate also a cultural link between the deaths of two young innocents, without necessitating the intentional slaughter of infants.

Many studies on pregnancy, childbirth, and menstruation in the Hebrew Bible center on the issue of purity. Whether the woman is impure due to childbirth or menstruation depends on a variety of factors, such as the gender of the child born or the timing of menstruation (recognizing that not all uterine bleeding is normal menstruation) and even the ideological goal of the author. Philip draws upon works outside the Torah, providing a study on these factors from the perspective of philology and comparative cultural analysis, within the ancient Near East[112] that attempts to update the more monolithic methodology of Douglas.[113]

## Healers

Unlike Egypt and Mesopotamia, the Canaanites did not have a specialized vocabulary for different types of professional healers. Priests associated with the various gods carried out most of the healing. The one exception to this may be the term *mulahhishu*, which essentially means "exorcist." But, based on its use in the Ugaritic texts, it is best thought of as someone who concentrates on incantations against snakebites. Although the documents are few, it appears the *mulahhishu* did not carry any priestly functions. This is

111. Philip C. Schmitz, "Phoenician-Punic Religion," in *The Cambridge History of Religions in the Ancient World*, ed. Michele Renee Salzman (Cambridge: Cambridge University Press, 2013), 205–34.

112. Tarja S. Philip, *Menstruation and Childbirth in the Bible: Fertility and Impurity* (New York: Peter Lang, 2006).

113. Douglas, *Purity and Danger*.

in contrast to the *tʿy*-priest, also found in the Ugaritic texts. The *tʿy*-priest is another type of exorcist but not exclusively medical. Apart from the medical incantations, other texts referring to the *tʿy*-priest describe his function as an official or minister during sacrifices. His function may have been to ensure that the sacrifice or patient is in a state acceptable to the gods.

According to the Hebrew Bible, healers among the Israelites came from two basic groups—the priests and the prophets. Since illness is a message from God, it stands to reason that the healers would divide along the same lines as those who act as communication points between God and the Israelites. The difference then is the focus of communication. The priest maintains communication within the camp (horizontal), while the prophet concentrates on the relationship between the congregation and God (vertical).

**Priests**

Some scholars take issue with the assertion that priests heal, noting that they do not apply any somatic treatments or charged substances to those suffering physical ailments. One must remember that healing can be both instrumental and symbolic and that reintegration within a community also constitutes a form of healing. It is the ritual of sacrifice that reintegrates the formerly afflicted with the human and divine communities and that fulfills the role of healing in medical anthropology. With this perspective, it is easy to see the priest's role as healer.

Another counterintuitive claim is that the Israelite priest focuses on the human community, the camp, since the main function of the priesthood is performing sacrifices, undoubtedly a form of communication with God. Yet closer examination of the instructions to the priest in Leviticus shows that he directs his proclamation (diagnosis) of clean or unclean to the camp. His actions center on determining whether someone can live within the camp or otherwise participate in the obligations of the human community. The healing ritual of sacrifice overseen by the priest has the purpose of reintegrating the person first with the camp, before being reinstated to the congregation. Additionally, to understand the message from God, the priest inspects the body of the inflicted as a form of mediumistic divination. All of these point to the priest as focusing on the human element of communication between humans and God.

## Prophets

The Israelite prophets practiced healing with a focus on cohesion of the community between humans and God, the congregation. Given that prophets do use instrumental or somatic treatments, this may also seem like an odd claim. The method of divination here is key. Prophets use intuitive or ecstatic divination, which means they receive an understanding of the message encoded in illness, without having to inspect the body of the afflicted. From the beginning, the prophet focuses on communication directly with God. The message from God always comes down to the divine relationship with the afflicted, even if he carries the blame for the camp's behavior toward God. Where the priestly instructions do not give a reason for why someone suffers a skin infliction or a discharge, the prophetic episodes of healing all involve a disruption between God and the congregation (they have broken one of the stipulations in the Mosaic covenant) as the disease etiology. Consequently, prophetic healing centers on communicating back to God through prayers and use of somatic treatments. At no point does the prophet ritually act to reintegrate the afflicted with the human community. The prophet declares only whether someone will live, thus indicating the person's final relationship in the congregation with God. It must be remembered that, for the ancient Israelites in the Bronze and Iron Ages, there was no expectation of an afterlife or final judgment in the Christian sense. Death meant separation from God and the congregation. Thus, the healing of the prophet depends upon demonstrations of obedience from the patient in order to secure consideration from the divine.

# 5. Hittite Medicine

## Location and History

The Hittites were located in the Anatolian peninsula (modern Turkey), which consists of a high central plateau bounded by the Pontus Mountains to the north and the Taurus Mountains on the south. This peninsula essentially separates the Mediterranean from the Black Sea, connected only by the narrow passage of the Bosporus. Although Anatolia had continuous occupation since the early Neolithic period, with settlements such as Çatal Huyuk (7000–5600 BCE), the Hittites came to prominence during the Bronze Age with two distinct phases, the Old Kingdom (1650–1400 BCE) and the New Kingdom (1400–1200 BCE). For many years, scholars dismissed the Hittites as a small tribe on the fringes of Israelite society, since the only information known about them came from their mention in the Hebrew Bible, with figures like Uriah the Hittite, whose wife Bathsheba had an affair with King David.[1] In 1876, A. H. Sayce pioneered the idea that the Hittites existed as a major empire in their own right rather than being a subordinate Canaanite tribal entity. They called themselves "the people of the land of Hatti."[2] The modern use of the term Hittite is a holdover from the biblical texts, which translated Hatti as Heth, thus Hittite. Recent philological studies have revealed that the Hittites consisted of an Indo-European language group, with Hattian, Hurrian, and Luwian being the most prominent languages. Overall, eight different languages are represented in the Hittite archives.[3] They used a cuneiform script for their language, and many tablets have been found that are bilingual with Akkadian. Despite over a

1. 2 Sam 11.

2. Trevor Bryce, *Life and Society in the Hittite World* (Oxford: Oxford University Press, 2004), 3.

3. Bryce, *Life and Society in the Hittite World*, 5.

hundred years of recognition of the Hittites as a significant empire, very little scholarship on them is available in English.

Merchant colonies from Assyria settled in central Anatolia during the early second millennium (2000–1750 BCE), with the most significant one at Kanesh (modern Kültepe), linking the Assyrian capital Assur with the Black and the Aegean Seas.[4] By the seventeenth century BCE, an independent kingdom arose, referred to now as the Old Kingdom (1650–1400),[5] with a capital at Hattusa (modern Boğasköy). This empire reached into Syria and perhaps as far as the Tigris River in Mesopotamia. The Assyrian Colonial period, as well as contact during the two Hittite empires, would explain some of the affinities between Hittite and Mesopotamian culture. Similarly, the power of the Hittite Empire brought it into the sphere of Egyptian foreign relations. The Amarna archive attests to correspondence between the pharaohs Amenhotep III and Akhenaten with the Hittite kings Tudhaliya I (ca. 1400 BCE) and Hattusili II (ca. 1360 BCE).

As we shall see, the Hittite court employed both Egyptian and Mesopotamian healers at various times, and they also adapted Mesopotamian medical prescriptions. To the west, the Hittites also forged trade networks with the Mycenaeans, likely acting as a conduit of medical knowledge between the cultures of the ancient Near East and the Aegean. A general political collapse that swept the ancient Near East and Mediterranean around the year 1200 BCE also brought a fiery destruction of the capital city, Hattusa, and the end of the Hittite Empire. Ramesses III takes credit for the destruction of the empire in 1175 BCE, but the accuracy of his claim is not clear, since excavations at Hattusa indicate an internal struggle between two branches of the ruling dynasty that could have just as easily led to the New Kingdom empire's collapse.[6] During the Iron Age (ca. 900 BCE), a resurgence of Neo-Hittite and Syro-Hittite kingdoms began, which brought the Hittites into contact with Israelites to the southeast, while, to the west, relations began with the Ionian Greek city-states along the coast of Asia Minor.[7] The rise of

4. Mogens Trolle Larsen, *Ancient Kanesh: A Merchant Colony in Bronze Age Anatolia* (Cambridge: Cambridge University Press, 2015).

5. One must take care not to confuse the Hittite Old Kingdom with the Egyptian Old Kingdom.

6. Hermann Genz and Dirk Paul Mielke, "Research on the Hittites: A Short Overview," in *Insights into Hittite History and Archaeology*, ed. Hermann Genz and Dirk Paul Mielke (Walpole, MA: Peeters, 2011), 1–29.

7. These Ionian city-states and their medical culture will be considered under the chapter on Greek medicine.

the Neo-Assyrian Empire under Sargon II caused the final destruction of an independent Hittite kingdom by 708 BCE.

## Religion and Culture

A number of Hittite texts boast of Hatti as the "land of a thousand Gods." The Hittites readily adopted the gods from places they conquered as a way to show their power, essentially claiming that these gods decided to join the Hittite side of battle. This attitude of gods changing sides is fairly common in the ancient Near East and expressed in stories from the Hebrew Bible, such as Yahweh Elohim siding with the Aramean general Na'aman to punish the Israelites. The process of adopting various gods resulted in many deities sharing the same name with just an appellation of local origin attached, such as Storm-god[8] of Nerik, Storm-god of Samuha, or Storm-god of Manuzziya. The Hittite pantheon had room for a plethora of deities, since they saw the gods as having a protective function, even on what we today might consider a minute scale. They included among their gods not only the ubiquitous protective deity for a city or a king, as one would expect, but they also referenced Protective Deity for a bedroom within the palace.[9] When writing about their deities, the Hittites adopted the Sumerian logogram DINGIR. But where its Mesopotamian context limited its use to just gods, the Hittites expanded it to characterize also demons, natural features, and parts of temples as possessing qualities of divinity.[10] Quite often, liturgies were done in foreign languages for these gods as a way of appeasing them.[11] This practice demonstrates a sensitivity to the gods' origins and their feelings about it rather than trying to force them into a specific cultural mold. Just because a god came to your land, it does not mean that god accepts everything about your society, in particular your language. We have seen a variation of this in the use of Canaanite incantations in Egyptian therapeutic texts, where the Egyptian gods, for "an unexplainable reason," preferred the Canaanite language.

8. Quite often the deities did not have a specific proper name but simply were called by the natural element or duty most associated with them.

9. Gary Beckman, "Hittite Religion," in *Cambridge History of Religions in the Ancient World*, ed. Michele Renee Salzman (Cambridge: Cambridge University Press, 2012), 85–101.

10. Beckman, "Hittite Religion," 85–101.

11. Bryce, *Life and Society in the Hittite World*, 136.

## Cosmology

The fluidity with which the Hittites moved between languages and deities also made them comfortable with a particular god possessing both male and female aspects. This gender fluidity reflects a necessity to change roles in differing social contexts and can especially be seen in their use of Ištar.[12] The Mesopotamian goddess Ištar first appeared in Hittite texts during the Assyrian Colonial period centered at Kanesh; it then spread westward by the mid-fifteenth century BCE.[13] When Ištar represents love and sex, the Hittites depict the deity as female, but Ištar becomes male when representing war and is shown with a lion and a mace. Ištar could also change people into women while fighting on the battlefield.[14] The sun goddess Arinna also changes to male when certain prayers to her retain their Mesopotamian origin, as dedications to the sun god Shamash. This ability to change gender in certain contexts has important implications for the Hittite concept of physiology.

The continuous conquering and accruing of gods meant the Hittites lacked a dogmatic religious system or even a hierarchical pantheon until the work of the priestess Puduḫepa, the Hurrian wife of King Hattusili III (1267–1237 BCE). She tried to enact reform and rationalize the pantheon, especially by syncretizing Hurrian and Hattian gods, as a way to solidify control and ensure loyalty to the king. The Assyrian priestess Enheduanna had used this same tactic of codifying the Mesopotamian pantheon to promote her father Sargon's reign (ca. 2280 BCE). The new hierarchy placed the sun goddess, Arinna,[15] as the chief female deity and the storm god, Teshub, as the chief male deity.[16] This is an interesting grafting, since Arinna is Hattian, while Teshub is Hurrian.[17] This system overlays an older cosmology that understood the universe as divided into three realms: sky represented by the eagle, earth by the bee, and the underworld signified by the snake. The three realms appear to have worked in conjunction rather than being ruled by a supreme deity adjudicating conflicts among them. The Hittite adoption of El the Creator, as Elkuniršа, a simple proper name, exhibits this lack of familiarity with a hierarchy among the supernatural realm.

12. Bryce, *Life and Society in the Hittite World*, 142.

13. Bryce, *Life and Society in the Hittite World*, 147.

14. Bryce, *Life and Society in the Hittite World*, 147.

15. Technically the name is Sun-goddess of Arinnu.

16. Bryce, *Life and Society in the Hittite World*, 137.

17. The Hepat is the Hurrian name for the sun goddess, while Taru is the Hattian name for the storm god.

It is not clear how far the Hurrian and Hattian syncretization impacted society beyond the royal court and vassal kings. Although this system became the official religion of the Hittites, there is no evidence of a royal administration enforcing it. No records have yet been found that attest to a different popular or folk religion competing with this system. Any attempt to force Puduḫepa's hierarchy would likely have encountered resistance from various localities not wanting to lose their character. Such royal tolerance for local variations would be of necessity in such a vast empire. The more expedient tactic would be to introduce the system as a cosmology the gods obviously want, by their backing the king, Hattusili III, and letting others follow to curry royal favor. The following king, Tudhaliya IV (1237–1228 BCE), had a different approach for pulling together a falling empire. He surveyed and rebuilt many temples across the empire as a way to ingratiate the king to the local elites.[18]

Although the Hittites eventually accepted a hierarchy to their gods, they still worked with the idea that the gods formed a council, especially when overseeing matters like the signing of a treaty; this is similar to the Canaanite conception of the divine realm and community cohesion. Like much of the ancient Near East, though, the Hittites understood the gods as ruling over human subjects. But there existed a reciprocal relationship between them based on a sense of duty, obedience, and consideration for everyone in the community relationships. The gods would maintain justice and order, while humans provided sustenance in the form of sacrifices.[19] The gods created humans, fashioned from clay by a mother goddess, to perform services.[20] This is less about contractual obligations and more about properly fulfilling roles.

The Hittites recounted a number of creation myths. In one of them, the moon god mated with a cow in order to create humans but had taken pity on the cow for its labor pains and so sent the Mother Goddess to act as a midwife. This story lends a sacred character to the practice of midwifery.[21] The significance of the moon god as a warrior is not lost in the connection with childbirth; the two are seen as an equivalent struggle. Another text has the storm god as the one who sent the mother goddess, since he headed up the pantheon. Some prayers refer to the sun goddess as the father of all humans, which seem to be borrowed from Mesopotamia.

18. Bryce, *Life and Society in the Hittite World*, 138.

19. Bryce, *Life and Society in the Hittite World*, 139.

20. Beckman, "Hittite Religion," 85–101.

21. Jackie Pringle, "Hittite Birth Rituals," in *Images of Women in Antiquity*, ed. Avril Cameron and Amélie Kuhrt (London: Croom Helm, 1983), 128–41.

Although not a creation story, the *Myth of Telepinu* is important for the study of medicine. It is a typical etiological story explaining the presence of seasons as the earth went dormant while Telepinu, son of the storm god and Hannahannas, went missing. The description of the world's state in his absence has the gods starving, since nothing can be harvested and sacrificed; this disrupted state includes pregnant animals (and humans) who cannot deliver. Telepinu returns after a bee stings him but also tries to soothe the pain with its own wax. The bee representing the earthly world spurs the divine to act properly. One particular version of the tale has the healing goddess Kamruspa alleviate Telepinu's anger after he is stung. This story seems tied to a ritual, as evidenced in passages that describe the anger being released through doors, windows, and gates, and down roads away from civilization, like a scapegoat ritual.[22]

Just as the gods ensure justice for humans, many Hittite myths espouse the idea that the king is responsible for the welfare of his subjects, bridging the supernatural and natural worlds through deeds, rather than his physical being sharing more with the divine than his subjects. In this capacity, the king is technically the high priest for every cult dedicated to the worship of a god or goddess. In practice, one man could not fulfill all the duties of every position, so the king delegates many of these duties to the rest of the priesthood. Scholars tend to divide Hittite priests into three groups: those overseeing the official state cults, local cults, and finally, "experts in special religious procedures,"[23] most likely meaning those who take oracles and perform sacrifices. One could assume that this category of "special religious procedures" included healing practices. But in extreme cases of a plague sweeping through the empire, the king may resume his position and intercede with the gods to effect healing for the entire community of subjects.

The gods would mete out punishments if humans violated their relationship with the gods. Divine justice, for the Hittites, could be slow and extend into the next generation, as demonstrated by a plague that started during the reign of Shuppiluliuma I (1344–1322 BCE) and stretched into the reign of Mursili II (1321–1295 BCE). A prayer of Mursili II highlights the fact that he did not sin, thus bringing the plague upon the Hittites,[24] as well as the fact

22. Harry A. Hoffner, *Hittite Myths* (Atlanta: Scholars Press, 1998).

23. Caroline Zimmer-Vorhaus, "Hittite Temples: Palaces of the Gods," in *Insights into Hittite History and Archaeology*, ed. Herman Genz and Dirk Paul Mielke (Walpole, MA: Peeters, 2011), 195–218.

24. KUB 14.8; cf. Exod 20:5. See Bryce, *Life and Society in the Hittite World*, 140.

that no workers were left to provide sacrifices to the gods.[25] The gods' lengthy punishment acted to destroy community cohesion rather than restore it. This text also shows that Hittite prayers often take the form of a legal defense, much like passages in the story of Job asserting that he had done nothing wrong to warrant the illness and other calamities. Yet, as far as scholars can tell, the Hittites had no such explicit system of covenants between gods and humans as in the Hebrew Bible.

The multiplicity of Hittite gods, as in other polytheistic societies, meant that for many problems, including ones of illness, people had to consult oracles to figure out which gods needed to be appeased for favorable outcomes. Many texts record the questions and answers used at these oracles. Interestingly, they kept asking the same question until the gods gave a positive answer. In the case of Mursili II, he consulted a series of oracles to stop the plague, resulting in a series of prayers to the various gods responsible, since it had a multifaceted etiology. Some of the more prominent style of oracles included birth and astronomical omens, especially for casting the horoscope of a child. Dream omens could be evoked with the practice of incubation by the priests. One should note that, other than using sleep to communicate with the gods, this incubation is different from the practice in the Greek asklepieion, in which the patient receives the dream.[26] Specialized diviners asked leading questions, accurately read the signs, and then translated them into the final yes-or-no answer. Some popular oracle rituals were casting lots on a board with aspects of life drawn on it and placing a snake in a water basin marked with sections of life, sin, temple, house, and prison. Watching the snake's movement through the sections could reveal a more complex situation and answer than the simple yes-or-no format.[27] Excavators have found clay liver models akin to the ones used in Mesopotamia, indicating that the Hittites also practiced extispicy, but the expense of the practice would have limited it to just the wealthy class.

Unlike other ancient Near Eastern and Mediterranean cultures, the Hittites do not appear to have many gods specifically tied to healing. Like the other societies, however, any god could be capable of healing. A few notable deities appear frequently in prayers and mythic stories that make them important to the overall study of Hittite medicine. Interestingly, most healing deities are female, while other aspects of Hittite society were fairly misogynistic.

25. KUB 24.3; cf. the Mesopotamian myth *Enuma Elish*.

26. Bryce, *Life and Society in the Hittite World*, 150.

27. Bryce, *Life and Society in the Hittite World*, 151.

## Hittite Gods and Goddesses of Disease and Healing

### *Kamrusepa*

The most obvious healing deity is Kamrusepa (Hurrian), also known as Katahipuri (Hattian). She appears in the tale of *Telepinu* as assuaging the anger of Telepinu after being stung by a bee. Most notably, prayers often link her to giving the gods and humans the necessary rituals for healing, in particular the use of sacrificial animals.[28] Her origins are not clear; she may be a personification of smoke used in divinatory practices tied to sacrifices,[29] but the name could also refer to a still unknown city.[30] Overall, she is seen as a goddess of magic and a midwife, as well as the guardian of herds and households.[31]

### *Hannahannas*

Hannahannas also appears in the tale of *Telepinu* as a mother-goddess figure; the name essentially means "grandmother," who sends out the bee to find and bring back Telepinu to save the world from its paralyzed, dormant state. She is mostly associated with childbirth. In some cases, the figures Kamrusepa and Old Woman appear to be representations of Hannahannas. She is said to wander among humans, because as the gods divided up and claimed cities for themselves, not a single one was left for her to claim as a patron. This may represent the overall protective nature of Hannahannas toward humans, as opposed to being centered in a particular place.

### *Old Woman*

The appellation Old Woman appears as a variant of Hannahannas. But this term is also employed for any female practitioner of magic and midwives. The Hittites connected the special or unique knowledge women gained through childbirth with the ability to access and manipulate cosmic power to some extent.

28. Alfonso Archi, "Kamrusepa and the Sheep of the Sun-God," *Orientalia* 62 (1993): 404–9.
29. Pringle, "Hittite Birth Rituals," 128–41.
30. The Indo-European linguistic element *-puri* can refer to a city, which would be in keeping with the naming practices of other Hittite gods, such as Arinna.
31. Bryce, *Life and Society in the Hittite World*, 149.

### *Arinna*

The sun goddess Arinna sat at the head of the Hittite pantheon (starting in the thirteenth century BCE). This position gave her considerable power over other deities and cosmic forces, which could be drawn upon during cases of illness. She is not a healing deity *per se*, but her position in the hierarchy makes her a powerful ally in combating illness, as noted in prayers. In contrast, mythic tales do not use Arinna in a healing capacity.

### *Ishara*

Some texts refer to Ishara or Sawusga. She is likely a Hurrian adoption of the goddess Ištar, through contact with the northern Canaanite/Syrian city-state of Ebla. Originally a goddess of love, she takes on the role of one who sends disease for breaking an oath and also the one to cure it. She appears to be associated mostly with diseases displaying the symptom of abdominal distention.

### *Storm God of Hatti*

Like Arinna, the Storm God of Hatti is another deity directly addressed in prayers for healing. His position at the top of the pantheon gives him considerable power, but interestingly, this is not his function in these prayers. The Storm God of Hatti appears to be invoked only when the cause of disease is the violation of a treaty or when humans have other political concerns, as attested in prayers of Mursili II. Unlike Arinna, a proper name for the storm god is not used, although other types of prayers refer to him as Teshub or another linguistic variant. This might be a particular habit of Mursili II rather than a significant feature of the god in a healing context.

### *Assembly of the Gods*

The assembly of the gods is another group invoked in healing prayers when the cause of the illness is political in nature. Since the assembly is quite often used as witnesses to oaths and treaties, it is only natural that they would cause an affliction when the oath is violated and therefore would also be the proper deities to address in order to alleviate that same affliction. We see this in the prayers of Mursili II, who notes that the twenty-year plague decimating Hatti directly results from Shuppiluliuma's betrayal of a loyalty oath and from his usurping the throne from the legitimate heir, Tudhaliya the Younger. Other prayers to the assembly name gods, including specific names, such as Iyarri of war and pestilence (Akkadian Erra) and Kamrusepa.

### *Telepinu*

Telepinu seems to be a type of grain or storm god and is categorized by scholars as one of the "disappearing gods" in Hittite cosmology. This is slightly different from the agricultural dying and resurrecting gods encountered in other cultures, such as Greece or Canaan. He does not struggle with death, like Baal.[32] Telepinu's place in medical practices comes from the tale of the same name, in which he needs healing from Kamrusepa in the form of alleviating his anger and bringing him back to civilization. His return to the community of the gods restores the natural processes of the world, such as rain and childbirth. Because of this story, he is a powerful ally addressed in prayers for healing.

## Sources

### Texts

For many years, the nearly twenty-five thousand tablets discovered during the excavations of the ancient capital Hattusa were our only written documents for the Hittites and do contain some medical texts. Sources from this archive are normally referred to as KUB (*Keilschrifturkunden aus Boghazköi*), followed by a catalog number. Laroche's *Catalogue des textes hittites* (CTH) originated in 1971 and is an ongoing collation of all known documents, maintained at Emory University. Scholarly consensus understands that many of the tablets from Hattusa (Boğasköy) come from a scribal school at the capital, which used medical texts as teaching tools. Many of them are obvious translations from Babylonian, with glosses in one of the Hittite languages.

32. Stories about the storm god Teshub fighting death and a serpent do have parallels with stories about Baal.

Some also appear to be of Hittite origin. Other scholars see some texts as written by healers for their own edification rather than for scribal students.[33]

Starting in 1990, archaeologists discovered over three thousand tablets at Sapinuwa (modern Ortaköy), which served as a residence for some Hittite kings during the fourteenth century BCE. Most of these are still in need of publication, especially with transliteration and translation. Their contents could possibly have more medical-oriented instructions or literary stories. Smaller archives have been found at the ancient cities of Sarissa and Tapikka, but publications from Sarissa seem more rapid.[34]

Unfortunately, no English translations exist for the Hittite medical texts, except for a few tablets in specific articles. Two German-language publications collate all the known KUB texts. Burde's 1974 publication, *Hethische Medizinische Texte*, gives an overall view of healers and a discussion of the goddess Ishara along with the German translation of many tablets. More recently, in 2003, Haas published a compendium of medical prescriptions divided into categories based on types of therapies, such as human substitutes in rituals or the use of colored threads.[35]

The medical texts can be divided into two types: omen texts and recipe texts. This falls along the same lines as the Mesopotamian medical texts. The recipe texts describe treatments for wounds, eye diseases, intestinal and throat problems, as well as the preparation and administration of the drugs.[36] Rituals often complement the somatic therapeutic procedures. One should not assume that Hittite medicine is based on only magic rituals with seemingly no medical benefit, as judged against modern medicine. A number of prescriptions have only somatic treatments. The prescriptions, in order to have enough efficacy to be a part of a codified repertoire, must have had some sufficiently active ingredient. It should also be remembered that, like all ancient societies of the Near East and Mediterranean, the Hittites likely thought of the use of these somatic treatments as part of, if not all of, the necessary physical rites to effect healing. These somatic or instrumental healing techniques function as both demonstrating obedience and potentially accessing power, like *heka* and *kišpu*, in neighboring medical cultures.

33. Federico Giusfredi, "The Akkadian Medical Text KUB 37.1," *Altorientalische Forschungen* 39 (2012): 49–63.

34. K. Aslihan Yener and Harry A. Hoffner, eds., *Recent Developments in Hittite Archaeology and History: Papers in Memory of Hans G. Guterböck* (Winona Lake, IN: Eisenbrauns, 2002).

35. Volkert Haas, *Materia Magica et Medica Hethitica* (New York: de Gruyter, 2003).

36. Bryce, *Life and Society in the Hittite World*, 164.

Apart from the obvious medical texts, other types of sources may be used to understand the overall character of Hittite medicine. Literary texts, such as the tale of *Telepinu* described above, give an image of healing rituals. The tale's use in subsequent incantations draws upon the power of cyclical time to effect healing. The story of Ullikummi depicts rituals surrounding childbirth and refers to a collective name for goddesses overseeing the birth, the Irsirra. The *Voyage of the Immortal Soul* sheds light on the Hittite understanding of the relationship between a person, anatomy, and the gods. Important texts can also be found in the eight prayers of Mursili II trying to alleviate a plague sweeping slowly through Hatti. Letters also attest to the exchange of medical personnel between the Hittites and the Egyptians and Mesopotamians. Additionally, archives not directly associated with the Hittites, such as the Amorite texts from Alalakh in southern Anatolia, can reveal Hittite divination practices tied to their medical system.

### Archaeology

As outlined earlier, the excavations of several Hittite cities have revealed texts related to medicine. Unfortunately, no sites specific to healing activities, such as shrines or workshops for preparing drugs, have come to light. Neither has a priest or other healer's house been discovered. Along these lines, no specific artifacts, like a medical kit, have been found. The lack of material evidence means scholars must rely solely on the textual descriptions for recreating the Hittite medical system. As we have seen, these texts usually reflect the royal perceptions rather than a spectrum across Hittite society. These problems notwithstanding, a general picture can be developed of the Hittite conception of the principles behind human physiology, disease etiology, and the restoration of health.

## Cultural Concepts

There are too few sources to construct a solid, single image for a Hittite ideology concerning anatomy and physiology. Information within the sources appears at times contradictory, likely because they speak to a particular time and place across a varied empire. Despite these difficulties, a general understanding of the Hittite explanatory model of illness can emerge, though much work still needs to be done on the subject.

## Anatomy and Physiology

Artistic images can help us discern the underlying concepts of Hittite theories on anatomy and physiology. The earliest statues from the Assyrian Colonial period (1950–1750 BCE) have a flat, idol-like appearance, highly stylized rather than trying to portray realism. Females are depicted with broad hips following a triangle shape of the pubis. Most artistic representations from the Hittite Empires, though, tend to show dynamic movement of the figures instead of static positions.[37] Scenes of battles and hunts are common, as are processionals. The reliefs at Alacahöyük (fourteenth century BCE) show a mixture of gods, royalty, priests, and workers, depicting different levels of society. The communicative aspect of Hittite art means that certain forms became codified and replicated across various media of reliefs, figurines, and seals.[38]

The replication of forms highlights certain physical aspects valued by the society, at least in a religious context, given the nature of the art. Large facial features (the eyes, nose, and ears) figure into most of the art pieces, but their bodies tend to be fairly proportioned. There is no type of exaggeration of anatomical features, such as sex organs, as would be found in fertility statues. Quite often they are clothed, thus obscuring most of the body. But the flowing lines of the clothing meld into the flowing lines of the limbs, underscoring the overall sense of movement in the scenes. Dynamic movement may reinforce the cultural value of fulfilling roles and performing socially expected duties. The hidden-body motif might explain the large facial features, as the senses of sight, smell, and sound act as the key physiological elements used in communication both with the divine and other humans.

Human and animal combinations do exist, such as sphinxes and bull-men. These are likely borrowed from Egypt and Mesopotamia, respectively, but do not figure as prominently in Hittite art as in their original cultural contexts. Hittite artists rendered the zoomorphic aspect of the gods by having the human figure stand atop their representative animal, like a lion for Arinna.

Literary texts can also provide clues to Hittite anatomy and physiology, such as the *Voyage of the Immortal Soul*. This tale recounts the soul of the deceased in different bucolic places, with a prayer for it to be carried back to where it belongs by either a bee or an eagle, depending on locations. The

37. Jeanny Vorys Canby, "Hittite Art," *Biblical Archaeologist* 52 (1989): 109–29.

38. Piotr Taracha, "Sculptures of Alacahöyük: A Key to Religious Symbolism in Hittite Representational Art," *Near Eastern Archaeology* 65 (2012): 108–15.

story does not specify the exact physical location of an afterlife but claims the soul should reside with the Mother Goddess, with the curious line, "What things are dear to her are 'opened' upon the eight body parts."[39] We have no explanation as to where on the body the Hittites make the division into eight parts or their significance. No known mortuary practices correspond to this division. The few bodies that have been found show no such physical division, so it is completely symbolic rather than instrumental.

This number eight stands in contrast to healing rituals found in many prescriptions, which mention a division of the body into twelve parts. Although the rituals specify twelve anatomical structures needing the removal of illness, the exact body parts have variation, with the most frequent being: head, throat, ear, arm, hand, finger, fingernails, rib, foot, toe, toenails, bones, ligaments, and blood, plus several other untranslated terms.[40] The named parts do not necessarily correspond to symptomatic areas in the specific medical cases. This may or may not indicate a separation between religious and medical ideologies or personnel. Another possibility is a heterarchical system in which one set of body part divisions has primacy in a purely religious context, while the importance shifts to other body parts when weight is given to its medical context. Thus, no significant division exists between religion and medicine (or their personnel), but particular contexts simply alter the emphasis.

Regardless of the number, the practice of dividing up the body shows that the Hittites understood the body as compartmentalized, much like creating compartments or sections on divinatory instruments, such as water bowls and liver models. This could mean that they also saw the living human body as sectioned into areas that convey messages to and from the gods. Additionally, every person had a protective deity and a fate deity, the latter acting as a type of guardian angel; the relationship between the protective and fate deities is still unclear.[41] As far as the texts show, these deities oversaw the body and person as a whole, rather symbolically watching over particular parts of the anatomy.

According to some stories, Ištar possessed an interesting power over human physiology—the ability to change someone's gender on the battlefield.[42] This indicates that the Hittites did not see the physical body as limited

39. Hoffner, *Hittite Myths*, 33.

40. Hans G. Güterbock, "Hittite Medicine," *Bulletin of the History of Medicine* 36 (1962): 109–13.

41. Beckman, "Hittite Religion," 85–101.

42. This is more amply attested in Mesopotamian texts, where she can change genders in other non-battlefield contexts, with perhaps some of her temple personnel being androgynous.

and fixed by obvious anatomy but actually quite malleable. Social roles were subject to gender coding, such as the male warrior, but the Hittites also accepted the warrior aspect of the goddess Ištar. To this end, the social role and one's relationship with the divine determined gender more so than the physical body. One assumes that such mythological gender changes resulted in anatomical changes. In practice, this may indicate that certain people were allowed to assume opposite gender roles without subsequent physical alteration, perhaps with the exception of castration. No evidence has come to light showing individuals doing so either socially or physically, as we have for Egypt and Mesopotamia. The question for medical practices then becomes to what extent this shift carried through treatment measures, since some of them were gender coded. Rituals for male patients would need male animals or representations; the same held for female patients.

Hittite medical cases seem to show that they work with a conception of anatomy and physiology different from those of other ancient Near Eastern cultures; they lack a sense of the body parts having a distinct identity from the person. Yet prescriptions akin to those from Mesopotamia do show the body parts as distinct, willful entities. One can try to make a division between native Hittite and non-native medical practices, but the fact that the Hittites fairly easily adopted the medical practices from cultures that had an understanding of a symbiotic anatomy indicates that it also fit their conception of anatomy and physiology. The fluidity of the cosmological relationship between the Hittites and their gods carried over to the nature of the human body. At times, their body parts can engage in their own relationship with the divine realm just as, at times, the gods wish to hear ritual incantations in Akkadian.

According to the prayers of Mursili II, illness, especially on a large scale among the people, causes anguish, so part of healing must be the removal of that anguish. This parallels the story of Telepinu in which his anger must be mitigated by the healing goddess Kamrusepa. Although our textual sources do not link such emotions to body parts, like liver or nose, as in other ancient Near Eastern cultures, there is a strong sense of the connection between the body as a whole and an emotional state. Without describing the precise mechanism(s) as to how one's emotions interplay with the physiology, therapeutic prescriptions, in addition to the literary tales, demonstrate that both need to be addressed, and perhaps the emotional part more so in order to heal the physical body. This emotional component underscores the impor-

---

The Hittites have adopted this aspect of the goddess in literature, but there is no evidence her priests in Hatti assumed an androgynous appearance.

tance of the relationships and community cohesion between humans, gods, and the body in Hittite medicine.

## Disease Etiology

Like all the other ancient Near Eastern cultures, the Hittites understood disease as a message from the gods, often sent as a correction to disruptions in relationships. Beckman notes that suffering and diseases were caused by "dislocation of an individual human or deity from his or her proper position in the cosmos."[43] The disruption means that one cannot perform his or her social role, which has a rippling effect in the social networks. This is exemplified on a larger cosmological scale when the storm god Telipinu disappears, causing the earth to become paralyzed, essentially dying. Most notably from the surviving royal documents, this disruption occurs when the political relationships between humans then carry over into their relationships with the divine. The medical texts tend not to give a specific disease etiology, but the types of rituals used in their therapeutic sections suggest an attempt to correct disruptions to community cohesion, at least between the human and the divine worlds.

Although disease ultimately comes from the gods, a disease itself can lead to further cases of illness through the notion of contaminated objects. The Hittites express this theory of contamination with the idea of impurity, that which is not acceptable to be in the presence of the gods. Anything that has had contact with a patient must be destroyed to avoid spreading the disease by transmitting its inherent impurity. Legal cases attest to the worry about careless handling of impure substances that can spread disease. If the owner of a sick cow leaves lying about the objects used in its healing and someone else's cow comes into contact with it, thus contracting the same illness, the owner of that second cow can rightly collect damages from the owner of the original sick cow.[44] Similarly, the objects and clothes used in rituals for impotence must be cast into a river in order to prevent contamination. The ability to contaminate with impurity plays an important part in the healing of King Mursili II. He had to avoid re-

43. Gary Beckman, "From the Cradle to the Grave: Women's Role in Hittite Medicine and Magic," *Journal of Ancient Civilizations* 8 (1993): 30.

44. Yitzhaq Feder, "Defilement, Disgust, and Disease: The Experiential Basis of Hittite and Akkadian Terms for Impurity," *Journal of the American Oriental Society* 136 (2016): 99–116.

touching things, especially objects used in food preparation, up until the end of his treatment/purification so as not to recontaminate himself.[45] This also shows that healing does not rest solely on the clearing of physical symptoms. Despite an appearance of being healed and returning to some normal actions, the impurity of the disease and its corollary, the sick role, still remain until ritually removed.

In addition to accidental contact with impurity, disease can arise also from the deliberate use of sorcery, a breakdown of cohesion within the human community. Hittite laws prohibit such acts of sorcery. Some medical cases indicate, though, that the Old Woman[46] can send the curses back on behalf of the patient as an acceptable form of retribution for malicious sorcery.[47] The most frequently cited causes of disease in the written sources are divine displeasure and malicious sorcery. Mursili II's prayer to Arinna shows that accusations against an enemy can send the plague. He hopes that, by pointing out the sins of the Kingdom of Mitanni, the goddess will transfer the plague to them. Other prayers specifically direct that gods should destroy the one person, or town, that is the sinner, not the whole country. This attitude helps shed light on the Hebrew Bible passages in which Abraham tries to save Sodom and Gomorrah for the sake of one good person. Although illness as a divine punishment can affect entire populations for the actions of one, such as a king, the converse is also true, namely, that the gods can single out one person to suffer a physical ailment.

Regardless of the exact cause of disruption and illness, a person can be caught in a catch-22 situation. He cannot adequately provide for the gods because of an illness; thus, he will continue to suffer with the illness for not appeasing the gods. Mursili II particularly notes this situation in his prayer asking the gods to release Hatti from the plague, which is preventing the entire community from properly offering sacrifices to provide for the gods. The Hittite explanatory model of illness straddles a fine line between, on the one hand, ailments as an appropriate sign of disruption to community cohesion, necessitating the healing process of obedience and consideration, and, on the other, the presence an illness in itself being the root cause of community disruption. The balance between the human-human and human-divine relationships further complicates navigating healing strategies. The apparent

45. Bryce, *Life and Society in the Hittite World*, 169.

46.A term for a midwife, as well as a practitioner of magic, derived from one of the names for the goddess Hannahannas.

47. Bryce, *Life and Society in the Hittite World*, 209.

lack of body parts being their own entities helps simplify the process of restoring health, in comparison to other ancient Near Eastern cultures.

### Restoration of Health

Bryce employs an outdated assessment that the Hittites treated injuries with a practical/somatic approach, while the more complicated or chronic illnesses were attributed to malevolent supernatural forces necessitating magic rituals using spells, incantations, or direct appeals to the gods.[48] He does acknowledge the beneficial effects of magic in psychosomatic illnesses and that some of Hittite *materia medica* may have had efficacy comparable to modern medical treatments. But this perspective ignores both the gods as a source of trauma and the ritual aspect to somatic treatments demonstrating obedience, as well as the necessity of social and cultural cohesion implicit in the restoration of health.

Healing is accomplished through two complimentary pathways: the use of charged substances and their ritual application. These appear as the use of somatic treatment methods with the incantations during physical rites. They demonstrate the afflicted's obedience to the gods, allow the gods to communicate their consideration, and act to restore the afflicted to the necessary communities. A prescription of a plant-based recipe applied as a drink, enema, and ointment for a child with abdominal pain, accompanied by prayers and washing, exemplifies this process.[49] Mursili II's prayer against the plague requires the congregation to recite part of the prayer, indicating that community cohesion was necessary for healing, especially if illness affected the community as a whole.

Rituals lie at the heart of Hittite therapeutic tactics. Bryce recognizes that rituals restore people to their proper functioning in a particular sphere of life, such as birth and puberty.[50] But they also serve the same purpose in matters of healing, namely, to remove the sick role. Ritual texts appear as step-by-step instructions that must be performed precisely, lest one risk starting all over again. Even the procurement and transport of materials had to be precise. Rituals could be in open-air temples, like the official court shrine at Yazilikaya, or inside a patient's home. The cost of treatment rituals can be tailored for a

48. Bryce, *Life and Society in the Hittite World.*

49. Güterbock, "Hittite Medicine," 109–13.

50. Bryce, *Life and Society in the Hittite World*, 201.

patient's financial ability.[51] If one cannot afford a donkey, a clay one can substitute for the ritual.[52] Substitution was an important concept not just for the poor to participate in rituals, but also the transferability allowed an object to transfer the burden of affliction, essentially allowing for a scapegoat.

Transference is the overall principle behind Hittite healing treatments. Almost all the rituals involve either transferring the disease/impurity to another object and discarding it or transferring the healthy properties of another person, animal, or a god to the patient. When a prescription calls for twelve parts of a ram to match the twelve parts of a patient in order to remove an illness from those areas, it is based on the transference of the negative substance. Similarly, Mursili II suffered an ailment described as his "mouth going sideways."[53] The cure involved loading onto an ox cart everything that he touched that day and burning it (ox and cart) as an offering to the storm god.

A ritual to cure impotence demonstrates both types of transference. A man walks with a spindle and distaff under a gate; as he passes through, they are replaced by a bow and arrow. An oral rite tells him they have taken away his femininity and restored his masculinity.[54] The spindle and distaff, as signs of femininity, absorb his inappropriate femininity, while the bow and arrow transfer to him their masculinity. The charging of these substances, essentially their transferability, occurs only by the power of the invoked goddess, who completes the healing process by appearing in a dream of the impotent man. Transferability, then, is not a passive act imbuing all objects. The impotent man is to repeat the ritual until such dream, which signifies his final acceptance in the community with both the divine and human (in this case, specifically with his wife or maidservant). A prescription for the infertility of a woman similarly focuses on the transferring of only positive elements. An Old Woman grasps the horn of a fertile cow and calls to the sun goddess, asking that fertility of the animal be transferred to the infertile woman.[55]

The idea of transferring the power of the gods worked across cultures as well. When Mursili suffered his facial condition, the Mycenaean kings along the Anatolian coast and the island of Lesbos sent him cult images as a healing technique. Similarly, Tushratta, the king of Mitanni, sent a statue of Ištar to help heal the Egyptian pharaoh Amenhotep III.

51. Bryce, *Life and Society in the Hittite World*, 203.

52. Sacrificial substitutions based on affordability can be found in Leviticus as well.

53. Possibly some form of facial paralysis.

54. CTH 406; see Harry A. Hoffner, "Paskuwatti's Ritual against Sexual Impotence," *Aula Orientalis* 5 (1987): 271–87.

55. KUB 7.53+(CTH 409) iv 7–14; see Bryce, *Life and Society in the Hittite World*, 166.

The Hittites understood that healing a particular illness meant community cohesion for only a limited time. If a person did not fulfill the promises made during the healing process, essentially not continuing their obedience, the gods may reconsider and resend an ailment. During the reign of Mursili II, his youngest son Hattusili became seriously ill. The goddess Ištar appeared in a dream to his older brother, demanding that Hattusili be dedicated to her in return for healing. Dedication to a god usually meant serving as a priest to the cult. Eventually, Hattusili III recovered and grew up to take the throne (1267–1237 BCE), but since he was not dedicated to Ištar, he suffered chronic eye and foot problems throughout his life. He went beyond the scope of Hittite medicine, seeking out Egyptian healers. His wife appealed to a higher authority, the goddess Arinna, beseeching her to appeal to the assembly of the gods, with promises of silver and gold votives.

## Illness

### Disease

Modern scholars cannot accurately determine the precise diseases afflicting the Hittites, apart from applying general statistics as to the frequency a particular illness occurs within an environmental region. The paucity of Hittite graves prevents paleopathological studies for either disease processes or trauma cases.[56] Excavators found only one significant cemetery at Alacahöyük (ca. 2500 BCE), predating the Assyrian Colonial period, but it did not contain enough bodies for a representative study.

Despite the many prayer texts of Mursili II concerning the fourteenth-century BCE plague that swept through Hatti, no precise description of symptoms has come to light. We cannot make a reasonable diagnosis as to the exact disease, although we know this is the same plague referred to in the Amarna Archive. This leaves physicians to create popular works claiming diseases, such as tularemia[57] or diabetic neuropathy,[58] based solely on ambiguous symptom descriptions. This ignores the fact that ancient

56. Genz and Mielke, "Research on the Hittites," 1–29.

57. Siro Igino Trevisanato, "The 'Hittite Plague' an Epidemic of Tularemia and the First Record of Biological Warfare," *Medical Hypotheses* 69 (2007): 1371–74.

58. S. Ozturk, "Description of Painful Neuropathy in Hittite Tablets," *European Journal of Neurology* 13 (2006): 139.

textual sources are mediated stories and not clinical descriptions in the modern sense.

Apart from the plague, even when analyzing individual cases in the Hittite medical literature, there are problems in accurately translating them. The text of KUB 37.1 is indicative of this issue. Originally, it was thought to be a treatment for baldness. But other scholars claim that it targets a dermatological illness like psoriasis or eczema,[59] while others explained it as a therapy for melancholia.[60] The problems with translation, as well as the paucity of textual sources, make it difficult to discern a pattern of cultural values that would influence symptom descriptions that we can more readily see in neighboring societies, such as the Egyptian focus on eye ailments and the Israelite concern for skin afflictions.

## Disability

Surviving documents addressing issues of disability are also scant. One should not assume that a lack of texts means the Hittites did not care for or otherwise neglect to integrate those with a physical impairment into the human and religious communities. There is some indication of social roles for the blind and deaf. The deaf did have a special function in some religious rituals.[61] It was likely that they could not serve as kings either for the overall empire or a vassal city-state. Within this limitation, they did work in a place called "the inner house," connected to the noble families, and carried titles such as "Head of Deaf People," indicating that these were not unique and rare positions for the royal court. But one should not assume the Hittites had a higher than normal frequency of deafness within the population.

It appears that the Hittites, like most of the cultures in the ancient world, understood a physical impairment, whether congenital or acquired, as yet another message from the gods that has a place in society. Hittite culture's emphasis on fulfilling duties and social roles would mean that as long as persons could carry out their expected obligations, then the modern concept of disability, dependent on physical perfection, really did not apply. We need to

59. Giusfredi, "Akkadian Medical Text KUB 37.1," 1, 49–63.

60. Haas, *Materia Magica et Medica Hethitica*, 120–21.

61. Berna Arda and Murat Aksu, "What the Hittites' Tablets Tell Us? A Short Historical View of Deafness on the Basis of Genetics," *Turkish Journal of Medical Sciences* 34 (2004): 357–58.

further investigate, though, as to how social roles and specific responsibilities changed in light of a physical impairment.

### Conditional States

Although rituals accompany every phase of life, from birth through puberty to death, the Hittites did not medicalize these life stages. Yet the ones concerned with birth do have a bearing on the study of medicine, due to the midwife, called an Old Woman, who acts also as a healer for issues apart from obstetrics. A common ritual has the Old Woman hand an axe and mace to a male child, while the female child gets a spindle and distaff. This is similar to the rituals for curing impotence in an adult man, indicating that the child is not born with an inherent disposition for masculinity or femininity based solely on anatomy but that the body must be charged with these specific powers. Whatever gender is born, the Old Woman then announces a prayer that the opposite gender may be born in a year.[62] Likely, this custom was thought to help maintain a balance of gendered social roles within the human community.

Birth takes place in the house of the expectant parents in a room called the "inner chamber."[63] It is not clear whether this is a play on the "inner chamber" of temples that would typically house statues of the gods or just a way to refer to the more private rooms of a house. Some royal births did occur in the temples. The parturient woman sits on a stool, with the midwife's stool facing opposite and a pillow between for the infant. Some texts indicate that a second midwife would stand behind the mother. Texts mention a bronze knife and four bronze pegs, but their role is not clear, and no such implements have been found in excavations. The knife may be for cutting the umbilical cord.

## Healers

Thirty-eight of the seventy-one named healers in the ritual texts are women (i.e., 53 percent), which is the highest percentage of female healers among ancient Near Eastern and Mediterranean cultures, with documentation of

62. Pringle, "Hittite Birth Rituals," 128–41.
63. Pringle, "Hittite Birth Rituals," 128–41.

both genders practicing medicine. The term for them typically is *hasawa*, which literally means "she of birth," indicating their obstetric function. The title Old Woman[64] is used for the more prominent healers, linking them to the goddess Hannahannas. Fourteen of these names are recorded as authors. Unlike later Hellenistic culture, in which male healers or philosophers expounded on the theoretical side of birth, leaving midwives to handle the practical or somatic aspects, the Hittite midwives were responsible for the incantations and rites. This places them in the same role as Kamrusepa, originating the necessary rituals for healing. Even the queen Puduḫepa labeled herself a midwife. The ubiquitous use of the title Old Woman/midwife likely became a verbal ploy to gain attention and favor from the gods, since they favored listening to midwives on behalf of newborns. This would explain the branching out of midwives into treating medical issues. Roman period sources in Greek refer to an *iatrina* in Anatolia, which seems to be a holdover from the Old Woman healer of the Hittite Empire.[65]

Scholars think these women kept a regular practice of healing instead of just being summoned when necessary, on rare occasions. Too often, people assume the midwife lives life in a domestic sphere, taking care of the home and only to "practice medicine" when a younger relative or neighbor needs assistance in birth. The reality is that the ancient world did not make a clear distinction between home and work, with women relegated to the home in a position without economic or social power. Men worked at home on the farm or a craft rather than being hired for a wage on a job outside of it, and their wives frequently worked alongside them, especially among the lower classes. This economic organization means that the Old Woman could work essentially as a professional healer. They likely practiced in conjunction rather than in competition with incantation priests, ritual specialists, diviners, and other types of healers. Hittite laws account for the need to properly pay healers, especially in cases of accidental injury or assault.

Another frequent term for healers in the Hittite documents is the borrowed Akkadian word *asû*. Ample court records from Hattusa attest to the fact that the Hittite kings did take on loan healers from both Babylonia and Egypt. A letter from 1270 BCE laments the unfortunate death of an *asû* from Babylonia, with curious excuses. Possibly, this healer married into the Hittite royal family, abandoning his position with the Babylonian king, thus causing grounds for an international incident. Another letter notes that Ramesses II

64. This is often written with the Sumerian logogram $^{\text{MUNUS}}$ŠU.GI.

65. Pringle, "Hittite Birth Rituals," 128–41.

sent healers to cure the infertility of the sister of King Hattusili III (1267–1237 BCE). Later, King Tudhaliya IV (1237–1209 BCE) asked Ramesses II that one of his healers be moved from the household of a Hittite vassal king to the royal court because previous healers have not helped. Interestingly, the correspondence with the Egyptians refers to the healers with the term *asû* rather than any of the Egyptian titles. This preference for an Akkadian title indicates that Hittite medical culture leaned more toward Mesopotamian cultural concepts. Yet there were still noticeable breaks between them, such as the Hittites lacking a sense of body parts as independent entities. How they reconcile borrowing Mesopotamian diagnostics and therapeutics based on anatomical independence still needs to be investigated.

Some texts do mention that the Egyptian healer is also a scribe. Güterbock interprets this as more in keeping with Egyptian medicine, whose healers frequently had scribal training or duties.[66] He also claims that the Hittite court used healers from Egypt and Babylonia because of their superior skills. This is an assumption based on the Hittite medical texts, focusing on the ritual aspects of healing and therefore not really effective. The explanation more likely comes from political considerations. Using healers from outside the Hittite Empire allows the royal court to avoid showing regional favoritism within their kingdom.[67] The link between choice of healers and wider political concerns appears more obviously when Kadashman-Enlil of Babylon sent an incantation priest and healer to Muwatalli II (1295–1272) at his request. During this period, the Hittites and Egyptians were embroiled in a war over control of the Levant, thus making Egyptian healers unavailable. Interestingly, healers labelled *asû* by the Hittites did take part in nonmedical rituals, such as one for the god Telipinu, with recitations, singing and accompaniment, and ecstatic dancing with needles.[68]

The text of KUB 17.28 attests to the patient himself acting as healer, without help from a specialized ritualist; the patient receives assistance only during the slaughter of an animal.[69] Two possible reasons might explain this exceptional incident. Either the man could not afford a ritual specialist/healer, or the ritual needed to be performed too quickly to call one. Since the patient could afford a ram for the ritual, the urgency of the latter might be

66. Güterbock, "Hittite Medicine," 109–13.

67. Giulia Torri, "A Hittite Magical Ritual to Be Performed in an Emergency," *Journal of Ancient Near Eastern Religions* 4 (2004): 129–41.

68. Beckman, "From the Cradle to the Grave," 25–39.

69. Torri, "Hittite Magical Ritual," 129–41.

the actual reason.[70] Yet an afflicted person can act as healer, since the gods send therapeutic answers in dreams. We know this from Mursili II receiving such dreams, but then again, he is technically a priest. It is not clear whether the average person has this dream ability apart from working in consultation with a healer, as in the case of the impotent man.

The literacy of healers, particularly the writing out of rituals and glosses on texts, indicates that they had some formal training, at least as scribes. Some male healers also carried the title of scribe. Other titles used by healers were "overseer of doctors, head doctor, and junior doctor," which may have been only for the court.[71] There is no evidence that healers organized themselves professionally in any type of guild. These titles, then, likely indicate a social ranking within the royal court. Another interesting title is "junior apprentice doctor." Such terminology would mean that healers learned their skills through a typical apprentice system rather than any specialized school.

Although Hittite medicine rests upon the ideology of community cohesion, a division between one type of healer focusing on communicating with or restoring cohesion among the human community and another type concentrating on the human-to-god relationship cannot be determined. This may be due to insufficient sources, but it is just as likely, perhaps even more so, that Hittite culture saw both human-human and human-divine communities as equally important in their explanatory model of illness; thus, simultaneous messaging and restoration was necessary. This then brings up questions about the reasoning behind the use of multiple titles, medical pluralism, within Hittite medical culture.

70. Torri, "Hittite Magical Ritual," 129–41.

71. Bryce, *Life and Society in the Hittite World*, 164.

# 6. Classical Greek Medicine

## Location and History

The modern student, upon hearing the phrase "ancient Greece," may equate this with the current nation-state of Greece in the southern Balkans, with its center at Athens. Yet two important differences exist between the ancient and the modern worlds of Greece. First, ancient Greece was not a unified political nation, but rather it was a collection of many autonomous city-states, or *poleis*.[1] Second, its geography extended on either side of the Aegean Sea. They shared a common culture, including recognized descent from Hellen,[2] religious practices, and language. It is on the point of language, though, that they subdivided themselves into four groups or ethnicities: Aeolians, Ionians, Dorians, and Achaeans.

The Aeolians settled in Thessaly and Boeotia, eventually spreading to Messenia on the southwestern tip of the Peloponnesus, as well as to the island of Lesbos. They spoke the Aeolic dialect of Greek, thought to be the oldest known form and attested in the poetry of Alcaeus and Sappho. The Ionians used the Ionian or East Greek dialect. They had their city-states on the central coast of Asia Minor, between Phocaea and Miletus and other nearby islands. This positioned them close to trade networks from the Black Sea and Mesopotamia, as well as made them militarily vulnerable to larger kingdoms, such as the Hittites, Assyrians, Lydians, and Persians. Ionian speakers could also be found in Attica, where Athens is situated on the triangular tip of the peninsula between the Island of Euboia and the Isthmus of Corinth. These widely dis-

1. *Polis* sg., *poleis* pl.

2. Hellen, the brother of Pandora, is credited with being the father of all the Greeks, hence their name Hellenes. Hesiod, *Catalogue of Women*; see Martina Hirschberger, *Gynaikôn Katalogos und Megalai Ehoiai: Ein Kommentar zu den Fragmenten zweier hesiodeischer* (Boston: de Gruyter, 2004).

persed settlements unified themselves in the Ionian League, a seventh-century military affiliation of mutual aid. The Dorians, speaking a West Greek dialect or Doric, concentrated in the Peloponnesus as far north as the city of Corinth, including in Sparta; they also spread to Crete and Rhodes and their surrounding smaller islands. The Achaeans also spoke a form of Doric originating in the northern part of the Peloponnesus but also settled in Argolis and Laconia.

The more prominent city-states sent out colonies that stretched from Iberia in the west to the eastern shores of the Ukraine and Georgia on the Black Sea. Each colony, though, was politically independent from its mother city or metropolis. Like the Ionian League, many of the city-states formed politico-military alliances, such as the Delian, Peloponnesian, and Achaean Leagues. Additionally, they would form an amphictyony, or religious alliance dedicated to taking care of important shrines, like Delphi. They also maintained religious and cultural contact through shared festival games, the Olympics being the most famous of them. Whereas the amphictyonies and games created a pan-Hellenic identity, the different military leagues could also foster internal tensions between the ethnic groupings. Greek philosophy arose in light of this duality of pan-Hellenism and ethnic rivalry. For many ancient Greeks, the pursuit of science and experimentation existed as a branch of natural philosophy rather than a contrast to it. Medicine itself formed an integral part of philosophical inquiry.[3]

## Religion and Culture

Because philosophical inquiry formed a cornerstone of Hellenic culture, debate surrounds the question whether the ancient Greeks actually believed in their gods.[4] The literature depicts a society intimately connected to deities, which is reinforced by the abundance of rituals performed at temples and shrines that peppered the landscape. Sparta had nineteen cultic sites, with another fourteen in its surrounding area.[5] The Greek geographer Pausanias described Athens as "far more zealous than other people in matters concerning the gods."[6] This demonstrates that the Greeks did believe in their gods.

3. Aristotle, *De Respiratione* 480b24–30.

4. For a concise discussion of the issue, see H. S. Versnel, *Coping with the Gods: Wayward Readings in Greek Theology* (Boston: Brill, 2011), 539–59.

5. Nicholas Richer, "The Religious System at Sparta," in *A Companion to Greek Religion*, ed. Daniel Ogden (London: Blackwell, 2007), 236–52.

6. Pausanias, *Description of Greece* 1.24.3.

Yet, starting in the sixth century BCE, there was also a tendency to explain the world according to natural laws rather than direct actions of the gods. Even the comedic works of Aristophanes began to question the gods' existence.[7] Many scholars resolve the paradox by explaining religion as a civic duty; one must participate in public religious rituals in order to participate in political life.[8] Actual piety or belief becomes a personal issue not always easily accessed in the historical record, especially for the lower and nonliterate classes. This approach creates a dichotomy between, on the one hand, the pantheon's "major deities" or Olympians, like Zeus, Apollo, and Athena, worshiped through state-sponsored activities, such as public sacrifices, and, on the other, the "lesser" but perhaps more popular deities that became integral to daily life, like Hestia, Hermes, and Pan.[9] But even with this division, one can see considerable overlap between "state" and "popular" deities. Evidence suggests that parallel rituals occurred in both urban and rural settings, in addition to the more distinct rites tailored to specific sites.[10] An ancient Greek essentially inherited his religious practices based upon, primarily, the *polis* but also his family or tribal grouping.

Students of Greek medicine should be aware of two pitfalls that can arise from the tensions between state-sponsored and personal worship, as well as between the reliance on supernatural explanations and on natural laws. First, one should not dismiss the state-sponsored rituals as hollow acts that citizens undertook merely for political reasons. These public rituals could only work to build community cohesion over centuries if most people actually accepted their premise—the gods exist. The archaeological and textual evidence of piety at the personal level indicates a belief in gods, so it would be logical for ancient Greeks to believe in the state-sponsored gods as easily as in their local nature deities. Second, one should avoid dividing the ancient Greeks into groups of the piously superstitious, on the one hand, and rational atheists, on the other. As we shall see, many of the philosophers that sought to explain the world through natural laws attributed everything to a single, unifying cause that ultimately equated with the gods. Thales, one of the earliest philosophers credited with introducing rational thought, claimed "everything is full of gods."[11]

7. Aristophanes, *The Knights* 30–34.

8. Jennifer Larson, *Ancient Greek Cults: A Guide* (London: Routledge, 2007), 1.

9. Some of these, such as Hestia and Hermes, may at times be considered Olympian. Within the system of twelve Olympian gods, each *polis* would favor a particular one or two as patrons.

10. Larson, *Ancient Greek Cults*, 9.

11. Aristotle, *De an.* 1.5, 411a8.

## Cosmology

Like in Egypt and Mesopotamia, stories about the gods, including creation myths, originated in a variety of locations throughout the Greek world. Popularity and use of one over another would depend on the political and economic dominance of the city-states, resulting in an ever-changing pantheon. Therefore, no single authority regulated religious dogma or practice across all the ancient Greek city-states. But certain features did coalesce over time, creating an overall understanding of how the universe worked. We can credit the eighth-century writers Hesiod and Homer with creating the most popular understandings of the Greek pantheon,[12] in terms of how the gods relate to each other as well as to humans.

For both of these poets, the gods have rather human characteristics, in that they feel lust, are jealous, quarrel, and cheat, among many other undesirable traits. Yet the world system is set up to favor those who do not give in to such temptations: "For this was the rule for men that Kronos' son [Zeus] laid down: whereas fish and beasts and flying birds would eat one another, because Right is not among them, to men he gave Right which is much the best in practice."[13] This parallels the concept of *maat*, seen in Egyptian cosmology. Whereas *maat* rules all the universe, including animals, the Greek ideal of right or justice is only among humans, making them distinct from animals. The Homeric epics illustrate, though, the clash between gods when one tries to right the errant ways of another, with far-reaching effects on humans, who in turn attempt to correct each other's wrong behavior.

> See how mortal men lay blame upon the gods! For they say that it is from us that all evil comes, and all the while they themselves by their own misconduct have trouble beyond what is ordained. . . . The punishment which must be exacted for this moral transgression[14] is the work not of the gods but of Destiny.[15]

12. Albert Henrichs, "What is a Greek God?" in *The Gods of Ancient Greece: Identities and Transformations*, ed. Jan N. Bremmer and Andrew Erskine (Edinburgh: Edinburgh University Press, 2010), 19–39.

13. Hesiod, *Theogony and Works and Days*, trans. M. L. West (Oxford: Oxford University Press, 1988), 45.

14. Aegisthus marrying Clytaemnestra, usurping the throne of Mycenaea.

15. Homer, *Odyssey* 1.32.

Homer equated Destiny and Right; either term referred to the fixed order of the universe, with each person and even the gods relegated to a particular, well-defined sphere.[16] Neither gods nor humans can change that order, but if they transgress it, then Right or Destiny will work to correct it. It is this Right/Destiny that is the natural order operating by understandable laws.

Greek philosophical culture investigated this pursuit of justice, which in itself can cause injustice, as described by the poets. If the gods have given justice as part of a natural order, how can humans come to understand not only justice but all aspects of that natural order? The philosophical inquiry into nature during the sixth century BCE gave rise to a particular study of medicine and its variant schools of thought. Prior to these Presocratic philosophers, we have only various mythological stories to draw upon for an understanding of medical culture. The gods and demigods closely connected to medicine should not be mistaken for an early, prescientific form of medicine that was jettisoned in the sixth century BCE. Although these medical links with the gods likely have their antecedents in Mycenaean (1600–1100 BCE) and possibly even Minoan (2600–1150 BCE) cultures, they carried through the classical era (480–323 BCE) and into the Hellenistic period (323–31 BCE). Whether these deities were invoked by healers and patients would depend on several factors, including their hierarchy of resort, as well as their particular school of medicine.

The epic poets attributed the sudden or dramatic onset of symptoms to the activity of the gods. This characterization would be in keeping, though, with the nature of the literary works.[17] Along with this literature, there is evidence from cultic sites that certain gods were thought to be intimately connected to both the cause and curing of illnesses. Inscriptions giving thanks for a cure (*iamata*) help discern the more popular healing deities, as well as dedicated temples and prolific myths. For the ancient Greeks, all of the gods have the ability to send or cure diseases, but some of the more notable figures are described below.

16. Michael Jerome Carella, *Matter, Morals, and Medicine: The Ancient Greek Origins of Science, Ethics, and the Medical Profession* (New York: Peter Lang, 1991), 8.

17. James Longrigg, *Greek Rational Medicine: Philosophy and Medicine from Alcmaeon to the Alexandrians* (London: Routledge, 1993), 13.

## Greek Gods and Goddesses of Disease and Healing

### *Apollo*

A common image of Apollo is that of the sun god driving his shining chariot across the sky or holding his lyre and his bow. It is the depiction of Apollo the Archer that connects him to medicine. According to the *Iliad*, his arrows sent a disease among the Greek army.[18] Like many ancient deities that caused plagues, he could also cure them, as he later did for that same Greek army.[19] This ability to cure disease, as well as generally protecting his worshipers, led the ancient Greeks to erect in front of their homes apotropaic pillars to Apollo. Tradition holds that he learned medicine from the centaur Chiron and that he fathered Asklepios with the nymph Koronis. He often has the epithets *iatros* (physician) and *paean* (healer) in addition to the localized identity of the healer Apollo Maleatas, who had sanctuaries northeast of Sparta and outside Epidauros on Mount Kynortion. Tradition has the famous physician Asklepios joining the Apollo Maleatas sanctuary at Epidauros. Inscriptions to Apollo Maleatas were found at the asklepieion at Epidauros.[20] Apollo's main cultic site at Delphi was also used as a healing shrine.

### *Artemis*

Artemis, the twin sister of Apollo, is depicted as the virgin huntress. Like her brother, her arrows are said to bring death. The death of Koronis, mother of Asklepios, are attributed to the arrow of Artemis. Because of her ability to bring death, she is viewed also as a healer; therefore, many healing incantations invoke her name.

### *Athena*

Athena is the goddess of wisdom and warfare and the patron of the city of Athens. She is depicted not only with helmet and spear but also with the aegis, a cloak decorated with the head of Medusa. Although the aegis can

18. Homer, *Iliad* 1.44–52.
19. Homer, *Iliad* 2.456.
20. Apollo Maleatas EAH.

strike fear in an army, the image of Medusa is apotropaic, perhaps based on the idea that her visage can scare away or overpower the disease-causing malevolence, thus making Athena a protective figure. Her many epithets included Hygieia (good health), and a shrine to Athena Hygieia stood inside the temple of Athena Nike on the Acropolis in Athens.[21]

### *Hygieia*

Hygieia is the personification of good health (*hygieia*). Early references simply name her the wife or daughter of Asklepios. A shrine to Hygieia existed in Athens as early as the seventh century BCE, which the temple for Athena Nike later absorbed. The Plague of Athens in the late fifth century BCE resulted in Hygieia becoming recognized once again as a distinct goddess, with temples at Epidauros, Corinth, Cos, and Pergamum.

### *Paean*

The word *paean* simply means healer but becomes a personification and a deity. Homer calls Paean the physician of the gods, healing both Hades[22] and Ares.[23] Hesiod also indicates Paean's status as an immortal and healer, on par with Apollo. Rather than developing a distinct cult, the name is used more as an epithet for other gods, such as Apollo.

### *Demigods/Heroes*

A common feature of Greek myths is the sexual activity between gods and humans, which created a class of heroes and mythical creatures. Herakles, a hero, born of the union between Zeus and the mortal woman Alcmene, possessed superhuman strength. Pasiphaë, the wife of King Minos, gave birth to the mythical creature, the Minotaur, after falling in love with the White Bull of Poseidon. The ancient Greeks also had the practice of recognizing

21. Susan Deacy, "'Famous Athens, Divine Polis': The Religious System at Athens," in *A Companion to Greek Religion*, ed. Daniel Ogden (London: Blackwell, 2007), 221–35.

22. Homer, *Iliad* 5.40.

23. Homer, *Iliad* 5.899.

through deification the superior ability of certain people who were seen as favored by the gods and having extraordinary talent, such as Asklepios. The fact that heroes had to die before becoming gods and being worshiped separated them from the Olympian or nature gods, but in cultic practice, sometimes the difference between a god and a hero is not always clear cut.

Evidence for hero cults date from the end of the Dark Ages (1100–750 BCE) or early in the archaic period (750–480 BCE).[24] They centered on the tombs, although over time, some cults spread beyond the initial tomb site, with myths developing that explain the hero's presence in the new location. As former mortals and therefore being sympathetic to humans, the heroes were often sought out in times of crisis for their beneficence, while other heroes acted as the cause of disease or misfortune, needing to be appeased, such as Orestes.[25] Often votive statues in the form of body parts would be left at the local shrines in order to effect healing. Athens in the fifth and fourth centuries had such sanctuaries dedicated to the local heroes of Amphiaraos, Amynos, and Hero Iatros.[26]

### *Melampus*

Melampus was a blind seer and grandson of Aeolus. The name Melampus means "black foot," a common way for the Greeks to refer to Egyptians.[27] Herodotus reflects this connection to Egypt in his claim that Melampus learned his medical skill there.[28] Yet older traditions have him learning medicine and prophecy directly from the god Apollo, or Chiron. Melampus is considered by the Greeks to be the first mortal to practice medicine. He used simple therapies[29] based on animals, minerals, or plants, such as black hellebore/ranunculus, to treat the madness of King Proteus's daughters. His sanctuary at Aegosthena in Attica held an annual festival, while other shrines were located at Argos and Orchomenos.

24. Gunnel Ekroth, "Heroes and Hero-Cults," in *A Companion to Greek Religion*, ed. Daniel Ogden (London: Blackwell, 2007), 100–114.

25. Hippocrates, *Sacred Disease* 4.34. In this context, "heroes" is often understood to mean the tragic hero Orestes.

26. Bronwen Wickkiser, *Asklepios, Medicine, and the Politics of Healing in Fifth-Century Greece: Between Cult and Craft* (Baltimore: Johns Hopkins University Press, 2008), 52–53.

27. Steven M. Oberhelman, "Melampus," in *The Encyclopedia of Ancient History*, ed. Roger S. Bagnall et al. (London: Blackwell, 2013).

28. Herodotus, *Histories* 2.48.

29. This is in contrast to compound medicines that require multiple ingredients.

### *Herakles*

As the son of Zeus, Herakles possessed superior strength. This image of physical perfection, coupled with tales of cleaning out the Augean stables, helped create the association of Herakles with good health and healing. His overall popularity, though, made him a natural object of appeal when using medical incantations. These incantations often took the form of threatening the disease to leave, comparing it to a notorious wild animal, such as the Nemean lion, making Herakles the one to defeat the disease. Some traditions also have the centaur Chiron acting as tutor to Herakles, furthering the association of Herakles with medicine.

### *Chiron*

Chiron, or Cheiron, was a centaur credited with the discovery of herbs having medicinal properties; he was, therefore, the first healer/physician. Some myths have Chiron teaching medicine to the god Apollo, as well as raising his son Asklepios. In other tales, he also taught medicine to Melampus, Jason, Herakles, and Achilles.

### *Asklepios*

Asklepios is first mentioned by Hesiod and Homer. Hesiod describes him as the son of Apollo and the mortal Koronis of Thessaly. Apollo delivered Asklepios by cesarean section[30] and then brought him to the centaur Chiron, who raised and trained Asklepios. Famed for his healing abilities, Zeus eventually killed Asklepios for trying to resurrect Hippolytus. He is often described as a chthonic deity based on his symbol of a staff with a single snake wound around it.[31] Various personifications accompany him, such as his consort Epione (the physician's gentle touch) and his wife or daughter Hygieia (good health), as well as the nymphs Akeso (relief), Iaso (healing),

30. Koronis, while pregnant with Asklepios, fell in love with the mortal Ischys. This so enraged Apollo that he killed Ischys with his bow, while Apollo's twin sister Artemis shot Koronis.

31. In the United States, the modern medical symbol of a staff with two entwined snakes is the caduceus, a sign of the god Hermes. Although Hermes had the ability like all gods to heal, he was not noted as a particular healing deity in antiquity.

and Panakeia (universal cure). Homer refers to Asklepios simply as a highly skilled mortal physician with two sons, Podalirius and Machaon, to whom he taught the art of medicine. Homer mentions the death of Machaon in the Trojan War, but Podalirius survived. Tradition holds that descendants of Podalirius split into three branches at Cos, Cnidus, and Rhodes, all areas renowned as centers of medical knowledge in the ancient world. Later aristocratic families from these areas traced their descent from Asklepios through Podalirius.

Asklepios was originally a local hero worshiped at an early shrine in Trikka, Thessaly, his traditional birthplace. The Plague of Athens in 430–427 BCE elevated the cult of Asklepios, and by 420, he was inducted into the pantheon of Athens. His cult had also spread to Corinth and Cos, where Hippocrates is said to have studied at its asklepieion in the fifth century BCE.[32] By the mid-fourth century, Asklepios had a shrine in Pergamum. The largest and most popular asklepieion was located at Epidauros in the Peloponnesus, which likely originated around 490–480 BCE. The nearby temple of Apollo Maleatas also contained offering bowls to Asklepios. His fame grew beyond the Greeks, with Rome adopting Asklepios in 292 BCE and even the Egyptians equating him with their deified healer Imhotep, maintaining active shrines into the sixth century CE. The dual nature of Greek medicine, being centered on both divine activities and human instrumental interventions, can easily be seen in these different descriptions of Aklepios's family. Apparent cognitive dissonance presented no problem for ancient people, who could just as easily believe in a multiplicity of creation stories.

## Philosophy

The stories of gods and demigods relating to medicine throughout Greek history likely predated Homer and Hesiod and linked to traditions from Minoan and Mycenaean culture. Unfortunately, no specific medical texts still exist that predate the Hippocratic Corpus (mid-fifth century BCE to mid-second century CE), which makes its claim to empiricism and non-reliance on the supernatural explanations seem fairly remarkable for the ancient world. Yet this "scientific" approach of Hippocratic medicine was not quite as sudden and unique as it first appears. It grows out of the tradition and as a reaction to natural philosophy. In order to understand developments in

32. Strabo, *Geography* 14.2.19; Pliny, *Natural History* 29.2.

Greek medicine, we must first look at how Greek philosophy explained the natural order and its relation to early Greek medicine.

In the Ionian city of Miletos off the coast of Asia Minor, natural philosophers developed explanations for phenomena such as earthquakes and thunder. Commonly referred to as the Presocratics, these sixth-century philosophers looked for a natural first cause that unified various phenomena of the natural world. Because they relied on a single cause, they also became known as Monists. This type of explanation pushed back religion in their chain of events but did not eliminate it. The divine essentially manifested in orderly and intelligible laws. They sought a rational system; since everything had a "nature," or *physeis*, it was only a matter of figuring out how that nature works.[33] This included the human body and disease. Yet this did not mean that their inquiry followed the modern scientific method or that they completely eliminated the supernatural from their rational explanations. The Presocratics did eschew direct divine intervention, but this is not the same as denying the existence of gods or their role in the overall universe/cosmology.

Thales (624–546 BCE), born and raised in Miletos, possibly by Phoenician parents, is credited with being the first philosopher to investigate the natural world without relying on supernatural explanations deriving from descriptions of the gods, as provided by Homer and Hesiod. He focused on mathematics and astronomy, postulating that the earth was a floating sphere. Consequently, water became the underlying principle of all created matter. Although he avoided divine intervention in his theories, he did espouse the soul as the cause of movement and that all things have a soul. His inquiry into natural causes led other philosophers to seek a single, unifying principle to the natural world.

Longrigg claims Miletos's economic prosperity and lack of a strong priesthood, unlike its non-Greek neighbors, allowed it to develop an inquisitive and rational culture.[34] This says more about the culture of secular capitalism surrounding twentieth-century scholarship than the environment of sixth-century BCE Miletos. Its Hittite, Egyptian, and Babylonian neighbors did not have strong central religious authorities either. Even the Israelites/Judahites were in flux, since their central temple in Jerusalem, destroyed in 586 BCE, was not rebuilt until 516 BCE, and the Hebrew Bible was not yet codified. The trade networks that benefited Miletos also brought wealth to

33. Longrigg, *Greek Rational Medicine*, 1–2.
34. Longrigg, *Greek Rational Medicine*, 29.

their trade partners in the rest of Asia Minor, as well as Egypt, Mesopotamian, and Canaan.

Unlike the other natural philosophers, Anaximander (610–546 BCE) claimed that the first principle was not a thing such as air, water, or fire. To have one element as the prime cause would automatically negate the existence of others, because things existed in paired opposites. He described the underlying cause of all things as indefinite. It was not created but always existed, and it cannot change or die, thus making it divine. Anaximander possibly derived this idea from the Egyptian concept of *nun* (potential) which is fluid and unbound.[35]

Anaximenes (585–525 BCE), a student of Anaximander, adopted the idea of change but saw air as the principle cause rather than something indefinable. Air could change form based upon its rarefication (thinness) or condensation (thickness). He explained that air can change temperature, depending on whether one breathed through an open mouth, making it warm, or through pursed lips, making it cold. He would further explain that the rarefication of air caused fire, while its condensation would create water or even stone.

Heraclitus (535–475 BCE or ca. 500 BCE) lived in Ephesos, the wealthiest city in Asia Minor after the Persian destruction of Miletos in 494 BCE. He is an exception to the rule of Presocratics coming from Miletos. He saw order in thought, speech, and experience, while human rationality expressed the unity of the cosmos. From this, he concluded that the soul was cognitive rather than simply an animating force in people. Change or flux also revealed the underlying unity of the world. He described fire as the physical embodiment of this principle of flux. In light of these early philosophies, a variety of medical texts arose in the fifth century BCE that drew upon ideas about single causes, the role of elements, and the need to balance opposites; these texts also acknowledged the divine in the Greek explanatory model of illness.

35. Bill Manley, "Anaximander of Miletos," in *The Encyclopedia of Ancient History*, ed. Roger S. Bagnall et al. (London: Blackwell, 2013).

## Sources

### Texts

Nearly three hundred papyri with medical content are published in *Corpus dei papiri Greci di medicina*. Many of these consist of *materia medica*, with the recipes organized by the type of affliction and the affected body parts. They likely had practical use intended for healer, patient, or both. Whereas Egyptian and Mesopotamian medical culture produced similar therapeutic texts with little to no theoretical explanations, the ancient Greeks did the exact opposite, in that a large number of medical texts focus on the theoretical underpinning of how the body works, its physiology, in relation to the greater natural world. From this theoretical basis, many Greek healers judged the efficacy of certain medical practices.

The theoretical nature of these texts helped train future physicians but also acted to assert a particular physician or philosophical school as an authority in the field. Through this struggle for authority, particular "schools of medicine," such as Sicilian, Cnidian, Hippocratic, or Asklepian, developed, centering on prominent areas and figures. This also created a dichotomy between healers that advocated a more pragmatic, experienced-based form of medicine (Empiricists) and those who relied on theoretical precepts (Dogmatists). Yet, in practice, the Greek patient did not have to choose between the different schools of thought but could easily move between them in seeking treatment. It is important to understand that each school strived for an intellectual authority among physicians. They did not seek to "corner the market" in acquiring patients. In this regard, Greek medical pluralism was akin to the rest of the ancient world.

Many of the medical texts from the early philosopher/physicians have not survived, but we know of their theories from references by later writers, such as Aristotle (384–322 BCE), Theophrastus (371–287 BCE), and Galen (129–216 CE). So influential was the philosophical tradition from Ionian Miletos that later medical texts from Cnidus and Cos, such as those in the Hippocratic Corpus, were written in Ionian Greek rather than the Doric form native to those areas.[36] For most texts, it is easier to trace them by their authors rather than by their titles, especially since many of them shared the same title, *On Nature*.

36. Longrigg, *Greek Rational Medicine*, 33.

Alcmaeon (ca. 450 BCE), a noted physician, was from the Achaean colony of Croton on the southern tip of the Italian peninsula. It is debated whether he was a student of Pythagoras. We have no surviving texts from Alcmaeon, but Aristotle, Theophrastus, and Diogenes Laertius (third century CE) refer to the medical teachings in his work *On Nature*, indicating that they likely had copies of it. Alcmaeon ascribed to a theory of opposites such as wet/dry and hot/cold and that good health came from a proper balance or equality (*isonomia*) of these qualities. Disease resulted when one of them gained supremacy (*monarchia*). He also acknowledged external causes for disease that affect the balance of these qualities. Most likely his theory of balanced opposites influenced the Hippocratic humoral theory.

Anaxagoras (500–428 BCE), originally from Clazomenae on the Ionian coast of Asia Minor, is credited with bringing eastern Aegean philosophy to Athens. His works survive only as fragments preserved by later writers, most notably Simplicius from the sixth century CE. Anaxagoras is most noted for work on astronomy and nutrition. He coined the term *sperma* as a technical term for the "seeds" that made up all matter.

Empedocles (490–430 BCE), born in Agrigentum in Sicily, traveled extensively throughout the various Greek city-states. Two of his poems have survived, *Purifications* and *On Nature*, which boast of his ability to cure old age and describe his theories on certain medical topics. This led later writers such as Diogenes Laertius (early third century CE) to claim that Empedocles was a practicing physician who could cure diseases.

Democritus of Abdera (b. 460 BCE) was a Thracian philosopher/physician credited, with Leucippus, as founding the school of Atomists, later called Epicurianism. He wrote many medical texts on prognosis and dietetics, which survive in some fragments, as well as the work *Medical Opinions*, which is now lost. His influence on medical practices reached into the medieval period, when several later treatises became falsely attributed to him. His work on diets espoused a sound regimen to prevent disease, maintaining that health lies in a person's own hands.

Diogenes of Apollonia[37] (ca. 425 BCE) likely came from the Greek settlement on the Black Sea, near the Pontus. According to Galen, Diogenes was a practicing physician advocating diagnosis by examining the tongue and complexion. His writings survive only as fragments reported by others,

37. He should not to be confused with the later biographer of Greek philosophers, Diogenes Laertius. Additionally, his origin in Apollonia should not be mistaken for the city of the same name on the island of Crete.

including the sixth-century writer Simplicius. Confusion exists across these sources about whether Diogenes wrote one work, *On Nature*, or a series of four different treatises.

The matter of Hippocrates and the writings attributed to his name can cause considerable confusion. Hippocrates was an historical figure who later became deified, especially around the city of Cos. Unlike other deified heroes, such as Herakles and Asklepios, whose very existence may be questioned because of the mythic tales surrounding their lives, there is enough evidence to verify the existence of Hippocrates. Yet we cannot attribute all the texts comprising the Hippocratic Corpus to him. The popularity and respect given to Hippocrates made the use of his name a way to claim authority for the ideas of anonymous writers. Attaching the name of a recognized authority was a common tactic throughout the ancient Mediterranean and Near East, not just for medical treatises but for any literary work whose author wanted to give it clout.

The earliest known biography of Hippocrates, by Soranus of Ephesus, dates to roughly the first or second century CE. Galen's extensive references to Hippocrates also provide considerable information. Our earliest mention of Hippocrates, though, comes from his contemporary Plato, whose dialogues *Protagoras* and *Phaedrus* attest not only to Hippocrates's fame as a physician but his accepting payment for treatment.

Hippocrates was born in 460 BCE on the island of Cos into the Asklepiad family. Although *asklepiad* was used as a general term to describe any physician, in the case of Hippocrates, he was a member of the Coan family branch of Asklepios, an aristocratic family who traced their descent through Asklepios's son Podalirius. Like most people of the ancient world, Hippocrates trained in the family business. His medical education would come through the family itself, since no medical school *per se* existed.

This presents an interesting situation in that the Asklepiad family formed its own guild (*koinon*).[38] Typically, the paying of guild fees determined guild membership, and the guild saw to the training through an apprenticeship system. But for the Asklepiads, one must also be a family member through the male line in order to be a part of the guild. An inscription found at Delphi refers to an oath that members of the Coan and Cnidian[39] family

38. Susan M. Sherwin-White, *Ancient Cos: An Historical Study from the Dorian Settlement to the Imperial Period* (Göttingen: Vandenhoeck & Ruprecht, 1978), 257.

39. The branch of the family from Rhodes seems to have died out earlier; Galen mentions the disappearance of Asklepiads from Rhodes but gives no reason how or why.

branches must swear in order to retain privileges at the shrine to Apollo on Delphi.[40] "Decree of the *koinon* [guild] of the Asclepiads of Cos and Cnidus: if the Asclepiad, having arrived at Delphi, wishes to consult the oracle or sacrifice, he must first swear that he is an Asclepiad by male descent. . . ."[41] What is not known is the relationship between the Asklepiad family *koinon*/guild and the shrine to Asklepios at Cos, run by a priesthood.[42]

Ancient stories about Hippocrates have him learning medicine by reading the cures mentioned in the votive inscriptions (*iamata*) at the Asklepios shrine in Cos. Anti-Hippocratic polemics also claim that Hippocrates burned down the shrine in order to avoid charges of plagiarism. Excavations at Cos have not yet revealed such votive inscriptions. Archaeological activity has focused on the eastern portion of the ancient city, whereas the Asklepios shrine in the time of Hippocrates would have been further to the west.[43] Apart from the Hippocratic stories, such inscriptions at Cos are mentioned by Pliny the Elder (23–79 CE) and other writers from the Roman period. Similar votive inscriptions have been found at the Asklepios shrine in Epidauros. Jouanna claims that the tradition of Hippocrates studying the votive inscriptions originated with the priests at the Coan Asklepios shrine in order to appropriate Hippocrates's fame and authority.[44]

Between 430 and 420 BCE, Hippocrates moved from Cos to Larissa in Thessaly. A plague broke out across Thessaly in 419 BCE, originating among the tribes in Illyria to the north. As it spread, the Illyrian tribes asked Hippocrates to help, but he refused to aid "barbarians" and treated only the Greeks within Thessaly. A similar story is told about the Persian king Artaxerxes I (464–424 BCE) inviting Hippocrates to work as his court physician, but he refused on the grounds of his loyalty to the Greeks. Other stories circulated about the summoning of Hippocrates to help cure an important figure, such as Democritus of Abdera. Although fictional, it is known that disciples of Hippocrates did work in Abdera. Confusion between the activities of Hippocrates and his disciples also colors his time in Thessaly. The writers of the

40. Vivian Nutton, *Ancient Medicine*, 2nd ed. (London: Routledge, 2013), 70.

41. Translation from Jacques Jouanna, *Greek Medicine from Hippocrates to Galen* (Boston: Brill, 2012), 115. Jouanna disagrees with Sherwin-White's theory that the Asklepiad family formed a unique type of guild.

42. Sherwin-White, *Ancient Cos*, 277; Jacques, *Greek Medicine from Hippocrates to Galen*, 113.

43. Jacques Jouanna, *Hippocrates*, trans. M. B. DeBevoise (Baltimore: Johns Hopkins University Press, 1999), 19.

44. Jouanna, *Hippocrates*, 19.

*Epidemics* volumes claim that Hippocrates went as far north as Odessus[45] and south to Corinth. This is more an indication of the geographical extent of his disciples than of his actual movements. Hippocrates passed away in Larissa sometime between 375 and 351 BCE; various traditions say that he died at either eighty-five or 109 years of age. By the first century BCE, a cult festival at Cos developed honoring the day of his birth, thus elevating him to a deified hero like Asklepios before him.

Approximately sixty texts make up the Hippocratic Corpus, ranging in date from the earliest, *On the Sacred Disease*, written around the mid-fifth century BCE, to the latest, *Decorum*, composed between the first and second centuries CE. The majority of the texts date from 420–350 BCE. The entire corpus can be divided into three main groups of authorship: the Coan school, the Cnidian school, and an unidentifiable group. In addition to claiming authority from Hippocrates, their use of a rational form of medicine to explain the interaction of disease and human physiology according to natural laws makes the texts a unified corpus. Ancient writers of medical glossaries, such as Erotian (first century CE), give a counting and list of titles slightly different from the corpus recognized since the nineteenth century CE by Émile Littré and F. Z. Ermerin in their compilations and translations. Jouanna gives a complete listing of the sixty texts, including a brief summary along with a discussion of authorship and dating for each one.[46]

The following selections highlight a few treatises representing a continuity with the previous philosopher/physicians. They may be in agreement, building on previous theories, or pointedly disagreeing with their predecessors. The varied nature of the Hippocratic Corpus is due to its texts' wide span of time and place for composition. Yet, even within one text, the author can contradict himself. This should not be taken as a lack of intelligence or hypocrisy on the part of the author. Inherent contradictions reflect how the author, although trying to break with traditions, is still in many ways bound by the ideology of Greek medical culture. *On the Sacred Disease* stands as a prime example of this tension between tradition and innovation in the Hippocratic Corpus.

*On the Sacred Disease* concerns the nature of epilepsy.[47] The opening of the treatise dismisses the disease's divine origin as an invention of charlatans

45. Now the modern city of Varna, Bulgaria.

46. Jouanna, *Hippocrates*, 373–416.

47. Use of the phrase "sacred disease" with highly particular symptom descriptions outside of just this text indicates that it was the name of a specific disease rather than a general classification of disease types.

who wish to disguise their own ignorance with pretend piety and superior knowledge. If such a physician fails, it was the will of the gods. The existence of the gods is not in question in *On the Sacred Disease*. The author, echoing Thales, declares all diseases as sacred, since they arise from the natural world created by the gods. "The disease called sacred comes from the same causes as the other diseases from what enters and exits the body, from the cold, from the sun and from the continuous and ever-changing winds, which are all divine things."[48] Therefore, one particular disease should not be singled out as sacred.

The science-religion dichotomy falsely attributed to the Hippocratic Corpus originates with late nineteenth- and early twentieth-century translators omitting from various texts key phrases indicating the authors' belief in the gods.[49] The treatise goes on to explain that the natural origins of the disease derive from blocked air passages to and from the brain. In this system of natural laws, failure to heal the disease results from it becoming entrenched over a long lapse of time.[50] This shifts blame to the patient for not consulting a proper physician early enough, which means it secondarily acts to undermine competing schools. Yet most ancient patients would not have read this, so it only negates a branch of medicine among practitioners. The author's main intent is to carve out a niche of authority in a society that does not have an accreditation system for physicians. The authority of physicians, especially over other natural philosophers, depends on their skill of argumentation in these types of treatises. Rather than a science-religion dichotomy, some Hippocratic texts line up a division between any form of natural philosophy and empirical medicine.

While these Hippocratic physicians insert themselves into the philosophical arguments on the body and natural laws, the treatise *Ancient Medicine* argues against the idea that medicine is subject to philosophy, and the practice of starting with a philosophical principle such as hot, cold, or dry is faulty. It specifically targets Empedocles by name. Instead, the author prefers a more empirical approach, and only through the study of medicine and the body can one derive natural laws. The text asserts that there are all types of qualities, such as salty, bitter, sweet, and acidic. When they are properly mixed, it is not a problem. But when one is isolated, it causes illness. This

48. *Morb. sacr.* 18; translation from Jouanna, *Greek Medicine from Hippocrates to Galen*, 107.

49. Jouanna, *Greek Medicine from Hippocrates to Galen*, 111.

50. *Morb. sacr.* 2.

is the same principle as *isonomia* and *monarchia*, used by Alcmaeon. This shows that while the author wishes to break with philosophical traditions, he is still beholden to them.

The treatise *On the Nature of Man* similarly argues against the philosophical idea of reducing humans to one element, specifically targeting the successors of the Monists, such as Hippon and Diogenes of Apollonia. The author asserts that only substances found in humans should be analyzed, such as blood, phlegm, and yellow and black bile. He also matches these fluids or humors with the four seasons. Although he claims to avoid philosophy, the text describes the need of the four humors to be in a balance, which again follows the philosophies of Alcmaeon and Empedocles.

*Epidemics* is a seven-volume work whose books can be broken down by date and authorship into three main groups: *Epidemics* 1 and 3; *Epidemics* 2, 4, and 6; and finally, *Epidemics* 5 and 7. According to some modern scholars, they serve as a model of clinical observation,[51] giving symptom details and some patient identification without resorting to supernatural causes.

> In Meliboa a youth, who had been feverish for a long time as a result of drunkenness and much sexual indulgence, took to his bed. His symptoms were shivering, nausea, insomnia and lack of thirst.
>
> On his first day, there passed from his bowels a large quantity of solid stools with much fluid. During the following days he passed a large quantity of watery to greenish excrement. His urine was thin, sparse and of bad color. His respiration was at long intervals and deep after a time. There was a rather flabby tension of the upper part of the abdomen extending laterally to both sides. Cardiac palpitation was continuous throughout. The urine was oily.
>
> Tenth day: he was delirious, but calm, well-behaved and silent. Skin dry and taut; stools either copious and thin or bilious and greasy. . . .
>
> Twenty-fourth day: died.[52]

But this rhetorical style matches many of the therapeutic texts from Mesopotamia and Egypt, which also catalog symptoms. Whereas *Epidemics* presents the information of specific case histories in narrative form, the Egyptian and Mesopotamian texts group them according to general symp-

51. Longrigg, *Greek Rational Medicine*, 99–100.

52. *Epidemics* 3.16.

tom classifications organized by anatomy and disease etiology, which is more akin to the structure of the modern Merck Manual. It should be noted that the diagnoses in *Epidemics*, though absent divine names, still rely on cultural precepts about drinking and sex, as well as philosophical understandings of physiology. This underlying moral attitude puts it in line with other types of medical systems that see illness as a punishment for transgressions that disrupt community cohesion. This compares to Democritus of Abdera's assertion that the body can impeach the soul for neglect, as well as to Homer's equating Right and Destiny. It is not a system in which the gods consciously target an individual for transgression but that the natural laws of the body ensure that a mechanistic punishment automatically occurs as a response to a moral transgression.

Two texts that reinforce the religiosity of the Hippocratic physicians are *Regimen* and the *Hippocratic Oath*. *Regimen*, dating from the end of the fifth or beginning of the fourth century BCE, analyzes the proper balance between diet and exercise for good health. Interestingly, the author claims he can give a prognosis prior to an actual illness, which is dependent on one of two classes of dreams. The first order of dreams is divine, to be handled by specialized dream interpreters. The second order of dreams comes from the soul, which reveals the state of the body and should be treated by the physician. Although the body functions according to natural laws, the physician's actions are a complement to the acts of the gods, not a replacement.

More famously, the *Hippocratic Oath* directly invokes the gods: "I swear by Apollo physician, by Asclepius, by Health, by Panacea, and by all the gods and goddesses, making them my witness, that I will carry out, according to my ability and my judgment, this oath and this indenture."[53] This highlights the position of the physician as essentially an agent of the gods; it is the physician who best understands the nature of the world and the human body that the gods created, and the gods guarantee that the physician behaves accordingly.

Asklepieia,[54] shrines to Asklepios, could be found throughout ancient Greece servicing local areas, but four temples stand out as significant centers of healing: Cos, Epidauros, and Lebena on Crete in the archaic and classical periods, while Pergamum flourished in the Hellenistic and Roman eras. Forty-eight inscriptions (*iamata*),[55] plus some fragments attesting to the

53. Jouanna, *Hippocrates*, 269.

54. *Asklepieion* sg., *asklepieia* pl.

55. *Iama* sg., *iamata* pl.

efficacy of the treatments, were found at Epidauros, while ancient authors such as Pausanias and Strabo refer to the ones not only at Epidauros but also Cos and Pergamum. Edelstein and Edelstein published English translations of the Epidaurian *iamata*.[56] They can also be found in their original Greek in the collection *Inscriptiones Graecae* (*IG* $4^2$).[57] Although some of the inscriptions describe symptoms, their main value to the study of medicine is in their reference to the healing practices at the asklepieion, especially in terms of the patient's perspective and patient-healer interaction.

Healing at the temples followed, with some variation, the pattern of ritual bathing for purification, sacrifice, and sleep (incubation), followed by reporting of the dream to a priest who would then prescribe treatment based upon his interpretation of the dream. The *iamata* narrated fantastical healing stories, such as curing a woman of a five-year pregnancy, but they focused mostly on the dream, which frequently involved conversations with the god Asklepios or him directly healing the ailment and the patient making promises of thanksgiving offerings. One story in particular describes how the sons of Asklepios tried to cure a woman of tapeworm by cutting off her head. When it suddenly dawned on them that they could not reattach it, they sent for Asklepios, who surgically restored her head, then cut open her stomach, removed the tapeworm, and sutured her abdomen. Another common feature of the dreams is the presence of snakes, a symbol of Asklepios, who would lick wounds or otherwise effect healing. Inscriptions also record the thanksgiving offering of individuals as a type of receipt, in case Asklepios forgets and mistakenly causes a recurrence of the ailment. The *iamata* also portray skeptics whom Asklepios afflicts with lameness or blindness for their apostasy. They then go through the process of incubation, becoming cured after seeing the error of their ways, and present a thanksgiving offering.

Many of the inscriptions indicate that the patients suffered from chronic diseases. It would be easy to conclude from this that incubation and healing by priests was an act of last resort for those left desperate by rational medicine. Yet the evidence from the various medical texts, as well as archaeology, shows that rational and "temple medicine" were not in direct competition for patients. The choice of healing strategies likely centered on availability

56. E. J. Edelstein and L. Edelstein, *Asclepius: A Collection and Interpretation of the Testimonies I–II* (Baltimore: Johns Hopkins University Press, 1998).

57. This compilation of Greek inscriptions across varying topics began in 1825, continuing to this day, with some items now digitized.

and tradition. Not every city-state had a physician. The cultural practice of beseeching and thanking the gods in a case of almost any misfortune and subsequent recovery would make the activities at the asklepieion simply a natural undertaking, without indicating a conscious and deliberate preference for a type of medicine or an act of desperation when reaching the end of a hierarchy of resort.

These texts serve a propagandistic function for the temples but should not be discounted as mere inventions or taken as exaggerated accounts of "faith-healing" for minor illnesses, as when Dillon asserts the asklepieion had no relation with the Asklepiad family of physicians, and the priests did not practice any form of rational medicine.[58] The asklepieion at Epidauros lasted roughly eight hundred years, treating a wide array of illnesses. In order for the temple to function as a major healing center, their success rate must have been greater than random chance of minor ailments healing on their own. In all likelihood, the priests practiced a form of rational medicine based on diet regulation, as mentioned in some of the texts of the Hippocratic Corpus when discussing the asklepieion. Although one might contrast incubation to the rational medicine of the Hippocratic Corpus, the text *Regimen* did espouse a form of dream interpretation.

The work of Herman Diels (1848–1922) and Walther Kranz (1884–1960) serves as another important source for the study of ancient Greek medicine. They edited a modern compilation of textual fragments from the Presocratic philosophers, *Die Fragmente der Vorsokratiker*, which were embedded in the writings of later classical authors. These texts are typically referred to by their DK number. For example, Alcmaeon's explanation of the physiological psychology of sight is preserved in DK 24A5. Diels and Kranz provide the original Greek along with German translations.

Texts from the ancient world were not published within separate divisions between topics, as in a modern bookstore. Literary works such as history, poetry, and dramatic plays could contain important medical information. The overall literary context of a culture could affect the writing of direct medical treatises. A particularly moving description of a plague in a particular context, like a history, can find its way into the symptom description of an illness when one would expect a more clinical assessment. This is a result of ancient authors often trying to bring to the fore an underlying cultural value rather than relating "accurately observed facts," expected in

58. M. P. J. Dillon, "The Didactic Nature of the Epidaurian Iamata," *Zeitschrift für Papyrologie und Epigraphik* 101 (1994): 239–60.

modern medical writing. The phenomenon of mediated tales is not limited to religious or literary writings.

As we have seen, the earliest accounts of a medical nature come from the poetry of Hesiod and Homer, linking the gods to disease, trauma, and healing. Famously, in the opening of the *Iliad*, Homer attributes the plague striking the Achaeans to the displeasure of the god Apollo. Similarly, healers staunch bleeding wounds with incantations.[59]

With the development of writing history, it would seem the Greeks moved away from a divine cause for disease. But Herodotus, the traditional father of history, uses only supernatural origins, while other parts of his history reference earlier physicians, such as Democedes in Croton (Italy) in the late sixth century. Thucydides's plague account refers to people seeking aid from priests rather than physicians.[60] Diodorus attributes a plague in Athens to natural causes,[61] much in the same vein as Thucydides, but he also understands a plague among Carthaginians as divine retribution,[62] showing an ambivalent attitude. In these contexts, it appears the divine origins of disease stem from an author's moral attitude toward his subject. This provides information on the fluidity of disease etiologies. Although a physician may prescribe therapies based on the natural philosophy of disease debated in medical treatises, his patient may understand the cause and efficacy of treatment by an entirely different set of rules derived from other cultural spheres.

Similarly, dramatic plays give insight not so much for the practice of medicine in itself but how the wider culture understood the relationships between diseases, patients, and healers. In Sophocles's *Philoktetes*, the title character suffers in exile from a putrefying snakebite after unwittingly trespassing, thus violating temple grounds. The play has no physician character, but the work does give a window into the inherent tensions with the belief that illness is a divine punishment communicating a breakdown in the human-divine relationship.

Beyond the content of the plays, Mitchell-Boyask studies the relationship between the cults of Asklepios and Dionysus in the wake of the Athenian plague.[63] Their temples were spatially aligned, and the ending of the

59. Homer, *Odyssey* 19.455–58.

60. Thucydides, *History of the Peloponnesian War* 2.47.

61. Diodorus Siculus 12.45.2 and 12.58.

62. Diodorus Siculus 14.70.4.

63. Robin Mitchell-Boyask, *Plague and the Athenian Imagination: Drama, History, and the Cult of Asclepius* (Cambridge: Cambridge University Press, 2008).

festival celebrating Asklepios overlapped with the beginning of the Dionysian festival, for which the plays were written.

## Archaeology

The Athenian asklepieion was built in 420 BCE with the official importation of the cult of Asklepios, likely in response to the plague that struck Athens in 430–426 BCE. Its foundation played an integral part in Pericles's building program, revitalizing the Acropolis with many images of Greek victories over the Persians, juxtaposed with heroic age themes, such as winged Nike (victory), whose temple was also built around 420 BCE. These scenes and the temple buildings stood as metaphors for the might of the new Athenian Empire. The Athenian *polis* sponsored the public cult festival for Asklepios at the asklepieion just as they did for the festival to Dionysus. It is not known whether the theater at Asklepios's temple complex in Epidauros was influenced by the linkage of Asklepios, Dionysus, and the theater in Athens. Comparatively, the private cultic practices of the asklepieion as a site of incubation appear to have been less important in Athens than at other temples to Asklepios in the Greek world.

The site of Epidauros is a good illustration of the typical ancient Greek temple complex. It is best to keep in mind that temples to a god were not just one large building. The complex at Epidauros contains the shrine to Asklepios but also one for Artemis, as well as a theater, banquet hall, gymnasium, and stadium. Originally excavated in 1881–1928 by Panayotis Kavvadias, the reports suffer from flaws typical of early archaeology, such as the misidentification of structures. Most studies of Epidauros in the fifth and fourth centuries BCE focus on the architecture and the social aspects of its construction. The asklepieion's largest construction phase occurred in 365 BCE as a result of the increasing popularity of Asklepios across the Greek world and the resulting influx of wealth. It appears that construction matters were handled by local city elites rather than simply the temple priests. Tomlinson provides the most comprehensive assessment of the site.[64]

Epidauros, a coastal city situated fifty miles from Athens and eighteen from Corinth, was not large by ancient Greek standards. Its Dorian population made its links with Corinth and Sparta through the Spartan Alliance appear fairly natural. Originally, the shrine to the local hero Maleatas

64. Richard A. Tomlinson, *Epidauros* (London: Granada, 1983).

synchronized and developed into the healing cult of Apollo Maleatas. The later temple complex to Asklepios developed nearby with the story that he died at Epidauros. An inscription at the asklepieion asserts that Koronis, Asklepios's mother, was the daughter of Malos, the first to build a shrine to Maleatas at Epidauros, making her a native of Epidauros rather than from Trikka in Thessaly. Following from this, the inscription ultimately claims that Asklepios was born in Epidauros in an attempt to give the local asklepieion primacy among his various healing shrines throughout the Aegean.

Another popular healing site connected to the worship of Asklepios is the island of Cos, located off the coast of Asia Minor, with its asklepieion situated in the northeastern portion, on a hill overlooking the modern city of Kos.[65] Excavations have revealed Mycenaean cemeteries on the island, but the area of most importance for the study of medicine was settled by Dorians during the Greek Dark Age (1100–750 BCE). In 366 BCE, a new political state was founded with the city of Kos, which became prominent in the Hellenistic period.

This asklepieion lay about two miles to the northwest of the original ancient city. But by the first century CE, the city expanded, so the temple eventually resided in a suburb. The temple complex was built over three terraces, with the highest most being an original shrine to Apollo Pythios, dating from the late fifth century BCE. This temple included a cypress grove that lasted well into the Hellenistic period. Only in the fourth century, with the founding of the new *polis* Kos, did the temple dramatically expand to its second and third terraces. City elites carefully planned this expansion of the temple, with its construction between 300 and 242 BCE.

Archaeological evidence of the asklepieion that predates the Hellenistic period is scant. Unfortunately, in the nineteenth century CE, a lime kiln was fed with many local stones, likely bearing inscriptions (*iamata*) attesting to activities at the asklepieion in the fifth and fourth centuries BCE. Additionally, most excavations of ancient Kos have been carried out to the east of the temple area.

In addition to major sites, individual artifacts can provide significant information for the history of medicine. Although there are substantial finds of medical instruments from the Roman period, nothing to date has surfaced of ancient Greece. This might be due to the itinerant nature of Greek physicians, who likely visited patients at their homes or worked out of their own

65. This study follows the convention of referring to the pre-Hellenistic city, state structure, and island by the spelling Cos while using Kos for the Hellenistic and modern entities.

domestic space, whereas the Roman artifacts are associated with substantial army installations. The shrines to Asklepios and other healing deities have not yielded medical instruments as such, which is not surprising given the nature of therapeutic tactics at the temples. The vast number of artifacts such as vases, reliefs, votives, and coins from ancient Greece, especially the classical period, would make a cataloging of them too difficult in this type of study, but we will highlight a few items and their significance.

Knowledge of what medical instruments looked like comes from vase paintings and wall reliefs. Unfortunately, no systematic study exists collating and assessing the various vase paintings and wall reliefs dealing with medical topics. Many studies on medicine in vase painting note a popular theme of Achilles using bandages. The physician's work space is depicted with hanging votives in various reliefs. It is difficult to tell whether these scenes take place in a physician's home or workshop. Reliefs showing similar hanging votives in temples further complicate the historical interpretation of location.

Votives are three-dimensional statues of body parts left as thanksgiving offerings at the asklepieia and other healing shrines. They could be of any part of the anatomy, such as legs, arms, hands, feet, partial torsos, eyes, noses, and ears, quite often depicting some aspect of the symptoms, such as swollen veins in a leg. This aspect allows for some estimation of what types of disease process or symptoms affected the patients, but no specific diagnosis can be made from them. Votives were typically made of terracotta, marble, or various metals, and they were also painted. Interestingly, they used white for the skin of females, with red for the males. Many have holes in them for hanging, reinforcing the interpretation of reliefs and vase paintings showing asklepieia with such votives hanging in the background. Curiously, more votives were found in Athens and Corinth than at the larger temples in Epidauros and Cos. It is not clear when exactly the patient made the votive offering, whether it was before or after healing.

Votives have several meanings in the process of obedience and consideration: they act as a thanksgiving reminder to the gods for the healing, a prayer to avoid reaffliction, and as a type of receipt for the god, essentially reminding Asklepios that the person has already suffered and made redress. The disassociation of the afflicted body part from the body of the patient could also serve as a type of scapegoat ritual, removing the illness and thus making the patient whole. The idea that the patient must undergo dismemberment before achieving healing and reintegration parallels the idea of dismemberment as a form of punishment but with a positive outcome, allowing for removal of the sick role and reestablishment of community cohesion. The process of fragmentation and reassemblage as a healing for both the illness and the social stigmas attached to it could be explained with the *iamata* stories of patients having their heads cut off and reattached or their chest opened and stitched together again,[66] since these are surgical procedures not actually carried out by the ancient Greeks.

Coins are another avenue by which one can investigate common cultural attitudes relating to medical practices. Ancient Greece was the first society of the Mediterranean basin to use a monetary economy. Each *polis* could mint its own coins showing various heroic and mythological images as well as local kings. In addition to these typical politico-religious motifs, they would also use images associated with medicine, such as Asklepios and members of the Asklepiad family, as well as Chiron. Medicinal plants could also be depicted but usually in association with mythic figures or from cities boasting that particular plant as a commodity. These types of artifacts could help trace the economic aspects as well as indicate the influence of medical families on local power structures.

## Cultural Concepts

The various sources express different ideologies among the *iatroi*, as well as common patients (a perspective lacking in many cultures), which inform the Greek explanatory model of illness. Students of the history of medicine must remember that even the Hippocratic Corpus did not use a post-Enlightenment scientific method separating natural and supernatural worlds. The divine realm was a significant environment affecting the human body.

### Anatomy and Physiology

Modern studies on the history of medicine typically cite Erasistratus (304–250 BCE) as the father of physiology. They work from the current definition of physiology as the functioning or vital processes of the structures of the human body.[67] But he is a Hellenistic physician, so to credit him with the

66. Jessica Hughes, "Fragmentation as Metaphor in the Classical Healing Sanctuary," *Social History of Medicine* 21 (2008): 217–36.

67. Stedman, *Stedman's Medical Dictionary*, 1084.

origins of physiology obscures the work of earlier Greek physicians and philosophers.

Our modern word comes from *physiologia*, meaning "inquiry into nature," undertaken by the Presocratic philosophers. They investigated physiology not from the standpoint of how the human body worked as a system unto itself but as a manifestation of the natural laws governing the entire world. When changes occurred within their natural philosophy, so too did their understanding of the functioning of the human body. The ancient Greeks did not have one authoritarian theory of the body's functioning. Because of this and the fragmentary nature of early medical writings, we can reconstruct only parts of their physiological theories. By comparing their physiologies, we can derive patterns that highlight the values the ancient Greeks imparted to the body.

Before the philosophical investigation of nature, the poet Hesiod outlined the different ages of humans, in some instances giving their composition or basic anatomy, as well as an explanation for disease etiology.[68] He begins with the Golden Age, which lacks a physiological description, but notes this is the time of Pandora. Because of her actions, sickness can now affect mortals. Next is the Silver Age, in which people were made of silver. Hesiod points out that they do not have the same type of bodies as the people of the Golden Age, but it is unclear exactly how they differ besides the obvious components of gold and silver. During this time, childhood lasted for a hundred years, but then they have a short span for adult life. They possessed a witless personality, committed crimes, and refused to sacrifice to the gods. This indicates thoughts about children in the eight century BCE. He designates the third age as the Bronze Age,[69] when people were made out of ash trees with hearts of adamant. They appeared as unshaped hulks with great arms and strength. Interestingly, his poem *Theogony* uses similar descriptions for Kronos's generation, the Titans. The fourth time period is the Age of Heroes or demigods, populated by people made from pastured earth. Some of them died in war, specifically noting the Trojan War, while others still live at the ends of the earth, apart from men. The last or Iron Age is Hesiod's own "race of men," doomed to always toil and suffer but with some good.

Hesiod explains that the end of each age occurred because they did not respect the gods, their parents, and each other. In essence, this is ac-

68. Hesiod, *Theogony and Works and Days*, 109–201.

69. Hesiod's Bronze and Iron Ages are time frames different from the modern use of the phrases by historians and archaeologists.

knowledging the need for community cohesion among human-human and human-divine relationships, as well as the process of obedience and consideration important to the explanatory models of illness across the ancient Near East and Mediterranean. Hesiod predicts that the present Iron Age will end similarly. This scheme presents human anatomy as a reflection of moral character, with humans as a species growing and developing over the ages. His most admirable stage, the Age of Heroes, can be thought of as akin to young adulthood. In this one, the people developed from "pastured earth," which highlights the positive connection between humans and the natural world, although he has no concern to explain the mechanism by which this connection is maintained throughout their lives. The gods simply imparted Right/soul to humans, making them distinct from animals and closer to the gods. The most important aspect to human anatomy, physiology, and life itself is a proper relationship with the gods and their family/community. This parallels similar concepts of anatomy and physiology in ancient Egypt, Mesopotamia, and Israel without ascribing to a symbiotic physiology in which anatomical parts have a will or the ability to consciously act independently of the human.

As natural philosophy and medicine developed from the sixth to early fourth century BCE, the importance given to the relationships between humans and gods no longer had center stage.[70] A focus on the mechanisms of the body as a functioning of natural laws and a manifestation of Right, Mind, or soul also gained prominence. Here, we can start to see the first evident pattern in Greek physiology.

Alcmaeon rejected the idea that all matter comes from a single entity. He also advocated an empirical approach to medicine, since humans have to interpret the evidence of the visible world, unlike the gods who directly know the truth. Some ancient authors claim Alcmaeon practiced dissections, but his teachings regarding the brain, optics, and embryology derived from his theoretical position about the brain rather than direct experimentation. His philosophical pursuit of eight key questions became the standard by which subsequent physicians/philosophers investigated medical issues.[71] The following is a list of the questions and his answers to them:

70. Due to a lack of information between the eighth and sixth centuries BCE, the Greek Dark Age makes tracing this shift nearly impossible. Any theory would be based more on conjecture than evidence.

71. Longrigg, *Greek Rational Medicine*, 54–57.

1. What is the nature of semen: it is a substance that comes from the brain.
2. What is the basis of reproduction and cause of sex differentiation: both parents contribute seed, with sex determined by who contributed the most.
3. What part of the body is first to develop: the head develops first.
4. What is the mode of nourishment for the embryo: the embryo's nourishment is through the whole body of the embryo.
5. What is the seat of the intellect: the head is the seat of the intellect.
6. What is the cause of sleep: withdrawal of blood into veins causes sleep.
7. What causes the sterility of mules: male mules have a fineness and coldness to their semen, which causes sterility, while female mules have sterility due to the failure of their wombs to open.
8. What is the physiological psychology of perception:[72] channels connect the sense organs to the brain, which does the actual perception of objects.[73]

With this assessment of sense perception, Alcmaeon gives the basis for organs and the person being one and the same rather than two distinct entities. We cannot definitely determine whether Alcmaeon started this connection between the mind (as person) and body parts or whether he simply elucidates a long-held Greek cultural belief about the relationship between people and their bodies.

Anaxagoras theorized that all matter initially existed as a great mass and that the Intellect (*noesis*) set it into motion. The spinning of the great mass caused the seeds to separate out into their distinct entities. Anaxagoras's answers to the standard eight questions posed by Alcmaeon reflect this theory of distinct seeds from an original mass.

1. The nature of semen is that all parts of the body are present in the seed.
2. Only males produce seed, while females provide place of development. Gender is determined by location; the right testicle and right side of womb produce males, while the left testicle and left side of the womb create females.
3. The brain develops first in the embryo.
4. Nourishment of the embryo occurs through the navel.

72. Essentially, the means by which an object acts upon the senses, such as the eyes, allowing for the specific perception of that object.

73. Theophrastus, *De sens.* 25–35. DK 24A5.

5. The brain is the seat of intellect.
6. Sleep comes from weariness of bodily activity.
7. No surviving references give Anaxagoras's explanation for sterility in mules.
8. Sense perception occurs when opposites act upon the sense organ; so, for example, eyes can perceive only what is not like them. Since eyes are dark, they cannot see at night, which is similarly dark.[74]

This perspective allows for organs to be separate from the individual, since it is their nature, not the person, that facilitates or hinders their functionality. Yet the organs have an automatic, passive mechanistic system as a response to the environment rather than the body parts exerting an independent will actively choosing a response that characterizes the relationship between body and environment in other ancient cultures.

In his writings, Empedocles asserted that the Olympian gods are really just temporary combinations of elements, which he limited to earth, air, fire, and water. The body itself came from combinations of these elements in different proportions, such as bones containing fire but no air. In this manner, all humans share in part of the divine; they are made up of the same materials, which recalls creation myths from Mesopotamia. Yet, unlike its ancient Near Eastern counterparts, this does not necessitate humans as special in some way. It is not clear whether Empedocles or his immediate disciples had a diminished view of the gods based on the idea that deities and mortals are made of the same substances.

His idea of matter consisting of combinations also led to his poetic descriptions of the initial creation of human anatomy, in which different body parts tried various pairings, such as a hand on top of the head, until they hit upon the best combinations, like a hand at the end of an arm. Some scholars assert Empedocles's use of combinations arose from the human-animal hybrids depicted in Mesopotamian art.[75] He focused on the four humors of black and yellow bile, blood, and phlegm, combining them with Alcmaeon's theory of balancing opposite substances. Empedocles also theorized that the body had an innate heat (fire/blood) that was kept in balance by the cooling

74. Theophrastus, *De sens.* 27–37 and 59. DK 59A92.

75. Stephanie Dalley, "Evolution of Gender in Mesopotamian Mythology and Iconography with a Possible Explanation of ša rēšēn, 'The Man with Two Heads,'" in *Sex and Gender in the Ancient Near East*, ed. S. Parpola and R. M. Whiting (Helsinki: The Neo-Assyrian Text Corpus Project, 2002), 117–22.

function of respiration (air/lungs). These ideas of innate heat and a balance between the four humors carry through Greco-Roman medicine. Although he did not write a direct medical treatise, he did give answers to Alcmaeon's eight basic questions in his poetry.

1. Semen is a form of blood.
2. Both parents contribute seed, but sex is determined by whether the womb is hot or cold.
3. The heart develops first in the embryo.[76]
4. Nourishment for the embryo happens by four vessels (two veins, two arteries) going through the navel.
5. The intellect comes from the blood around the heart.
6. Sleep derives from a cooling of the heat within the blood.
7. Sterility in mules comes from the hardening of the mixture of male and female semen.
8. Sense perception comes from something fitting into the passages of the sense organs, which have varying widths. An object that fits in the passages for the nose would not fit into the passages for the eyes; thus, one cannot see a smell.[77]

It is not clear whether this mechanistic explanation meant that Empedocles understood organs as entities distinct from the self. But if the idea of body parts looking for the correct partners is accurately ascribed to him, then it is likely he thought of them as separate from the individual.

The exact date and locality of Hippon (fl. 460–450 BCE) is unknown, with some placing him in Sicily. He revived Thales's idea of water as the basis of all matter, with a focus on medicine more so than other areas of natural philosophy. He posited that disease arose from a drying up of the body's natural moisture. Although mostly dismissed by Aristotle for his derivative theories, Hippon's idea of moisture in the body did influence subsequent Greek medical thought. His writings do not survive, but later references provide Hippon's answers to some of Alcmaeon's eight questions:

1. Semen's nature is moist and flows from the marrow.
2. Both parents contribute seed, with the child's sex determined by who contributes the most.

76. This is in contrast to other treatises, which focus on the head.
77. Theophrastus, *De sens.* 1–2 and 7–24. DK 31A86.

3. The head develops first in the embryo.
4. Nourishment of embryo is through its whole body.
5. The head is the seat of the intellect.

The last three questions on the cause of sleep, sterility in mules, and the physiological psychology of perception have no known answers.

The Atomists, following Democritus of Abdera, claimed all matter as coming from small, imperceptible, and indivisible particles or atoms, which were not so much things as physical individuals who can form aggregates. Additionally, these atoms/individuals could not fuse but only mildly attract or repel. From this, we can conclude that healers ascribing to the theory of atoms would view body parts as distinct, separate entities aggregated to the individual but still lacking an independent will. Democritus also gave importance to the role of air (*pneuma*).

Since atoms have individuality and people are responsible for their own health, Democritus claimed the body can impeach the soul for neglect, as it prefers to overindulge in luxuries such as wine. This is one of the rare instances in which Greek conceptions of the body express an idea close to the symbiotic physiology of Egypt and Mesopotamia. He held that the soul is material like the body.

Some ancient sources claim that Democritus carried out animal dissections to further his theories, but no real evidence exists of this. It appears that his theories derived more from deduction and observation of animals than through a practice of dissection. For example, he postulated that animals have multiple births due to multi-chambered wombs. Subsequent Hippocratic medicine explains human twins, drawing upon this theory of multi-chambered wombs.

Democritus's answers for some of the standard eight questions, as recreated through subsequent sources, are:

1. Semen develops from the whole body, especially the principle parts of bone, flesh, and sinews.
2. Both males and females produce seed, while gender is determined by whether the mother's or father's prevails.
3. The navel, external parts, head, or belly develops first.[78]
4. The embryo is nourished by sucking on a bit of flesh in the womb.

78. Although this includes the head, like most treatises, it also incorporates the belly, which is roughly the area of the liver, the seat of thought and emotion in ancient Near Eastern cultures.

5. Intellect is in the brain, while reasoning is in the thorax.
6. Sleep is caused by separation of finer particles exceeding the rate of production of psychic heat, thus cooling the body.[79]
7. Sterility in mules comes from the malformation of genital passages, because of their artificial creation.
8. Sense perception depends upon the air between the object and the sense organ becoming compressed and an imprint of the object being formed on the sense organ.[80]

Although the explanation of sense perception sounds simply mechanistic, the underlying theory of atoms as individuals indicates that this really describes how distinct entities create predictable relationships.

Diogenes of Apollonia agreed with Anaximenes that the first principle was air (*pneuma*), defining it as eternal yet always changing its state. Since air is the first principle, the intellect or soul (*noesis*) is air, while blood contained an innate heat. He also followed Empedocles's ideas of balance and humors. From this, Diogenes posited that good health results from air mixing with blood in the right amount, which can create a white foam appearance or semen. This mixture can also carry the soul/intellect (*noesis*), whereas blood alone does not. Failure for air and blood to mix results in the blood coagulating and, in turn, causes illness. Intelligence depends on the amount of cool, dry air, while the more moisture something has is likened to being drunk and therefore less intelligent. He explained that children are more moist and hence less intelligent. Like many of the natural philosophers/physicians, he used deductive reasoning from the principle of air for his theories. Diogenes's answers to the standard eight questions are:

1. Semen is aerated foam of the blood.
2. Only the male produces seed.
3. Development in the embryo starts with flesh, then bones, then sinews and other parts of the body.
4. Nourishment for the embryo comes through certain protuberances within the womb.
5. Air around the brain or the heart[81] is the seat of the intellect.

79. This idea is drawn from Leucippus and thought to be held also by Democritus.

80. Theophrastus, *De sens.* 49–58, 60–83. DK 68A135.

81. Secondhand reports from Theophratus and Aetius have the air around the heart as the seat of intellect.

6. Sleep comes from blood filling the veins and forcing air into the chest and stomach.
7. No surviving documents provide evidence for his answer to sterility in mules.
8. Sense perception comes from movement in the air immediately surrounding the sense organs and the brain.[82]

It is unclear whether Diogenes is like Empedocles, giving a mechanistic basis for organs and the self to be integrated or whether there is an underlying theory akin to what the Atomists held, seeing the body parts as distinct.

Greek interest in the origins of humans is demonstrated not only by Alcmaeon's original eight questions but the fact that his successors continually debated the answers to them. The study of human reproduction represents a microcosm of the origin of matter for the entire universe, the macrocosm. The items not concerned with reproduction—that is, the seat of intellect, cause of sleep, and physiology of perception—indicate that these are the aspects of the body the Greeks understood as making one human; they are the ways in which the soul/mind manifests and interacts with the rest of the body. Interestingly, they are not in agreement as to the extent to which one's body parts are integral to one's soul or mind.

Although Alcmaeon, Anaxagoras, Hippon, and Diogenes have different theories about the first principle, their unifying anatomical structure is the brain. Empedocles stands apart in that he gives prominence to the heart. Yet they all work with a physiology based on passages in the body that allow for the movement of the substances air, blood, phlegm, and black and yellow bile. This appears to be a coincidental similarity to the Egyptian physiological system of *mtw*, or vessels. Just like the Greek physicians differed on the first principle, they also gave varying emphasis to these substances that had to be in certain proportions or balance with each other. They did not think of the body as a system of organs but rather as a body of fluids.[83] This contrasts with the modern conception of a physiology wholly dependent on the anatomical structures.

Another important concept for ancient Greek physiology is the idea of movement. Because movement was the key to understanding natural laws and the formation of the world, movement also played a significant part in human physiology. This led the physicians to analyze influences on move-

82. Theophrastus, *De sens.* 49–58, 60–83. DK 68A135.

83. Horstmanshoff, King, and Zittel, *Blood, Sweat, and Tears*, 5.

ment, such as temperature and diet. They understood that the movement of food and water through the body essentially shared similar pathways as the vital fluids black and yellow bile, phlegm, and blood, as well as the element air. Nutrition then became a focal point for prevention and treatment of diseases.

For the Hippocratic Corpus, there was no direct answer to the original eight questions of Alcmaeon. Several texts do investigate similar topics. *Eight Months' Child*, *Generation*, and *Nature of Child* focus on embryology, while *Fleshes* discusses the formation of certain anatomical structures, as well as the functioning of the senses hearing, smell, sight, and speech. Interestingly, most of the physicians, including Hippocratic ones, see both males and females contributing seed for the formation of a child, whereas Anaxagoras and Diogenes claim that only males contribute the essential seed for human reproduction.

The Hippocratic authors worked with the same basic physiology that the other physicians used. They understood the movement of substances kept in a balance as the most important aspect of a healthy, properly functioning body. Yet they do begin to codify the four humors of blood, phlegm, and black and yellow bile rather than including air or other elements. They also place a greater emphasis on diet and environment as affecting their movement. The text *Airs, Waters, and Places* goes so far as to postulate variations in physiology (and personality) for people in Asia, Europe, and Scythia, depending upon those particular geographical environments. Descriptions of physiology closely tied to anatomical structures appear to be a later, Hellenistic addition to the Hippocratic Corpus, with the texts *Anatomy*, *Places in Man*, and *Glands*. The dating of *Glands* is debated; if it is an early text from the fifth century BCE, it would be one of the first to mark a shift toward an anatomical-based physiology that will take hold more strongly through the Hellenistic period, lasting into late antiquity.

The anatomy of the Hippocratic Corpus displays an interesting mix between, on the one hand, the rationalist idea of mechanical explanations based on observations devoid of the supernatural and, on the other, a simple adherence to traditions grounded in the supernatural. The most obvious example is their explanation of the "wandering womb" for certain gynecological issues. In some respects, it is a simple mechanical issue of the womb drying out and floating upward, strangling other organs. Binding treatments rely on this mechanistic explanation. Some passages have it seeking out moisture, which indicates at least an instinctive animalistic level of volition. Treatments by aromatic fumigations reinforce the notion of an independent entity with a sense of smell.

It appears that, prior to the Hellenistic period and the increased reliance on anatomical knowledge from dissections, some Greeks worked with a conception of anatomy and physiology closer to the symbiotic physiology seen in Egypt and Mesopotamia. The extent to which the Asklepiads followed any of these ideas about anatomy and physiology or have their own theories is not entirely clear. Parts of the Hippocratic Corpus may give some indication of the Asklepiads incorporating elements of various explanatory models of illness.

## Disease Etiology

Like their ancient Near Eastern neighbors, the Greeks understood disease as ultimately originating with the gods. Hesiod's description of Zeus's retribution against humans for accepting fire from Prometheus and by giving a gift to Pandora serves as a form of disease etiology:

> For formerly the tribes of men on earth lived remote from ills, without harsh toil and the grievous sicknesses that are deadly to men. But the woman [Pandora] unstopped the jar and let it all out, and brought grim cares upon mankind. Only Hope remained there inside in her secure dwelling, under the lip of the jar, and did not fly out, because the woman put the lid back in time by the providence of Zeus the cloud-gatherer who bears the aegis. But for the rest, countless troubles roam among men: full of ills is the earth, and full the sea. Sicknesses visit men by day, and others by night, uninvited, bringing ill to mortals, silently, because Zeus the resourceful deprived them of voice. Thus there is no way to evade the purpose of Zeus.[84]

In this passage, Hesiod makes several salient points about illness. It balances out the power humans have with mastery of fire, silence makes it unavoidable, and it acts of its own volition like an animal following natural laws. The first and second points explain why humans must suffer disease, but the third point creates an ideological space for later rationalist medicine, based on natural philosophy, to develop a practical disease etiology. Illness as a form of direct communication from the gods, given for specific disruptions to community cohesion, does not have much of a place in this particular cosmology.

84. Hesiod, *Theogony and Works and Days*, 39–40.

Yet Hesiod also offers a disease etiology that relies on direct involvement from the gods as a form of punishment:

> But for those who occupy themselves with violence and wickedness and brutal deeds, Kronos' son, wide-seeing Zeus, marks out retribution. Often a whole community together suffers in consequence of a bad man who does wrong and contrives evil. From heaven, Kronos' son brings disaster upon them, famine and with it plague, and the people waste away. The womenfolk do not give birth, and households decline, by Olympian Zeus' design. At other times again he either destroys those men's broad army or city wall, or punishes their ships at sea.[85]

Within one text, *Works and Days*, Hesiod establishes a disease etiology as both natural and understandable, as well as a supernatural event necessitating a close look at personal relationships in order to effect healing.

This latter conception is reinforced by the stories of Philoktetes's festering snakebite wound, which resulted from his accidental defiling of a religious shrine. The supernatural disease etiology is not limited to poetry and plays. Incantations demonstrate the belief that many diseases come from direct attacks and possession by demons, which cause the patient to cry and behave like an animal. The *iamata* from Epidauros attest to similar ideas about a supernatural origin for ailments. Supplicants, such as Kaphisias, originally mocked Asklepios's ability to heal the lame, only to immediately suffer injuries causing lameness.[86] Other supernatural entities, like Medusa, may cause illness. Additionally, the personification of disease as its own entity with volition allows it to carry a demonic name, such as Antaura, rather than a diagnostic title.

In parallel to the idea of disease stemming from the gods is the conception of illness deriving from a disruption of the body's natural balance of substances. It must be remembered that this is not a competing notion but a complementary one, a refinement of how the gods send disease. As the author of *On the Sacred Disease* outlines, all diseases are sacred, so to approach one with that perspective but not others is counterproductive. For the rationalist physician, the sacredness of all illnesses is just the beginning of disease etiology, not the end point on which to base therapies. By understanding that diseases have divine origins, it means they fall into the same category as the primary manifestation of divinity—the natural laws.

85. Hesiod, *Theogony and Works and Days*, 44.
86. Case 36; see Edelstein and Edelstein, *Asclepius*.

From this, we can see that disease etiology in ancient Greek rational medicine has two components: (1) the underlying natural philosophy such as the presence or absence of a first principle or the idea of balance; (2) the mechanistic manifestation of these philosophical ideas, such as the coagulation of blood, the blockage of air, overheating, and the like. It is the specific mechanical manifestation that gives rise to specific diseases. The first component, though, allows for the external world to affect the body, which handily follows the exact same set of natural laws governing the body. Natural laws then become the basis of treatment, with the art of diagnosis and prognosis relying upon the combination of natural laws at work in and on the body.

The process of proceeding along natural laws for disease etiology applies also to trauma. The *iatros* of somatic medicine does not investigate why the wound happened, since his expertise does not address the socio-religious motivations of the gods. Directions in *On Wounds in the Head* do require the physician to ask how the wound was acquired in order to determine a specific course of inspection and treatment. In the treatment of trauma, the interplay of disease etiology and natural laws is evident when addressing the buildup of pus and the drying out of bones. Natural laws prompt the warning that treating children is more problematic since children's natural abundance of blood makes their bones moist and thinner in comparison to adults. Similarly, natural philosophy indicates that patients with head injuries are more likely to survive in winter than summer because of the influence of the environment.

The division between types of healers based on the community to which healing efforts communicate still holds true among the Greeks. The *iatros*, whether Hippocratic, an Atomist, or even an Asklepiad, focuses on building cohesion among the human-human community by removing the sick role. The role of the gods is not dismissed but acknowledged generally as underlying the natural principles of medical practices. The priests working in the asklepieia bring the human-divine community cohesion to the fore with their healing techniques. But like other ancient cultures with medical pluralism, the Greek patients did not have to choose and use one healing strategy exclusively.

## Restoration of Health

Because the ancient Greek *iatros* worked with a physiology and disease etiology grounded in the idea of balancing humors, dietetics became the primary therapy for restoring the balance, especially among the Hippocratic authors.[87] Yet, alongside the manipulation of diets, other treatments, such as incantations, address more directly the supernatural aspect of the ailments. The use of certain treatments does not divide neatly between somatic and religious-based medicine; many therapies overlap in practice, even though healers from various epistemological schools of thought may give different explanations for why they are effective. Note that the Greek word *pharmakon*, from which the modern term "pharmacy" developed, could mean "spell" or "charm." Similarly, root-cutters recited incantations with their therapeutic preparations, which indicates a performative, ritual aspect even to somatic treatment measures. This parallels similar ritual acts in Pharaonic medicine, such as using *materia medica* as a method of communicating obedience to the gods.

For somatic healers, obedience to the gods meant understanding and working with the natural laws governing the world. Like the humors in people, foodstuffs have properties of hot/cold and dry/moist that follow the natural laws. By eating certain foods, one can manipulate the qualities of humors in the body. If you have too much moisture, then you can eat a dry food to absorb the moisture or otherwise draw it out as a purgative. The author of *Regimen on Acute Diseases* sees diet as the best treatment and warns against the overuse of emetics that some like to do. Similarly, there is a caution against laxatives, to be used only when evacuation of the bowels is necessary and not as a matter of course. This may be an attack on an Egyptian style of medical treatment whose healers had much renown in the ancient world.[88] The text recommends *ptisan*, a barley-based drink; mead; and a honey-vinegar concoction. These drinks regulate the body's hot/cold and dry/moist properties. Hot compresses and plasters may also be applied with various ingredients to the same effect.

There is a caution against sudden changes in the diet. It acknowledges that some physicians make the patient fast, with the homeopathic logic that the body underwent a sudden change by becoming ill, so a sudden change is needed to bring it back to health. *Regimen on Acute Diseases* agrees that a sudden change precipitates illness, but it is precisely the suddenness that can

87. Longrigg, *Greek Rational Medicine*, 53.

88. The text also defends the art of medicine by outlining how it is not as capricious as augurs reading bird flights and animal entrails. The reference to divination by birds and entrails might indicate the author's knowledge of medical practices originating among the Etruscans/Romans as well as the Mesopotamians.

make an illness worse, so the body should not be subject to another threat through fasting. This may be a criticism of the fasting process required by some of the shrines to Asklepios. Even fifth-century BCE Greeks saw manipulation of one's diet as an old practice. *On Medicine* claims the first dietetic treatments arose from the simple act of cooking and observing how various foodstuffs affected people.

Incubation is the ritual process—carried out at the asklepieion for receiving a dream from the god Asklepios—that either heals or tells one how to become healed. Asklepieia existed in many cities, such as Corinth and Trikka, but the most popular were at Cos, Epidauros, Lebena, and later Pergamum, drawing pilgrims/patients from all over the Greek world. Incubation was not limited to the worship of Asklepios. Healing shrines with incubation, dedicated to Trophonios and Amphiaraos, were found at Lebadeia and at Oropos, near Athens. It is not clear, but very likely, that they practiced incubation at Delphi or the shrine to Apollo Maleatas.

The process involved a payment or fee to priests; initial sacrifice, preferably with a pig; a purifying bath, sleep, report of dream to the temple priests; and finally, a thanksgiving offering to the god. Many of the thanksgiving offerings were either roosters or votive statues in the shape of various body parts. Each shrine had some variation to these, since not all of them required fasting, and priests were not always present. Even without fasting, there would be a prohibition against drinking wine and eating goat meat and cheese for three days prior to the incubation, and an insistence on sexual abstinence. Scholars often interpret that the prohibitions on eating certain foods may have been a dietary treatment along the lines of those recommended by the Hippocratic authors; Hippocratic texts do acknowledge that healing at Asklepios shrines does have some beneficial practices in dietetics.

The sleeping arrangements were segregated by gender, with males on one side of the altar and females on the other. If the patient was unable to go to the shrine, a proxy could undergo incubation, such as a relative or the priest of the shrine. The exact rituals surrounding the sleeping itself is not known, other than the supplicant is to wear a white robe. One of the *iamata* reports that a man who tried to spy on the sleeping patients from a tree subsequently hurt himself falling out of the tree as a punishment from Asklepios. When dreams are reported to the priests, they are said to then enact certain therapies, but their exact nature is not known. Some reliefs depict priests holding snakes that lick diseased areas, but we do not know to what extent this is an accurate depiction of ritual practices or a visual metaphor.

The relationship between rational Hippocratic medicine and the incubation practices of the asklepieion is not entirely clear. Some modern scholars reject the idea that Hippocratic medicine started with the religious practices at the Coan asklepieion, in favor of it developing as a guild with Asklepios as their patron god.[89] Still others think neither the priests nor a guild gave rise to Hippocratic medicine but that it grew out of a pragmatic secular practice (*techne*) with religion mixed in later.[90]

Unfortunately, we have no surviving medical texts that include incantations, yet several sources indicate they were a common therapeutic strategy. The author of *On the Sacred Disease* does charge the "charlatan healer" with the use of them. We do have various magical papyri, as well as apotropaic amulets, charm plaques, and inscribed gemstones. Only a few survive from the classical period, with our largest collections dating to the Hellenistic and Roman periods. Many ancient Greeks would attach a plaque on or by the door with a general charm warding off evil spirits and misfortune. Given Hesiod's description of sickness as an entity that silently roams, sneaking up on people, these charms in a way serve as a preventative medical therapy. The incantations directly targeting medical issues typically take the form of a command telling the disease to flee because a god is pursuing it. The disease itself may be described as dreaded figures from mythology, like Medusa, or an animalistic demon, such as Antaura. These types of incantations have antecedents in amulets used in scapegoat rituals from Crete in the fourteenth century BCE.

Bandaging was one of the most popular therapies not only for stemming bleeding but also for the setting of bones. It should be kept in mind that no hard plaster casts existed in the ancient world. Texts have a great variety of recommendations for positioning the bones before bandaging them. Many are likened to the straight-arm stance of an archer or the bent arm of a javelin thrower, since they mimic what healers considered the "natural position." Other texts advocate not using these types of positioning references, because they cannot mimic a "natural position"; there is no such thing, since the arm habitually moves. Physicians would use large machines, such as pulleys and winches, to help align the larger bones in the hips.

Bandaging could get highly ornate, with different styles having different names. The Hippocratic Corpus chastises physicians more intent on the artistry of decorative bandages than actually helping the patient. It goes so far

89. Sherwin-White, *Ancient Cos*, 257.

90. Longrigg, *Greek Rational Medicine*, 22–25.

as to accuse some of applying bandages unnecessarily in order to show off their skill. This brings up the issue of bandaging having a ritual component either as a way of showing obeisance to the gods or assuring the patient that the physician possesses enough skill to manipulate the necessary powers for healing.

Coupled with bandaging were poultices that used various ingredients with similar properties to the nutritional regimen. Medicated bandages infused or extracted the needed qualities of hot/cold or dry/moist. The poultice was just one method of delivery for the *materia medica* adjusting the balance of humors. Yet the use of such aromatic bandages directly related to the therapeutic practice of fumigations. The Hippocratic text *Diseases of Women*, in treating "the wandering womb," recommends sweet smells to attract the womb back into its normal position, while other passages suggest simple bindings around the abdomen to mechanically force the womb into position. Interestingly, the Hippocratic use of fumigations works on the principle that the womb is a sentient entity capable of smelling.

Typically, though, fumigations had the patient inhaling the smoke or odor of strong substances, either pleasant or foul. The foul odor was meant to repel attacking demons, while the pleasant one could attract gods or other helpful sources. The practice grew out of purification rituals used for a variety of contexts, such as purifying sacred areas or removing a moral contagion or *miasma*, such as the bloodstain resulting from murder—all practices making an object acceptable to the gods. Odysseus undertakes a purification ritual based on fumigation after slaughtering the suitors of Penelope. Blood could carry the moral impurities, so blood rituals involved covering a person (or object) with blood and then washing it away. The applied blood picks up the stain (*miasma*) from the original blood, which can then be removed when the applied blood is removed. The shift of *miasma* from a contagious bloodstain to the modern use of a "bad air carrying a disease" appears to come from the Hippocratic physicians who criticized blood rituals. They shifted emphasis from the notion of moral bloodstain to a contagion effecting one of the underlying principles of the natural laws. The air then, rather than blood, became the vector of transmission. Impurity shifted from a breakdown of the human-divine relationship to a disruption within just the human community.

Blood, like diet, served as a therapeutic focal point for somatic healing, with bloodletting the most popular form of surgery. Iconography from as early as the fifth century BCE shows cupping glasses used in bloodletting. These cupping glasses became a typical sign of the physician. Given the physiological basis of balancing humors, including blood, it only stands to reason that bloodletting would be one of the tactics to regulate the properties of the body, especially heat. Hellenistic texts in the Hippocratic Corpus give specific instructions on how to practice such a delicate art. Incisions need to be a certain distance from the wound or infection so as not to further contaminate the affected area. Also, care must be shown so as not to remove too much blood, which would harm or even kill the patient. Bloodletting should be done only on those strong enough and one of the last resorts, though its usefulness in a variety of contexts, from fever to childbirth, added to its popularity.

Like bloodletting, the idea of applying direct heat, in the form of cauterization, to a medical problem drew upon the idea of physiology and disease etiology having a basis in the balance of humors. Burning key spots on the body, such as behind the ears, on the shoulder blades, thighs, buttocks, corner of the eyes, above the knee, and on the temples, can stop the flow of substances, especially bile and phlegm, thus healing illnesses relating to their imbalance. The ancient Greek physician considered it one of his most powerful tools but also the tactic of last resort, executed conservatively. *Epidemic* 5 records, as a warning, the death of a patient subjected to too many burns.

The ancient Greeks used trephination, a surgical procedure of drilling into the skull, as a way of treating head wounds by removing fragments of bone from skull fractures. The Hippocratic text *On Wounds in the Head* gives details of carrying out the procedure as well as advice on various complications. The text does warn that only a skilled physician should perform trephination and that most physicians would need to seek out an expert. This does not mean there were specialized surgeons like the modern neurosurgeon but that some physicians had more experience and better, delicate techniques that would not cause further harm to the patient.

The Hippocratic Oath explicitly states, "I will neither give a deadly drug to anybody if asked for it, nor will I make a suggestion to this effect. Similarly, I will not give to a woman an abortive remedy." This brings up the issue of abortion. The Hippocratic statement appears to echo the Pythagorean sentiment that life begins at conception. Yet other philosophical positions informing medical practices, such as those of Plato and Aristotle, support abortion as a viable treatment measure, whether induced medicinally or through the piercing of the ovum, due to the onset of life occurring either at birth or when the soul infuses the fetus in late term.

Carrick outlines nine basic reasons for aborting a pregnancy in ancient Greece and Rome: (1) the desire to preserve sexual beauty; (2) to avoid personal inconvenience; (3) to avoid poverty; (4) to limit competition for scarce resources; (5) perceived economic advantage of more male than female offspring; (6) to protect the mother's life; (7) to rid society of weak and thus worthless or burdensome citizens; (8) to conceal adultery; and (9) to protect the estate from doubtful legitimacy.[91] Although the sixth reason is a direct medical cause by modern standards—that is, restoring the somatic health of another—the other eight justifications demonstrate the ancient worldview that the removal of the sick role depends greatly on how the patient and the wider community perceive their ultimate cohesion.

Restoration of health involves a two-step process: (1) removal of the sick role; and (2) reintegration with the target community. The reliance on the somatic treatments of an *iatros*, which alleviate physical symptoms, satisfies the removal of the sick role, while the thanksgiving offering of votives fulfills the requirements for reintegration. But it seems that, during this period of classical Greek medicine, the two-step process collapses into one for healing by an *iatros*. The obvious removal of the physical ailment in itself allows for the reintegration into the human community.

## Illness

To understand the illnesses faced by the ancient Greeks, one can approach it from the perspective of paleopathology, using skeletal remains and coprolites, as well as textual sources. Skeletal remains from the archaic and classical periods are rare, due to the Greek cultural practice of cremation, as well as the natural decay of bodies. The environment, unlike dry Egypt, did not allow for much in the way of accidental preservation.

### Disease

Most of the paleopathological literature concerns itself with the plague that struck Athens in 430–426 BCE. Suggestions range from *Yersinia pestis*, also thought to be responsible for the Black Death of the European Middle Ages, to anthrax and scarlet fever. In 1994, a mass grave of 150 bodies was found at Kerameikos outside Athens, with vases that could be dated to

91. Paul J. Carrick, *Medical Ethics in the Ancient World* (Washington, DC: Georgetown University Press, 2001), 117–18.

430–420 BCE. Studies carried out on DNA extracted from pulp of teeth from these bodies found the presence of *Salmonella enterica*, the agent for typhoid fever.[92]

Investigation of primary sources shows that the ancient Greek physician focused on epidemics, as well as noncontagious diseases. The most detail on etiology, symptom description, and treatments can be found in the Hippocratic Corpus's *Epidemics* and *Disease* 1–4. Because the Hippocratic Corpus contains texts specifically addressing epilepsy, gynecology, and obstetrics, these become the focus of modern textual analyses of the disease processes effecting the ancient Greeks and read against what little physical evidence exists from remains. The problem with such studies is that they generally ignore the social aspect of illness elicited by questions as to how ancient Greek persons, not physicians, understood that they were ill or their beliefs about the cause of the illness and what constituted being healed. Someone can suffer from a disease process but not acknowledge the illness until it interferes with work or fulfilling civic obligations. Similarly, he or she may have physically eradicated the disease from the body but not think so until after making a thanksgiving offering to Asklepios. With this caveat about our paucity of information concerning the social aspect of illness, we can paint a rudimentary picture for some of the physical diseases suffered by the ancient Greeks.

Malaria was problematic for certain areas of lowland marshes or where irrigation practices created substantial bodies of standing water. In addition to the extensive concern about fevers in the medical texts, analysis of skeletal remains from the Middle Helladic period (1900–1600 BCE) showed malarial infections, especially for places like Boeotia, whereas Crete did not suffer from malaria epidemics.[93] In areas with endemic malaria, the population starts to form a genetic anemia that acts as a defense against the infection. Paleopathologists can tell whether malaria is newly introduced to an area, by the infant mortality rate until the genetic anemia takes root. Mycenae proper on mainland Greece seemed not to suffer much from malaria. By the early Bronze Age (1600 BCE), Mycenaeans instituted draining practices that reduced their chances of infection. It is thought that Greek colonization

92. Manolis Papagrigorakis et al., "DNA Examination of Ancient Dental Pulp Incriminates Typhoid Fever as the Probable Cause of the Ancient Plague of Athens," *International Journal of Infectious Disease* 10 (2006): 206–14.

93. Robert Arnott, "Disease and the Prehistory of the Aegean," in *Health in Antiquity*, ed. Helen King (London: Routledge, 2005), 12–31.

of the Italian peninsula in the eighth century BCE brought an increase of malaria to that area.

Apart from malaria, the two most prevalent disease processes evident from the skeletal record were scurvy and rickets. Scurvy speaks to a diet deficient in vitamin C, while rickets attests to significant physical labor for the children and lack of exposure to sunlight. The ancient population of Crete provides one of our more complete demographic studies on morbidity and mortality. From the Early Minoan (2100 BCE) to the Late Minoan (1300 BCE), there was a decrease in life expectancy for males, which seems to be a response to the increase in urbanization during that period. Female life expectancy remained fairly constant during this period, although it was lower than in males. Children had the lowest life expectancy with 56 percent not surviving past five years of age. Some early studies claimed the morbidity and mortality rates for women depended on the stress of child bearing. Paleopathologists now understand that insufficient nutrition during a female's childhood would make her more susceptible to disease in her early adulthood, as well as delay the onset of menarche or cause infertility. Thus, pregnancy could not be the explanation for the lower life expectancy of women. Cultural factors, such as a food-distribution system favoring males, were more likely the cause.[94]

## Trauma

No one type of injury stands out from the others in ancient Greece. Both *On Joints* and *Fractures* attest to a variety of trauma that can occur in both warfare and industrial/farming accidents. Treatment of such injuries focused on debriding the wound and maintaining the appropriate balance of dryness and moisture. Roughly 10 percent of the skeletal remains from Athens have fractures. Most were not deadly, showing signs of healing, although in a manner that would have left the person with a limp or other disability. The Hippocratic Corpus levies charges against certain physicians not properly setting and bandaging. Yet these skeletons appear as if no attempt was made to correct the fractures. Some scholars assume this indicates that many could not afford an *iatros* to properly set the bones. This situation speaks directly to the issue of acknowledging a physical ailment and thus taking on the sick

94. Kimberly Calnan Gray, "The Health Status of Bronze Age Greek Women," *American Journal of Archaeology* 98 (1994): 340.

role. Although having fractures, these people may have been able to fulfill their daily obligations, making it unnecessary for them to seek treatment rather than just being too poor to afford an *iatros*.

## Disability

Given the percentage of population suffering from improperly healed fractures, this also brings up the issue of ancient Greek attitudes toward disability. Greek art focused on healthy depictions of the body, paying little attention to deformities or disability, with the exception of dwarfism and some cases of obesity. Occasionally, the medical literature cataloged a few anatomical oddities.

Ancient Greek terminology for disabilities is usually pejorative and does not distinguish between congenital and noncongenital defects. Birth deformities were viewed as punishment from the gods toward the parents. Yet the parents did not face any social stigmas for raising the disabled child, such as barring them from political or religious life. Aristotle, however, proposed a law making it illegal to raise a deformed child. He also, ironically, concluded that the blind were more intelligent than the deaf-mute.[95] As far as we can determine, the ancient Greeks exposed children if the disability was visible from birth but not if it manifested later in infancy or childhood. Unlike Mesopotamia and Rome, monstrous births were not seen as an ill omen, except when reporting on non-Greek cultures, and even then it was limited to animals, not humans. The disabled would be used in scapegoat rituals in times of crisis, which would range from ritual expulsion to actual execution.

Socrates and Plato urged pity for those who acquired a disability, since it would be by luck or nature; if disability meant suffering a punishment, then everyone is to blame. Because illness or injury as a form of punishment was an acceptable etiology for many ancient Greeks, it was difficult for the average person to tell the difference between a "sinner" and simply one with "bad luck," in determining the cause of the disability. Treatment of those with disability varied in each *polis*. Athens seemed more tolerant of disabilities, enacting welfare provisions, while Sparta's law required the exposure of disabled infants. It is not clear how closely this law was followed in practice. The respect shown in Athens might have arisen from large segments of the pop-

95. Aristotle, *On Sense Perception* 1.437a16.

ulation left disfigured in the wake of the plague of 430 BCE, in addition to the 10 percent of the population suffering from improperly healed fractures.

Hephaistos, a lame but highly skilled blacksmith, figured prominently in the Greek pantheon. The occupation of blacksmithing was one of the few routes open to the disabled, so it stands to reason that the patron god would also be disabled. Their view of cosmology also required that a special gift be balanced, so the lameness of Hephaistos compensates for his extraordinary skill with dangerous substances. This parallels the idea that fire needs to be controlled or crippled to be useful. Disability, then, may act as a metaphor for the liminality of a profession incorporating magical properties, like smithing.

Interestingly, the story of Hephaistos's birth recalls the theme of proper roles, found in the Mesopotamian story of Enki and Ninmah creating disabled humans. Zeus bore Athena without the help of a female, and she stands as a model of physical and mental perfection, whereas Hephaistos was conceived by Hera without Zeus; therefore, he is not perfect. Hera tried to expose Hephaistos, but even she cannot kill a god. Contrary to the Greek artistic insistence on perfection, the existence of Hephaistos reinforces cultural roles for disability, ultimately recognizing that no population is perfect.

## Conditional States

Modern medicine treats stages of life, such as childhood, pregnancy, and old age, as conditions needing specialists. Ancient Greek medicine acknowledged children and the elderly as special cases adjunctive to their other concerns about illness. Pregnancy itself was less a clinical issue, left to the practice of midwives, than a field of epistemological discourse, like the formation of the fetus.

Ancient Greek culture did not value childhood as an important stage in life, with many biographies skipping over it. Formal burial sites have an underrepresentation of children. A few elite funerary reliefs for them depict the deceased children in an idealized adult form. This seeming disregard comes from the belief that children were animalistic, incapable of rational thought, which was valued as the pinnacle of Greek society. Yet art, literature, and personal letters attest to parents missing dead children. This disjuncture stems from their cultural precepts that did not allow for the outward expression of grief, especially for adult males.

From a physiological perspective analyzing human remains, the onset of puberty occurred roughly at the age of fourteen, although it varied according to the availability of proper nutrition and therefore social status. Culturally, though, adolescence for females ended with marriage and pregnancy, whereas for males it ended with thicker, coarser beard growth. It is interesting that the determination rested partially on a social-legal classification for one, while the other simply relied on a physical process. But during male adolescence among the elites, boys were expected to play a passive role in homosexual encounters. Families would show off young males at symposiums as a way of building alliances with the more powerful families. With full-beard growth, men could then assume the active role in homosexual relationships.

The medical literature describes children as having more blood and thus more innate heat than adults. Given the overall physical weakness and excess of blood in children, medical treatments could vary but not simply because the patient was a child. The physician's decision ultimately rested on the strength of the patient to withstand treatment measures.

Greek culture refrained from designating a definitive age as "old." Signs of old age included white hair or baldness, stooped stature, and a quivering voice, as well as menopause in women. Medical treatments had no significant shift based on old age. Most therapies in the texts are cosmetic treatments for signs of old age, especially targeting baldness. Old age did affect social status for males, based on the assumption of loss of rationality. In this regard, they are reverting to a status similar to the irrational child. For postmenopausal women, they gained certain legal freedoms and authority but did lose social status relative to married women of childbearing age. Ultimately, as long as persons could fulfill their social roles, we see no real marginalization of them. To this end, preventive medical therapies focused on diet and exercise as staving off the degradations of aging.

Pregnancy was not considered part of the physician's repertoire, except for treating infertility and an interest in reasons for the survival of premature babies. The Hippocratic physician writing *Diseases of Women* understood conception as a sign of health. In order to become pregnant, the womb must be in its proper place and open. Yet, almost in contradiction, giving birth purged the body, thus restoring it to a proper balance and therefore health. This indicates that the pregnancy itself was not considered a healthy state but one the body naturally corrects. Only when the body has difficulty expelling the natural but temporary buildup of substances in the female body is a physician required to intervene. Similarly, the text claims that marriage and its assumed consequence, pregnancy, can cure some diseases, such as the "wandering womb," by helping to settle and open it.

## Healers

Like many ancient cultures, the Greeks used a variety of terms for healers, with different shades of meaning. Although the term *iatros* translates to "physician," one should not make the mistake of equating this completely with the modern notions of physician. *Iatros* was not a regulated term referring only to those practicing somatic, Hippocratic-style medicine. It was frequently used for gods such as Apollo and Dionysus. Another general term for physician was *asklepiad*. Yet in certain contexts, it meant someone from the family of Asklepios at either Cos, Cnidus, or Rhodes. While these physicians may have undergone a particular form of education aligned with theories of Hippocrates, Empedocles, Democritus, or other famous writers of medical treatises, they did not have a monopoly on the terms meaning "physician." Quite often, someone who was simply apprenticed to a practicing physician could adopt the title when striking out on his own. Other healers, such as the priests of Asklepios, practiced in conjunction with these healers. Yet at times, it may appear that the ancient Greeks differentiated titles between one who focused on communication with the community (*iatros*), while the other concerned himself with the divine (*asklepiad*). The *iatros* did become the preferred term for all healers, regardless of their adherence to somatic natural laws or more direct religious practices, while the *asklepiad* diminished in use, due to its more restrictive meaning associated with the god.

Healers were not limited to males. Midwives, typically older and more experienced women, had no formal training yet cared for women during parturition. They could work with the *iatros* or asklepiad but not in the modern sense of calling in a "professional" physician in times of crisis. Midwives do not appear to have handled issues of fertility or other gynecological problems, but this image might stem from a paucity of medical sources mentioning them. A clearer picture may be derived from personal letters or literature, such as plays depicting the activity of "nurses." Like the midwives, with whom they may overlap in terminology, they were older, experienced women. In all probability, they acted as healers in their own right, as a first tier in the hierarchy of resort for most people, given their immediate presence in elite family structures.

# 7. Hellenism and Hellenistic Medicine: A Brief Introduction

The rise of Philip of Macedonia (382–336 BCE) and his son Alexander III, "the Great" (356–323 BCE), created a significant shift not only in Greek politics but also the territory of Greece. Magna Graecia occupied roughly the same geographical region centered on the Aegean Sea, with slight changes to include Macedonia to the north, nestled between Illyria and Thrace, while excluding the Italian peninsula and eventually the island of Sicily. Alexander the Great founded approximately seventy cities, all named Alexandria, mostly in the eastern part of his empire, as military bases. Some of them lasted, such as in Egypt, while others were viewed by locals as an imposition; thus, they did not survive long after his death. He also adopted the practice of installing governors or satraps from the Achaemenid dynasty on the Iranian plateau. Eventually, Alexander filled the positions with Macedonians rather than local Persians. This spread Greek culture into new areas, especially among the ancient Near Eastern polities in Mesopotamia, Egypt, and the Levant.

The Greeks of the classical period looked at Macedonia as a cultural backwater in comparison to the more dominant *poleis* in the Peloponnesus. Macedonian customs were slightly different from Hellenistic ones, such as the practice of polygamy and regional rather than city-state kingship. But for the most part, there was considerable overlap between them, especially in the worship of the Olympian gods, although Alexander additionally fostered his deification among the newly conquered territories to the east. As Philip and Alexander rose to power, the cultural connections between Macedonia and Greece were reinforced as the royal family tried to legitimize itself to the Greek population. The conquests of Alexander the Great spread this hybrid form, known as Hellenistic culture.

After the death of Alexander, the cavalry commander and regent Perdikkas tried to control the empire by dividing its territories among the generals already governing as satraps,[1] intending to keep the more powerful ones on the fringes. The kings back in Macedonia tried to assert control, but satraps like Ptolemy and Seleucus claimed that they did not have to respond to those who did not participate in the conquests. These successors set themselves up as absolute kings and encouraged worship of themselves among the local pantheons, as did Alexander. By 322, the Diadochi Wars (322–301 BCE) broke out among the various Alexandrian generals vying for control of parts of the former empire. Demetrios, the son of Antigonos I, the "One-Eyed," took Athens from general Kassandros and later held off Ptolemy in a naval battle in 306 BCE. This victory allowed Demetrios to declare himself king, establishing the Antigonid dynasty. Kassandros fought him back toward the eastern Aegean, but Demetrios reasserted himself and then tried to march on Macedonia itself in 294 BCE. Yet by 286, the general Lysimachos had control of Macedonia.

Antigonos II Gonatas (277–239 BCE), son of Demetrios, overthrew Lysimachos in 277, becoming king of Macedonia. He kept an active defense of the north through the use of border forts against Illyria, now inhabited by Celts, while also creating a defense against the possible incursions of Greece by the Ptolemies or Seleucids. Mainland Greece itself to the south had a rather passive form of governance, since the population was still mostly homogeneous. The city-states retained rulers as well as revived the Aetolian and Achaean Leagues, making them more amenable to act as a buffer against successors trying to move against the Antigonids. Internally, Macedonia was also rather quiet. This allowed the Antigonids to focus more on commerce, building up the wealth of various regions under their rule. Unlike the other generals turning into kings, Antigonos II did not actively foster a ruler cult.[2] More toward the west, Rome came to power, eventually conquering Greece and adopting many of its Hellenistic cultural traits.

## Religion and Culture

Many of the original Greek city-states surrounding the Aegean held on to their traditional beliefs, unlike the areas newly conquered by Alexander

1. Satraps, originally a Persian administrative unit, were adopted by Alexander the Great, who gave generals certain areas to govern as his main army moved eastward.

2. Winthrop Lindsay Adams, "The Hellenistic Kingdoms," in *The Cambridge Companion to the Hellenistic World*, ed. Glenn R. Bugh (Cambridge: Cambridge University Press, 2006), 28–51.

and incorporated into the Hellenistic successor states, which experienced a greater degree of cultural hybridization.[3] Exceptions to this generality exist, such as Delos, traditionally the center of worship for Apollo and Artemis, but its role as an important trading port led to the incorporation of temples for Sarapis and Isis from Egypt, Atargatis and Hadad from Syria, the Canaanite Astarte and Baal, as well as a Jewish synagogue. Eventually, the Romans brought their more traditional cultic practices to the island.[4]

In the classical period, religious practices tended to be dictated by the city-state in which one was raised. The rituals associated with particular deities were also tied to certain localities. The increased movement of peoples in the Hellenistic period separated people from specific cultic localities, leaving them free to adopt the religious practices of their new home. Conversely, cults whose practices could more easily tolerate geographical transfers increased in popularity. This is evident in some healing cults during the classical period, such as the cult of Asklepios. By the second century BCE, the asklepieion on Delos gave way to the popularity of the Sarapieion healing sanctuary.[5]

The favor of the ruling family and other elites acted as another important, determining factor for religious choices. The traditional Olympian gods found continued importance through such a system of patronage. Yet many ruling elites would follow other religious practices, if politically expedient. The Ptolemies adopted the local Egyptian cult of Isis as well as created the hybrid god Sarapis. Meanwhile, many Egyptian elites found favor with the new ruling Ptolemies by adopting the worship of Zeus or Herakles. Those not so closely allied with the ruling elites would likely continue with their more traditional religious practices. This situation is how merchant classes brought the worship of gods like Isis or Baal to Delos. The overlap between the deities was stressed, so that traders from Phoenicia simply gave Baal the Greek-styled name of Poseidon. It must be remembered that these religious practices in the Hellenistic period were, for the most part, polytheistic. With the exception of Judaism, the gods from various traditions, such as Dionysos, Isis, and Hadad, could be combined in a personal pantheon.

The Hellenistic world developed the practice of *asylia* or inviolability, in which a temple and its associated city-state gains prestige and royal recogni-

3. Jon D. Mikalson, "Greek Religion: Continuity and Change in the Hellenistic Period," in *The Cambridge Companion to the Hellenistic World*, ed. Glenn R. Bugh (Cambridge: Cambridge University Press, 2006), 208–22.

4. Mikalson, "Greek Religion."

5. Mikalson, "Greek Religion."

tion. This is done by the city and temple in question sending out delegates to the most prominent cities and capitals of empires asking for recognition of *asylia*. Once given *asylia*, the temple and its associated deity became a rather powerful cultural focal point. The asklepieion at Kos achieved *asylia* status, thus securing it as a major healing site.

Goddesses that personified aspects of healing and health, such as Epione (Soothing), the wife of Asklepios, and their daughter Hygieia (Health), remained part of the medical culture in the Hellenistic period, especially in literature and statuary. The popularity of Asklepios and use of the asklepieion aided the popularity of these personifications. Interestingly, Hygieia is always portrayed with Asklepios rather than his actual consort Epione. In some cases, the name Hygieia is grafted on to the identity of Athena. There are a number of possible theories for why Hygieia's popularity eclipsed that of her mother and other sisters.[6] Her representation of health likely spoke to those who already enjoyed good health and beseeched the gods for such continued prosperity, whereas the other deities signified the afflicted. This is in addition to those suffering from an ailment and seeking the favor of Hygieia. Although some might claim that, as a female deity, she incorporated female worshipers into the cult of Asklepios, this alone does not explain the Hellenistic world favoring her over the other female deities associated with Asklepios. Like the god Apollo, these personifications are the forces underlying the natural system the *iatros* drew upon to practice his art.

## Philosophy

The classical period of ancient Greece (480–323 BCE) included an impressive chain of teachers and peoples, starting with Socrates, passing on to Plato, and then Aristotle (384–322 BCE), who tutored Alexander III, "the Great." Aristotle dies the year after his pupil Alexander reinforces the dividing line of 323 BCE, which marks the shift to the Hellenistic world. Just as Alexander signified a significant change in the political map of the ancient Mediterranean and Near East, Aristotle's philosophies had a similar long-lasting and far-reaching impact on medical practices.

The successor empires to Alexander imitated his alliance with philosophy by a system of patronage for scholars, including physicians. These em-

6. Michael T. Compton, "The Association of Hygieia with Asklepios in Graeco-Roman Asklepieion Medicine," *Journal of the History of Medicine and Allied Sciences* 57 (2002): 312–29.

pires also created and competed for large libraries that became centers of learning for the elite classes. Although the idea of a preeminent philosopher as royal tutor developed from the relationship between Aristotle and Alexander, the practice of libraries had antecedents in the temple archives of both Egypt and Mesopotamia.[7]

These Hellenistic libraries aggressively acquired scrolls, fervently copied them, and attempted to create standard editions. Such practices also made them open to many forgeries. The philosophical nature of many medical texts made them more popular than the pragmatic engineering texts. Texts by popular figures and those copied as part of school lessons proliferated, which allowed some to survive the destruction of the libraries that occurred during the Roman conquests of the second and first centuries BCE and Christian riots of the late fourth century CE.[8]

Just as in the classical era, different philosophical schools influenced medical theory and practices during the Hellenistic period. Some of them, such as the Dogmatists and Methodists, became schools of medical thought rather than general philosophical schools. One should remember, the use of "school" in this context does not mean a set institution or curriculum but rather a loose grouping of like-minded people. Their arguments played out in treatises. It is unknown the extent to which the average physician exclusively followed a particular school of thought when practicing medicine. Pragmatism would dictate that a healer likely drew from a variety of theories as the situation at hand warranted. Let us then briefly look at the major philosophical/medical schools in Hellenistic Greece.

The label Dogmatism for a school of thought was created by later commentators on the Hellenistic medical texts. This group has also been referred to as "logical" or "the rationalists," since they emphasized the role of deductive and inductive logic to better understand observed phenomena and experiences. In part, the Dogmatists' emphasis on rational theory was meant to bring medicine into the philosophical realm rather than viewing it as simply a practical craft.[9] Although they subscribed to a basic humoral theory, they did not have precisely the same understanding of it. The number of humors could vary, such as Praxagoras identifying eleven instead of just

7. Paul T. Keyser and Georgia Irby-Massie, "Science, Medicine, and Technology," in *The Cambridge Companion to the Hellenistic World*, ed. Glenn R. Bugh (Cambridge: Cambridge University Press, 2006), 241–64.

8. Keyser and Irby-Massie, "Science, Medicine, and Technology," 241–64.

9. E. M. Craik, "Dogmatism, Medical," in *The Encyclopedia of Ancient History*, ed. Roger S. Bagnall et al. (London: Blackwell, 2013).

four.[10] The relationship between the humors, as well as to the environment, became known as the "hidden causes." Other schools of medicine, such as the Empiricists, denounced the existence of "hidden causes."

Empiricism is a school of medical thought developed from the work of Pyrrhon of Elis (365–275 BCE) and Philinos of Kos (ca. 250 BCE)[11] in response to the work of the Dogmatists. During the Roman era, medical Empiricists became a branch of philosophers known as Skeptics. They advocated observation and recording of repeated experiences rather than attributing physiological phenomena to "hidden causes," since by definition they cannot be observed. They avoided looking for disease causes overall, since no one can agree on them. Treatments could be quickly found without an etiology. According to some scholars,[12] Empiricists did not offer any new theories or therapeutic practices for medicine, but their rejection of hidden causes, while favoring the observable, is actually a theory that can affect symptomatology and thus therapeutic practices.

The claim that Empiricists lacked new theories likely stems from the fact that their writings typically had the form of case histories with a concern for drug therapies. They focused more on treating the symptoms, based on prior experiences and examination of all circumstances. Additionally, Empiricists rejected studying anatomy and physiology *per se* but encouraged an analysis of similar cases. As part of their eschewing of anatomy as a field of study, they rejected dissections by stressing the differences between living and dead bodies.[13] The similarities between the two types of bodies are not sufficient enough for proper comparison; plus, the act of dissection does not provide information on processes within the body, which is important to the Empiricist. They maintained that treatment of body parts should be done by analogy. This means that since an arm and leg are similar, they should have the same treatment.[14] Effectiveness of a healer ultimately rests on three principles: (1) accurate observation; (2) an extensive library or collective memory of case histories; and (3) knowing the limits and virtues of similarities.

Epicurianism grew out of the Atomists, who originated in classical Greece with Leucippus and Democritus. It became popular under Epicurus

10. Nutton, *Ancient Medicine*.

11. Keyser and Irby-Massie, "Science, Medicine, and Technology," 241–64.

12. Julius Rocca, "Empiricism, Medical," in *The Encyclopedia of Ancient History*, ed. Roger S. Bagnall et al. (London: Blackwell, 2013); Keyser and Irby-Massie, "Science, Medicine, and Technology."

13. Nutton, *Ancient Medicine*, 148–49.

14. Keyser and Irby-Massie, "Science, Medicine, and Technology."

of Athens (341–270 BCE). Epicureans understood the natural world as made up of individual and unobservable things—atoms. They are infinite in number but have specific properties of shape, size, spatial ordering, and orientation. They come together as aggregates to form things. The aggregates exist as two or more atoms staying in tension with one another, much like repelling magnets, so atoms can never actually fuse. When atoms separate, there is a void, but the void does not exist within an atom; an atom can never be split.[15]

Asklepiades of Bithynia (124–40 BCE) was the most prominent Epicurean who applied the philosophy to the practice of medicine. He rejected humoral theory in favor of a physiology reliant upon the aggregation of atoms. Disease etiology was based on the movement of atoms making up and within the body, especially how they constrict or open pores.[16] He is the first physician to outline a theory of acute and chronic diseases related to these pores. His reliance on the aggregation of atoms also meant that he saw no difference between the physical body and the soul. His ideas quickly developed into the Methodist philosophy of medicine that became popular within Roman culture. Unfortunately, none of his writings have survived, so the medical theories attributed to him are reconstructed by collating descriptions by other ancient authors.

Although Pythagoras lived during the late sixth century BCE, his ideas still could be found in later Hellenistic medicine. Namely, there was an emphasis on numbers, which influenced the medical idea of critical days. One should note the overlap with Mesopotamian medicine, in which specific days are important in therapeutic measures. Also for the Egyptians, the number of days plays a key role in diagnosis, especially when evaluating the progress of the illness or healing.

Older histories of Greco-Roman medicine identified a particular group as the "Sicilian School," defined in relation to the Dogmatists and Empiricists. Modern scholars slotted Aristotle and Diocles, among others, into this group. They were attributed with formulating the idea of innate heat; of the body containing the elements of fire, water, earth, and air; that the heart is the seat of intelligence; and that the blood carries nutrients. More recently, though, a particular style of "Sicilian" medicine is coming into question.[17]

15. The word "atom" literally translates as "uncuttable."

16. Pores in this context are spaces or voids within the body and not necessarily in the dermatological sense.

17. Marie Cronier, "Diocles of Karystos," in *The Encyclopedia of Ancient History*, ed. Roger S. Bagnall et al. (London: Blackwell, 2013).

## Influential Figures and Texts

Apart from the philosophical positions outlined above, a few key figures and texts are also important for the history of medicine in the Hellenistic period. They do not fit neatly into the geographical schema of the following chapters, since their careers and writings span various territories throughout the Hellenistic world. Porous borders still existed despite the political divisions of new empires.

Theophrastus (371–287 BCE) comes from Eresus on the island of Lesbos but moved to Athens, studying under Aristotle and eventually becoming head of the Lyceum. Many of his theories closely parallel those of Aristotle. He is said to have written about 227 works on a wide range of topics, but only fragments survive.[18] His work *On Sensation* is the most informative for the study of ancient medicine, providing us with descriptions of many of the medical texts outside the Hippocratic Corpus. *On Sensation* can be found in the modern compilation *Doxographi Graeci*. With his *History of Plants*, especially book 9, he is one of the first herbalists to influence later pharmacology texts.

Diocles of Carystus lived in the fourth century BCE. He is considered one of the most influential early physicians after Hippocrates and thought to follow theories similar to his. He wrote approximately twenty treatises[19] in the Attic dialect rather than the typical Ionian used for philosophical and medical treatises. Only fragments and titles survive, such as *Matters of Health* and *On Matters Related to Women*. Apollonius of Citium (first century BCE) is the earliest to mentioned Diocles's works on surgery, such as *On Things in the Surgery*. Later medical writings from Celsus, Galen, and Pliny the Elder, as well as many others into the medieval period, refer to Diocles. He favored both long-term medical experience (empirical) and basing ideas on an overarching theory of nature, leading later ancient authors to categorize him as a Rationalist.[20]

He is credited with being the first to write a systematic investigation of anatomy based on animal dissections and perhaps even coined the term "anatomy." He is mostly known for his study on dietetics. Some of his

18. *Enquiry into Plants* and *On the Causes of Plants* are the only works of his to survive almost entirely intact.

19. Philip J. van der Eijk, *Diocles of Carystus: A Collection of Fragments with Translation and Commentary* (Boston: Brill, 2000), vii.

20. Pseudo-Galen, *Introduction or Physician* 4 (XIV, 683K) and Galen, *On Medical Experience* 13.4–5; see van der Eijk, *Diocles of Carystus*, 13, 21.

works were intended for younger physicians, such as *Matters of Health to Pleistarchus*, but also to a wider, nonmedical audience, like *Archidamus*.[21] Fragment 109 from *Affection, Cause, Treatment* indicates his methodology: symptom description with explanation of underlying physiology, followed by empirical evidence; he includes agreement by other authors on similar cases.

Diocles divided the study of medicine into three categories: symptomatology, etiology, and therapeutics. Treatments varied according to the patient's age and constitution. The potentialities or powers within plants/drugs can change with these variables as well as by preparation. He advocated the idea that accumulation of experiences will make visible the hidden causes of disease. He gave teleological explanations for anatomy and held that the external climate influenced health. The soul or psychic pneuma derived from the heart, but use of one's full intellectual ability required it to interact with the brain. Treatments besides diet included bathing, venesection, exercise, emetics, and drugs, which may be pills or salves. Max Wellmann claimed Diocles was a student of Philistion and therefore part of a Sicilian School, whose existence is now in doubt.[22] The following is a list of possible works by Diocles: (1) *On Anatomy*; (2) *Archidamus*; (3) *Prophylactic Letter to Antigonus*; (4) *Cookery*; (5) *Affection, Cause, Treatment*; (6) *On Sexual Activity*; (7) *On Matters Related to Women*; (8) *On Evacuations*; (9) *On Bandages*; (10) *On Lethal Drugs*; (11) *On Treatments*; (12) *On Catarrhs*; (13) *On Vegetables*; (14) *On Digestion*; (15) *On Fevers*; (16) *On External Remedies*; (17) *On Things in Surgery*; (18) *On Prognosis*; (19) *On Rootcutting*; and (20) *Matters of Health*.[23]

Praxagoras of Kos (ca. 300 BCE) comes from the Asklepiads, a family of healers developed from priests of Asklepios. He had taught Herophilus. Although none of his writings survived, his influence on those whose texts we still have should be noted. Praxagoras quite often went against the dominant theories. He proposed eleven humors as a criticism of the four humors theory: sweet, mixed, clear, sour, salty, soapy, bitter, oniony, yolky, corrosive, clotting, and blood.[24] Additionally, he claimed that nutrition was inhaled *pneuma*, while digestion was a corruption of the process; this is in

21. This work explains the medical views of Archidamus, who is otherwise unknown; see van der Eijk, *Diocles of Carystus*. There is some speculation that Archidamus was the name of Diocles's father and is the physician being referenced in this work; see Nutton, *Ancient Medicine*, 123.

22. Van der Eijk doubts the existence of the Sicilian school; see van der Eijk, *Diocles of Carystus*, ix; contra Longrigg, *Greek Rational Medicine*, 162.

23. Van der Eijk, *Diocles of Carystus*, xxxiii–xxxiv.

24. Keyser and Irby-Massie, "Science, Medicine, and Technology."

contrast to theories of Empedocles and Anaxagoras, who thought essential elements were found in food.[25] To develop these theories, Praxagoras studied structures along with processes within the body, thus bridging anatomy and physiology, and in this manner he also tied together philosophers such as Plato and Aristotle with the anatomists from Alexandria.

He taught that the heart was the seat of the soul, where thoughts originated, and that the brain arose from the spinal cord as simply an appendage. Arteries arose in the heart, carrying pneuma, while veins had blood and originated in the liver. Veins get smaller and smaller, eventually turning into nerves that control movement in the extremities. He advocated taking the pulse as a diagnostic tool, despite thinking that the pulse and the heartbeat were independent of each other. There is no surviving description of exactly how his taking the pulse translated into a diagnosis or prognosis. Some claim he performed abdominal surgery in treatment of ileus.[26]

The ancient work *Problemata* is a collection of nine hundred questions and answers, falsely attributed to Aristotle. It was likely written around 250 BCE, with elements as late as the sixth century CE. It borrows heavily from the Hippocratic text *Airs, Waters, and Places*, which attests to the rising popularity of Hippocrates in the Hellenistic period.[27] The answers in *Problemata* follow Aristotle's theory of four qualities and elements as well as imbalances (excess/deficiency). Diet and exercise are the keys to preventing illnesses, but the text acknowledges that different types of people, based on environment, are prone to different types of imbalances. Plague attacks anyone already with compromised health. Treatments are also based on diet and drugs that restore balance (allopathy).

The Hellenistic botanists described plants with a focus on pharmacology, based on theories about similar properties between plants and the necessary therapies for specific ailments.[28] Mantias (120–100 BCE), the Herophilean who specialized in compound medicines, and Krateuas (100–60 BCE), a "root-cutter" who served under Mithridates VI of Pontos, are the two most prominent botanists/pharmacologists. Apollodorus (ca. 280 BCE) wrote the earliest study on poisons, which Nicander of Colophon (ca. 130 BCE) drew upon in his poetic works. The *Alexipharmaca* treats all types of poisons, while *Theriaca* deals only with poisonous animals.

25. Keyser and Irby-Massie, "Science, Medicine, and Technology."

26. Nutton, *Ancient Medicine*, 125–26.

27. Nutton, *Ancient Medicine*, 144–45.

28. Keyser and Irby-Massie, "Science, Medicine, and Technology."

## A New Culture of Medicine

The most significant contributor to Hellenistic medicine is Ptolemaic Egypt, which we will look at as a distinct entity. Although an itinerancy could be found among Hellenistic healers, such as Erasistratus, there was the distinction of different political authority between Ptolemies and Seleucids that could influence the medical arts; in particular, the Ptolemies seem to have briefly tolerated human dissection, whereas the Seleucids and much of the rest of the Hellenistic world did not allow such practices at any point in time. During the Hellenistic period, Greece proper did not have significantly unique developments but rather incorporated those from Egypt while continuing most practices from the classical era; thus, it will not be discussed in a separate chapter.

The intertwining of the medical cultures of the Etruscans and the Roman Republic and Empire will be analyzed as a part of the greater Hellenistic world, despite the history predating this form of Hellenism. Rome as a cultural entity presents a problem in that it expanded considerably from its city-state origins in the central Italian peninsula to incorporate a variety of cultural traditions across the Mediterranean basin. The most obvious for the study of medicine is the adoption and adaptation of Greek medicine as it was practiced in both classical Greece and the Ptolemaic kingdom in Egypt during the Hellenistic period.

Additionally, many medical practitioners traveled throughout the territorial holdings during both the Republic and Empire. Galen serves as an example of a preeminent Roman physician who was trained in Alexandria yet practiced predominantly in Pergamum, with only a brief stint working in the city of Rome itself. One could be a prominent physician without working in Rome or even the Italian peninsula. As we shall see, the physicians who focused on the epistemology of medicine are concentrated in the Greek-speaking eastern half of the Roman Empire.

The Roman political apparatus, especially under the Empire, lent a greater amount of cultural continuity, despite its legal differences enacted among the various provinces.[29] For example, the ability to gain Roman citizenship within Egypt was so difficult that the majority of the population were classified simply as Egyptian, regardless of their actual ethnic/cultural

29. Naphtali Lewis, "The Romanity of Roman Egypt: A Growing Consensus," in *On Government and Law: Collected Essays of Naphtali Lewis* (Atlanta: American Society of Papyrologists, 1995), 298–305.

makeup, yet ample inscriptional evidence shows that many inhabitants had multiple names, in Egyptian, Greek, Latin, or combinations thereof. Because of this situation, areas normally thought of as culturally different in previous periods, such as Egypt, will now be grouped under Roman medicine, but distinctions will be made if practices in one area differ from the rest of Roman territory.

The development of Judaism under the domination of Hellenistic polities significantly affected medical practices in the Levant, as well as the Diaspora, making a dedicated chapter on Second Temple and early rabbinic medicine appropriate. Medicine, as reported in the Jerusalem and Babylonian Talmuds, straddles the cultural and political boundaries of the Roman and Sasanian Empires, as well as local Hasmonean rule.

Similarly, the medical practices of the Persian dynasties of the Iranian plateau will be addressed under the Hellenistic world, since our evidence predominantly spans the period just prior to the Alexandrian conquest well into the Roman period.

# 8. Ptolemaic Egyptian Medicine

## Location and History

Ptolemy, a Macedonian, was appointed as a satrap, or governor, of Egypt under Alexander in 323 BCE. Upon the death of Alexander, Perdikkas, the *de facto* regent for Alexander's unborn son, began to divide the satraps among the generals, attempting to keep the more powerful ones on the fringes of the empire. Ptolemy chose Egypt, keeping a distance from Perdikkas, and later captured Alexander's funeral procession, thus being able to lay claim as an heir. By 305, he declared himself king of Egypt, taking the name Ptolemy I Soter. The Ptolemaic dynasty lasted until 30 BCE, with the death of Cleopatra VII and Egypt's annexation as Augustus Caesar's personal property.

Geographically, Ptolemaic Egypt covered roughly the same territory as Pharaonic Egypt, with its southern terminus at the first cataract marking the border with Nubia. Just as the New Kingdom pharaohs attempted to exert control over the Levant, the Ptolemies similarly clashed in the area with another Macedonian dynasty, the Seleucids. In Ptolemaic Egypt, the study of medicine with a subsequent writing of treatises seems limited to the city of Alexandria rather than being spread throughout the kingdom. Yet this does not preclude other cities as centers of healing, such as Memphis.

This also brings up the extent to which Alexandrian medicine was practiced across Egypt. We know from surviving texts in other regions that Alexandrian medicine influenced theorists and practitioners across the Mediterranean, but it seems limited to those who adopted Hellenistic culture in other aspects of their lives as well—essentially, those wishing to be a part of a dominant power structure. What has been left out of the historical and archaeological record so far is the incorporation of Alexandrian medicine among the lower classes traditionally blocked from participation in the Hellenistic courts. Whereas Pharaonic Egypt substantially shared the same culture among the upper and lower classes, Ptolemaic Egypt had a marked distinction between the Hellenistic ruling class and its Egyptian subjects. Traditional Egyptian power elites would be an exception. For example, the high priests of Ptah at Memphis, as well as the officials at the temple of Horus in Edfu, enjoyed normalized relations with the Ptolemaic dynasty.[1] We can only estimate that the Egyptian peasant under Hellenistic rule used Alexandrian medicine based on his proximity to Alexandria or a similar Hellenistic city. It also depends on how far he moved along the hierarchy of resort in seeking care and to what extent the upper levels of that hierarchy grafted on to the hierarchy of political power controlled by the Ptolemies. The ideas in Alexandrian medicine spread through the Hellenistic world after the expulsion of Alexandrian intellectuals by Ptolemy VIII in 145 BCE.[2]

## Religion and Culture

Alexander the Great founded the city of Alexandria, making it free from the entrenched Egyptian religious practices that would be found in older cities, such as Memphis, Thebes, and Heliopolis. Alexandria was a multiethnic city composed mostly of Macedonians, Greeks, Egyptians, and Jews. The Ptolemies allowed various religious practices rather than enforcing one Hellenistic mode.[3] This is in keeping with the conquest policy of Alexander, who allowed traditional religious forms as a way of placating the various regions. They invented Sarapis, a new hybrid god, indicating the combined religious sensibilities of the Greeks and Egyptians while elevating in status more traditional Egyptian gods, such as Isis and Imhotep.

Whereas ancient Egyptian religion formed the underpinnings of Pharaonic medicine, Ptolemaic or, more accurately, Alexandrian medicine is thought to have grown out of the cultural traditions of classical Greece. Debate surrounds the question of influence the long-standing traditions of Egyptian medicine had on the Alexandrian physicians.[4] Von Staden points out three issues complicating the matter: a significant chronological gap between the Pharaonic texts and the writings of the Alexandrians, uncertainty of terms used in the medical treatises, and the general overlap in "ideas,

1. Lang, *Medicine and Society in Ptolemaic Egypt*, 27.

2. Heinrich von Staden, *Herophilus: The Art of Medicine in Early Alexandria* (Cambridge: Cambridge University Press, 2007), 67–68.

3. Mikalson, "Greek Religion," 208–22.

4. Von Staden, *Herophilus*, 3.

insights, and therapeutic or preventive practices"[5] across the Mediterranean. Although no direct evidence exists pertaining to Egyptian medical practices between 1085 and 300 BCE, commentary on it by writers ranging from Herodotus to Diodorus Siculus gives no reason to suspect any appreciable change to Egyptian medicine during those intervening years. The use of *cippi* statues developing during the Late period may stand as an exception to this. Although modern scholars have difficulty in translating terms, this may not have been the experience of Alexandrian physicians who possibly witnessed more traditional Egyptian medicine in action or otherwise encountered these terms in context rather than as a sterile document in a "dead language."

Some overlap between both medical cultures is inevitable considering that both address the same topic, the human body, and therefore will make the same discoveries. In order to uncover an exchange between the cultures, especially the precise direction of Egyptian influencing Greek, one must analyze a specific idea or practice as to its theoretical or cultural basis and trace the likelihood of that idea being both in contact and adopted. For example, an Egyptian test for fertility calls for a woman to vaginally insert an onion overnight, with an examination of her breath in the morning. If it smells of onion, then she would be able to conceive. The idea is that the *mtw* are open, allowing for passage of the odor, which would also allow for the passage of semen. A similar prescription occurs in Greek texts but calls for garlic cloves; this rests on the idea that certain substances rise up toward the head, while semen forms in the head and travels downward. It is possible that one culture borrowed from another, given that both use the physiological concept of substances traveling within the body, but more investigation is need to determine whether it is coincidental.

One should not try to make sweeping generalizations about the whole of medical culture, such as declaring Egyptian medicine as grounded in magic whereas the Alexandrians avoided such practices, making any borrowing unlikely. This obscures the more rational/somatic aspects of Egyptian medicine as well as the religious beliefs fundamental to Greek medicine. Additionally, it ignores the ability of cultures to reinterpret and adapt practices that obscure its origins. More assured is the influence of Egyptian pharmacology on the *materia medica* of the Alexandrian physicians. This is not surprising given the availability of various plants and minerals both native to Egypt and part of the trade networks passing through the area.

There is the problem of Egyptian and Greek culture being fairly isolated

5. Von Staden, *Herophilus*, 5.

from one another early in the Ptolemaic dynasty. Initial crossover could happen more on the part of the Egyptians imitating the Greeks in hopes of gaining access to the new power structures. Manetho stands as an example of this. By the latter half of the dynasty, though, the Egyptian population gained ground, making the Greeks more apt to culturally borrow from the Egyptians. Although this tends to be the typical pattern for areas under an imperial colonial rule, it does not preclude the phenomenon of "intellectual tourism"[6] creating cross-fertilization among certain Greeks, which would prove significant for the history of medicine. Scholars and students of Ptolemaic medicine must be careful not to slavishly apply postcolonial theories, since Greco-Egyptian identity enjoyed a greater degree of fluidity than what is allowed for in the imperialism of the modern nation-state.[7]

The writing system for Ptolemaic Egypt was not straightforward. Hieroglyphs were still in use for monumental inscriptions and some sacred papyri. They also used Hieratic, a cursive form of Hieroglyphs, for many documents. In the seventh century BCE, the Egyptian language had evolved along with a cursive writing system, both called Demotic, which became the dominant form, especially for government documents, by the Ptolemaic period.

## Cosmology

The concept of *maat* as a natural order or balance to the universe remained a fundamental aspect to the cosmology of Ptolemaic Egypt. The ruling dynasty tried to insert themselves in this rationale for legitimacy by proclaiming their benevolence to the temples and Egyptian subjects, hence maintaining *maat*. Decrees such as the Rosetta Stone demonstrated this ideology among the ruling dynasty. Egypt held a special, quasi-mythical status among the classical Greeks, evidenced by the writings of Homer and Herodotus, who saw it as a place of great ideas, especially in terms of medical knowledge. But they also believed that Egypt suffered stagnation under its adherence to tradition,[8] which is why they would need Greek rule.

For modern scholars, the practice of incubation presents a problem if it is understood as completely synonymous with the Greek practice. Incubations in Ptolemaic Egypt were used mostly by people with ac-

6. Von Staden, *Herophilus*, 25.

7. Lang, *Medicine and Society in Ptolemaic Egypt*, 29–30.

8. Lang, *Medicine and Society in Ptolemaic Egypt*, 41.

cess to the temples, and dream interpretation allowed them to acquire a higher religious status. The common peasant typically was not "pure" enough to actually enter an Egyptian temple and likely continued the Pharaonic practice of submitting written questions and pleas for help to temple personnel, who would then return an answer after consulting with the petitioned deity. Papyri Leiden and Strassburg 21 preserve such petitions.[9] Thus, the traditional Egyptian temples and shrines for healing continued to be popular among the Egyptian population as well as an upsurge in consultations with Imhotep and Osiris. Yet shrines for newer gods associated with healing, in particular Sarapis, experienced frequent use under the Ptolemies. Although a number of the gods from the Pharaonic period, such as Thoth and Sobek, were still intimately connected with healing, let us look at a few of the more important deities consulted in Ptolemaic medicine.

## Ptolemaic Gods and Goddesses of Disease and Healing

### *Sarapis*

Sarapis is the hellenized form of the Egyptian Osiris, combined with aspects of Aphrodite and Dionysos. The name derives from "Osiris of Apis," the sacred bull at Memphis dedicated to Osiris. The Ptolemies legitimized their reign by associating themselves with the ruling triad of Osiris-Isis-Horus (Harpokrates). The original Pharaonic conception of Osiris understood him to be a resurrected god, but the hellenized form portrayed Sarapis as a more active healing deity in addition to his role as protector of the royal family. Herodotus relates the story of Cambyses's slaughter of the Apis Bull resulting in his insanity,[10] which would help popularize the medical connection of Serapis for later Greeks living in Egypt.

There was a tradition that Demetrios of Phaleron (307–280 BCE) wrote five books composed of cures based on interpretations of dreams from Sarapis. A sarapieion at Kanopos had supplicants sleep inside just like a typical asklepieion. Memphis has a similar sarapieion as well as a temple in Kanopos just outside Alexandria. The temple to Osiris at Abydos, although abandoned

9. Lang, *Medicine and Society in Ptolemaic Egypt*, 47.
10. Herodotus, *Histories* 3.30.1.

in the Ptolemaic period, has inscriptions dedicated to Sarapis from people still visiting it for medical issues.

### *Isis*

The goddess Isis was a personification of the throne, seen as a protective figure. Her original connection with healing came from the mythic cycle *The Contendings of Horus and Seth*, in which Isis gathers the scattered parts of Osiris and resurrects him in order to conceive Horus. Greco-Roman incantations depict her with Nephthys curing a headache for Horus.[11] Lang claims that the specific healing aspect of Isis declined during the Ptolemaic period in favor of a general protective figure, due to her expanding role over all in the religions of the Greco-Roman world.[12] Many areas had smaller shrines that attracted locals in times of need, including incidents of illness, as letters from farmers indicate.[13] She possessed different names depending on the region, such as Isis Nephorses in the Fayum, where she perhaps had the form of a crocodile god.[14] The largest temple to Isis in Philae has almost no references to her healing abilities and rarely sees supplicants from outside the area.

### *Imhotep*

Imhotep was a deified official from the Third-Dynasty reign of Djoser (2667–2648 BCE), who initially served as a royal architect. As a god, he was viewed as the architect of the cosmos who oversees order and harmony,[15] bringing him into the sphere of Maat. His sanctuaries at Thebes and Memphis were operational in the Ptolemaic period. The Ptolemies syncretized him with Asklepios, evidenced by a second-century CE papyrus.[16] Late Ptolemaic and Roman sources start to differentiate between the Egyptian

11. *PDM* XIV.1219–27.

12. Lang, *Medicine and Society in Ptolemaic Egypt*, 60.

13. Lang, *Medicine and Society in Ptolemaic Egypt*, 61.

14. Lang, *Medicine and Society in Ptolemaic Egypt*, 48.

15. Lajtar, *Deir El-Bahari in the Hellenistic and Roman Periods: A Study of an Egyptian Temple Based on Greek Sources* (Warsaw: Institute of Archaeology, Warsaw University, 2006), 57.

16. P. Oxy. XI 1381.

Imhotep-Asklepios and the Greek Asklepios, with Imhotep-Asklepios depicted in more traditional Egyptian scribal attire.[17] The name was hellenized to Imouthes in some sources. He was part of a dual sanctuary with Amenhotep son of Hapy at Deir el-Bahari, established roughly around 120 BCE. Wildung published a comprehensive study of Imhotep.[18]

### *Amenhotep son of Hapy/Hapu*

Amenhotep son of Hapy (1430–1350 BCE) was a deified official from the reign of Amenhotep III (1390–1352 BCE), whose mortuary cult at Thebes took on the character of a healing cult in the Ptolemaic period.[19] Like Imhotep, his role as a scribe, lector priest, and intermediary with the king demonstrates his access to power (*heka*) that lends to associations with healing. He acquired the title "god physician" (*swnw nfr*). His first mention as a god came in a Greek source from the third century BCE.[20] His association with healing, though, can be dated to 628 BCE, in a royal stela that links him to the healing of an eye ailment.[21] Shrines and inscriptions often associate him with Imhotep, especially at Deir el-Bahari, but they do not syncretize the two. This shrine was established around 300 BCE in an abandoned sanctuary to Hatshepsut.[22] Most inscriptions about him at Deir el-Bahari were written in Greek; thus, the concepts of *swnw* and *iatros* became conflated. Lajtar published the most comprehensive study of the site, but the majority of the inscriptions date to the later Roman period rather than the Ptolemaic dynasty.[23] The Ostracon of Polyaratos mentions seeking aid from Amenhotep after failure of physicians to cure an eight-year-long illness.[24]

17. Lang, *Medicine and Society in Ptolemaic Egypt*, 86.

18. Dietrich Wildung, *Imhotep und Amenhotep: Gottwerdung im alten Ägypten* (Munich: Deutscher Kunstverlag, 1977).

19. Lang, *Medicine and Society in Ptolemaic Egypt*, 56.

20. Lang, *Medicine and Society in Ptolemaic Egypt*, 83.

21. Lang, *Medicine and Society in Ptolemaic Egypt*, 84.

22. Lang, *Medicine and Society in Ptolemaic Egypt*, 87.

23. Lajtar, *Deir El-Bahari in the Hellenistic and Roman Periods*.

24. Lajtar, *Deir El-Bahari in the Hellenistic and Roman Periods*, 51.

### *Khonsu Neferhotep*

Khonsu Neferhotep was an oracular god from the Third Intermediate through the Greco-Roman period. He would declare that oracles will be fulfilled rather than originally pronouncing oracles himself. His popularity may indicate a new wrinkle in the hierarchy of resort or act as an expression of doubt as traditional Egyptian and Greek medicine began to combine. He enjoyed royal backing, as indicated by a record of Ptolemy II giving thanks to Khonsu for the healing of Philadelphos.[25]

## Sources

There is a problem with secondary source material blending Ptolemaic with Roman concepts, which makes it difficult to trace the cultural history of the two types of medicine. This problem arises from the primary sources themselves, since most of the medical treatises from Ptolemaic Egypt have not survived, except for a few fragments. Most Ptolemaic texts are known through references and quotations made by later writers, such as Galen, Diogenes, Celsus, or Tertullian. By grouping the sources according to particular authors as well as titles of texts, we can see a divide between the sources. The ones stemming from healers carrying on the Greek philosophical tradition of logical treatises are easier to group by the name of the author, whether attributed accurately or not. These frequently had an overlap in titles, since they may "argue" with one another over the same topics. The sources listed by their titles tend to draw more upon the traditional Egyptian style of medical texts, acting as practical manuals without necessarily an identified author. They have similarities also with the textual traditions associated with the Asklepiads, allowing them to function as bridges between Egyptian and Greek medicine. Additionally, there are modern collections of medical texts drawn from a larger body of nonmedical sources.

### Texts

The sources slotted into the traditional Greek medical treatises can be divided into two schools, the Herophileans and the Empiricists. Philinus of

25. Lang, *Medicine and Society in Ptolemaic Egypt*, 48.

Cos founded the Empiricists as an offshoot of the Herophileans in 250 BCE, but his writings, which were part of the Hippocratic corpus, have not survived. Herophilean physicians carried on for nearly three hundred years.[26]

Herophilus of Chalkedon (ca. 275 BCE) was a court physician in Alexandria who studied under Praxagoras and pioneered dissection. Scholars debate why the taboos against cutting into the human body did not apply to Herophilus. Possible reasons for it are: (1) personal choice based on the Pythagorean idea of the body as just a container for the soul; (2) Greek misunderstanding of Egyptian embalming practices; and (3) Greek disregard for Egyptian subjects as not human; therefore, taboos do not apply. Some think that Herophilus may have used criminals, but this may be a retrojection from dissection practices in early modern Europe. Through his dissections, Herophilus identified nerves as distinct organs with sensory and motor ones, named parts of the cranium, liver, and reproductive organs, which are still in use, and he discovered that the pulse originates in the heart.

Ancient authors attribute eleven treatises to Herophilus, but von Staden identifies only six of them as truly authored by Herophilus.[27] A few references from Pliny, Demosthenes, and Galen claim direct reading of Herophilus, while other writers know of Herophilus through doxographical works by writers such as Aristoxenus (*On the School of Herophilus*) and Alexander Philalethes. Herophilus wrote *On Anatomy* (only fragments exist, covering the head, reproductive organs, and vascular system), *On Pulses*, *On Midwifery*, *Therapeutics*, *Dietetics*, and *Against Common Opinions*. Doubt exists as to his authorship of the treatises *On Eyes*, *Against Hippocrates's Prognostic*, *Commentary on Hippocratic Aphorisms*, and *On Nutriment*. The latter work is now part of the Hippocratic corpus, but even ancient authors debated Herophilus's authorship. The text *Epistula Herophili ad regem Antiochum* is now known to be a medieval work.

According to Galen, Herophilus divided medicine into three sections: (1) knowledge of things related to health, dealing primarily with anatomy and physiology; (2) knowledge of things related to disease, which covers disruptions to the harmony of the body; and (3) knowledge of the neutrals, focusing on therapeutic measures encompassing pharmacology, surgery, and dietetics.[28] Although a later division, this is within the context of the clas-

26. Keyser and Irby-Massie, "Science, Medicine, and Technology," 241–64.

27. Von Staden, *Herophilus*, 72.

28. Pseudo-Galen, *Introductio sive medicus* 6 (XIV, 688K); see von Staden, *Herophilus*, 108–9.

sical and Hellenistic Greek philosophical tradition of creating knowledge taxonomies. Herophilus was never credited with writing a treatise for each of these; rather, this taxonomy can be derived from the aggregate of information found throughout his writings, such as *On Pulses* and *Midwifery*.

Erasistratus of Keos (ca. 294 BCE) was a contemporary of Herophilus who worked in Alexandria for a time, but that is not definitively known. Erasistratus supposedly also worked for the Seleucids in Antioch as well as spent time in Athens and Knidos. It is also thought that Erasistratus practiced dissections, identifying the cerebrum from the cerebellum as well as ventricles and valves of the heart. He divided medicine into different branches: therapeutics and semiotics (diagnostics), which were seen as conjectural in contrast to the scientific fields of etiology and physiology.[29] None of his writings have survived, but they are frequently referenced by later writers, such as Galen. Physicians following his methods existed as a "school" for about four hundred years. These later writers will refer to him and his disciples under the catchall "Alexandrian physicians."

Andreas of Karystos was a Herophilean who wrote *Narthex* about drugs and cosmetics, a treatise on difficult births as well as a history/genealogy of physicians. The ancient philosopher-healers Eratosthenes, Heraclides, and Soranus all questioned the accuracy of Andreas, while Celsus and Galen credited him with creating new machines to help set dislocated bones. Andreas acted as court physician to Ptolemy IV Philopater.[30] He is an interesting figure in puzzling out the relationship and argumentation between healers beyond just the philosophical differences represented by the dominant ideologies, such as Empiricism and Dogmatism.

*Oneirokritika* is the Greek term for dream books written in Demotic. Many dreams related to illness predict the onset and recovery but nothing of therapeutics. Dreams in these texts tended to be self-explanatory rather than symbolic and so did not need a specialized interpreter. In addition to dream manuals written on papyri, there are ostraca with inscriptions, such as those by Hor of Sebennytos (second century BCE), who lived and worked as a low-level official at a shrine to Thoth in Memphis. Some of his dreams related therapeutics for the queen and followed a format similar to

29. Pseudo-Galen, *Introductio sive medicus* 5; see Heinrich von Staden, "Body and Machine: Interactions between Medicine, Mechanics, and Philosophy in Early Alexandria," in *Alexandria and Alexandrianism* (Malibu, CA: J. Paul Getty Museum, 1996), 92.

30. Claire Gorteman, "Médecins de cour dans l'Égypte du IIIe siècle avant J.-C.," *Chronique d'Égypte* 32 (1957): 313–36.

the medical texts from the Pharaonic period, which include an incantation and *materia medica*.[31] Similarly, dreams relating to medical matters can be found in funerary stelae like that of Taimhotep (first century BCE).[32]

Deir el-Bahari is a funerary site, across the Nile from Luxor, for the Eighteenth-Dynasty monarch Hatshepsut (1473–1458 BCE). It was eventually abandoned but later housed a shrine for Amenhotep son of Hapy, an official from the reign of Amenhotep III, who had healing powers ascribed to him. By the reign of Ptolemy VIII Euergetes II (145–116 BCE), a shrine to Imhotep was also installed. An ostracon from 260 BCE is the first attestation of the site being used for a healing cult to Amenhotep son of Hapy. The site has five hundred inscriptions, two-thirds in Greek with the rest in Demotic. Only about fifty-five can be dated to the Ptolemaic period.[33] Most inscriptions follow the typical formula of the supplicant's name, possible occupation, and an appeal to the god, which highlights beneficent characteristics. Conspicuously, Imhotep appears only in the official hieroglyphic inscriptions and reliefs rather than the Demotic ones.[34] One particular ostracon carries the title "Instructions of Amenothes," which has Greek philosophical maxims recast as traditional Egyptian wisdom literature.[35] Although some inscriptions refer to same-day healing, others indicate there may have been incubation or at least dream interpretation carried out in conjunction with the Amenhotep shrine.[36] Definitive evidence of incubation at the site does not occur until the Roman period in the second century CE, with an inscription from the soldier Athenodoros.[37]

The inscriptions from the dual shrine are published by Latjar.[38] He breaks down the cultural characteristics of the people using the shrine, who come mostly from a status lower than those who would visit the healing shrine at Philae. Although inscriptions indicate that people appear in person, several reference a child or wife who did not come to the shrine, even though they still sought healing from Amenhotep and Imhotep.[39] Frequently, requests for healing were made through letters to the deities, which is unusual

31. Lang, *Medicine and Society in Ptolemaic Egypt*, 79.
32. Lang, *Medicine and Society in Ptolemaic Egypt*, 81.
33. Lang, *Medicine and Society in Ptolemaic Egypt*, 88–89.
34. Lang, *Medicine and Society in Ptolemaic Egypt*, 89.
35. Lang, *Medicine and Society in Ptolemaic Egypt*, 90.
36. Lang, *Medicine and Society in Ptolemaic Egypt*, 90–92.
37. Lang, *Medicine and Society in Ptolemaic Egypt*, 93.
38. Lajtar, *Deir El-Bahari in the Hellenistic and Roman Periods*.
39. Lajtar, *Deir El-Bahari in the Hellenistic and Roman Periods*, 51.

for Greek medicine but common enough in Egyptian New Kingdom practices.[40] The letters follow typical legal practices, with gods as a last-resort judge, but they also give detailed symptom descriptions.[41]

The Brooklyn Museum Papyrus,[42] written in Hieratic, lists snakes and other reptiles with the severity of their bites and includes a pharmacology. It follows the prognosis terminology of medical texts from the Pharaonic period, with the three classifications: "can be saved, nonfatal, and dies quickly." This type of encyclopedia of drugs will gain in popularity through the Roman period. Yet it had some popularity in Pharaonic medicine, as a section of the Ebers Papyrus attests.[43]

Greek papyri fragments from the Fayum, dating between the second and early third century BCE, appear to be treatises explaining the process of vision and outline surgeries on defects in the eyelid.[44] The problem with using the various papyrus fragments is that their translation and analysis overlap with the field of papyrology, so one must look beyond the study of the history of medicine to find sources. Since the 1990s, many relevant Greek papyri have been published in papyrological journals focused more on their translation and transmission than the specific content. For example, a study on the accuracy of translation from Egyptian to Greek for P. Oxy. 1381 actually had content on Imhotep-Asklepios, even though the article's author never addresses medical history.[45]

Galen refers to a text called *Euporista* written by Apollonios Mys (first century BCE), a student of Herophilus. It outlines common remedies available to those without access to an *iatros*. Such a document is a rarity that indicates a lower level on the hierarchy of resort available to people. The document sheds light on the relationship between what modern scholars call "professional" and "popular" medicine. Texts like *Euporista* would be useful for someone who is literate but not connected to a populous city containing an *iatros* or for one illiterate but with access to someone possessing reading skills.

40. Lajtar, *Deir El-Bahari in the Hellenistic and Roman Periods*, 53.

41. Lajtar, *Deir El-Bahari in the Hellenistic and Roman Periods*, 52.

42. Brooklyn Museum Papyrus 47, 218+47, 218.85, TM 58496; see Serge Sauneron, *Une traité égyptien d'ophiologie* (Le Caire: Institut française d'archéologie orientale, 1989).

43. Ebers 251.

44. P. Univ. Giss. 4.44 (MP³ 2375); see Marie-Hélène Marganne, *La chirurgie dans l'Égypte Gréco-Romaine d'après les papyrus littéraires Grecs* (Boston: Brill, 1998), 1–12.

45. Caroline Disler, "Oxyrhynchus 1381," *Target: International Journal of Translation Studies* 24 (2012): 225–52.

The Zenon Archive is a collection of papyri made by Zenon, who was in the employ of Apollonios, a financial administrator under Ptolemy II. The records span from 267 to 229 BCE, mentioning various physicians from Philadelphia in the Fayum who also have connections with Alexandria.[46] Some of the referenced physicians come from cities outside Ptolemaic Egypt, such as Rhodes or Cos. All of the healers have Greek names and were trained in Greek medicine, with no indication of incorporating traditional Egyptian medicine. Many of the letters indicate that an *iatros* was often involved in political matters beyond the physical care of the king and his court. It is interesting to note that this echoes the *swnw* accomplices of the harem plots from Pharaonic Egypt.

Apart from the Zenon Archive, letters from physicians as well as nonmedical people often refer to illnesses and can be a valuable resource. Some letters are requests for medical supplies, such as honey from Attica or wine from Lesbos, indicating not only *materia medica* but that there are preferred types of ingredients for the pharmacology. It is not clear whether these are thought to have a special property imbued by the location, making it a necessity for the prescription, essentially a charged substance for a physical rite, or whether these are just thought to be better quality, even though honey or wine from anywhere would actually suffice. One letter in Greek speaks of someone learning Egyptian writing and who will be employed by a healer specializing in enemas (likely the Greek approximation of the Egyptian title "Shepherd of the Anus").[47] Court letters also reveal the role of physicians, including the rare title *basilikos iatros* or "King's Physician," which parallels previous Pharaonic titles.[48] Some *iatroi* were involved in court intrigues, such as the assassination plot of Arsinoe. It is not clear the extent that these individuals acted as practicing *iatroi* or whether the Greek term simply functioned as a ranking title. This parallels the problem with the Egyptian title *swnw*.[49]

Two modern collections of Greco-Roman texts categorized as magical provide primary sources relating to medical issues: *Papyri Graecae Magicae* (*PGM*) and *Papyri Demoticae Magicae* (*PDM*). These texts range in date from the second century BCE to the fifth century CE. Many likely came from The-

46. Lang, *Medicine and Society in Ptolemaic Egypt*, 223.

47. UPZ I 148 = TM 3540; see Lang, *Medicine and Society in Ptolemaic Egypt*, 205.

48. R. S. Bagnall and P. Derow, eds. and trans., *The Hellenistic Period: Historical Sources in Translation* (Malden, MA: Blackwell, 2004).

49. Schol. in Theocr. XVII 128; see Gorteman, "Médecins de cour dans l'Égypte."

bes but do incorporate other areas of Egypt. Initial publication of the *PGM* omitted Demotic texts, while subsequent publications[50] reinstated the mixed used of Greek and Demotic, revealing a much closer relationship between Egyptian religion and the influx of Greek traditions. A few of the spells also contain a mixture of Babylonian, Jewish, and Christian religious elements in addition to the Greco-Egyptian ones. The *PGM* texts often call for a magical phrase or symbols written on papyrus and bound to the patient.[51] The *PDM* cases frequently invoke the gods either to provide therapy through a dream or to vanquish an enemy causing the ailment. Some also provide instruction for writing out a papyrus that is to be used as an amulet. Interestingly, these prescriptions acknowledge a cultural overlap in the origin of diseases as well as the use of different languages in therapeutic speech.

> To heal evil eye in a man: "Oh Amoun, this lofty male, this male of Ethiopia, who came down from Meroe to Egypt and who found my son Horus hurrying on his feet. He beat him on his head with three spells in the Ethiopian language. When he finds NN, whom NN bore, he will hurry on his feet, and he will beat him on his head with three spells in the Ethiopian language: *GENTINI tentina qyqybi akkhe akha*."[52]

This is an acknowledgment that the gods, despite hellenization, still prefer other languages for curing certain cases.

## Archaeology

Ptolemy made the city of Alexandria his capital in 311 BCE after a brief tenure in Memphis. The city had five zones, with the western one predominantly occupied by Egyptians and known in Egyptian as Rhakotis; this area housed the Sarapeion founded by Ptolemy III, replacing a smaller shrine to Isis and Sarapis. But it was not frequented as much as the one nearby in Kanopos.[53] No asklepieion existed in Alexandria. There is also no evidence of Egyptians working or studying at either the museum or the library.

50. Hans Dieter Betz, ed., *The Greek Magical Papyri in Translation, Including the Demotic Spells*, 2nd ed. (Chicago: University of Chicago Press, 1996).

51. *PGM* VII.193–214; see Betz, *Greek Magical Papyri*, 120–21.

52. *PDM* XIV.1097–1103; see Betz, *Greek Magical Papyri*, 247.

53. Richard A. Tomlinson, "From Houses to Tenements: Domestic Architecture in Hellenistic Alexandria," *British School at Athens Studies* 15 (2007): 307–11.

The museum essentially was a temple of the Muses (*mouseion*), founded by Ptolemy I Soter. Strabo described it as being a part of the palace complex, with a lecture hall and a common dining room.[54] The Ptolemaic kings appointed a priest of the Muses to oversee the museum. Assertions from early scholarship assume a close connection between the museum and Alexandrian physicians.[55] Yet no evidence exists of medical studies or Herophilus himself working at the museum in Alexandria. A second-century BCE inscription from Delos contains a reference to Chrysermus, with the titles "Superintendent of the Physicians" and "Supervisor of the Museum."[56] This inscription provides too scant information to determine whether this person was a practicing healer/theorist or simply an administrator without any medical training or knowledge.

When building the Temple to the Muses complex, Ptolemy I Soter charged the peripatetic[57] Demetrius of Phalerum (350–280 BCE) to build an extensive library in 295 BCE, the famed Library of Alexandria. As the library grew, a branch was created at the Sarapeion. Lang claims that the library was "closely connected to the best-known and most influential forms of medicine in Alexandria: that of the anatomists, the subsequent 'sects,' and the court physicians."[58] Other than likely containing copies of their treatises, as well as of other philosophers such as Aristotle, there is no clear evidence of a direct connection between them, which Lang later admits in the same work.[59]

The library was likely destroyed in 48 BCE by a fire that swept through Alexandria during a civil war between the forces of Julius Caesar/Cleopatra VII and her brother Ptolemy XIII. The Sarapeion branch survived until 391 CE, when Emperor Theodosius I in his zeal for Christianity ordered the destruction of all temples.

The Egyptian city of Memphis, originally founded in 2925 BCE, frequently served as a capital during the Dynastic period. Galen noted the Sanctuary to Hephaistos[60] as the birthplace of several pharmaceutical practices. The Sarapeion in Memphis dates from the fourth or third century BCE and remained in use until its Christian repurposing in the fifth to sixth century

54. Strabo, *Geography* 17.793–94.

55. Gorteman, "Médecins de cour dans l'Égypte."

56. Von Staden, *Herophilus*, 27.

57. Peripatetics are the philosophical disciples of Aristotle. Demetrius of Phalerum was from the first generation of peripatetics and may have been a student of Aristotle himself.

58. Lang, *Medicine and Society in Ptolemaic Egypt*, 249.

59. Lang, *Medicine and Society in Ptolemaic Egypt*, 258.

60. The Greeks syncretized their craftsman god Hephaistos with the Egyptian equivalent Ptah, who served as the patron deity for Memphis since its founding.

CE.[61] Although built on an already existing and sizable temple to Osiris-Apis, it had a much more Greek-styled entrance (in comparison to Alexandria). Its main function was to house the body of the sacrificed Apis bull. It is thought to be the only Sarapeion in Ptolemaic Egypt that did incubation, but no definitive evidence exists that sleeping at the temple was carried out for the purpose of healing dreams. An inscription attests to someone named Kres who could give dream interpretations in Greek.[62] The incubation practices at Memphis are used by scholars to suggest that similar therapies were carried out at other shrines around Egypt.

The ancient necropolis nearby, called Saqqara, also had a temple dedicated to Imhotep, which we know about from textual references, but it has yet to be found. This temple had an asklepieion attached to it, in which incubation was practiced. This is attested in letters and ostraca. Like its Greek counterpart, this sanctuary would accommodate visitors for days at a time.[63] Since the temple to Imhotep has not been found, it is difficult to see its physical proximity to the Sarapeion. An ibis gallery dedicated to Thoth has yielded finds significant to the history of Ptolemaic medicine, such as plaster casts or perhaps votives of body parts, such as torsos, legs, and hands. It is not clear whether these are practice casts from a workshop near the asklepieion.[64] Pharaonic medicine did not use votives, but they were common enough in classical Greece that the practice may have been imported, indicating that a hellenized population coming from as far as the Fayum used the shrine.

Texts in Demotic, Hieratic, Aramaic, and Greek from Memphis's West Dump argue against a purely Greek population. Within the four hieratic documents, one fragment of a medical papyri dating from the Persian period contains recipes and incantations.[65] A similar Ptolemaic-era medical fragment in Demotic was found at the South Dump.[66] Another document is a plea to Osiris-Apis concerning the behavior of a priest of Imhotep.[67] An adjacent building might have been an incubation site.[68]

61. Geoffrey T. Martin, *The Sacred Animal Necropolis at Saqqâra: The Southern Dependencies of the Main Temple Complex* (London: Egyptian Exploration Society, 1981), 1.

62. Lang, *Medicine and Society in Ptolemaic Egypt*, 69.

63. Lang, *Medicine and Society in Ptolemaic Egypt*, 75.

64. Lang, *Medicine and Society in Ptolemaic Egypt*, 76.

65. Martin, *Sacred Animal Necropolis at Saqqâra*, 62.

66. 72/3-DP17+56; see Martin, *Sacred Animal Necropolis at Saqqâra*, 57.

67. 71/2-DP146. Martin does not provide a translation but indicates that one was being prepared by H. S. Smith; see Martin, *Sacred Animal Necropolis at Saqqâra*, 62.

68. Lang, *Medicine and Society in Ptolemaic Egypt*, 73n108.

Near Aswan, Ptolemy VI Philometor (186–145 BCE) began construction on a temple dedicated to Horus and Sobek, known as Kom Ombo. Its wall relief shows many devices bearing a strong resemblance to known Roman surgical instruments. This is rather striking since no surgical instruments from the Pharaonic period have been discovered, and there is no depiction in wall reliefs or paintings from the Pharaonic period of surgery or surgical instruments. Images of castration are the only exception, but they show only a basic knife rather than a unique implement for medical procedures.

Egyptians used the dual shrine of Imhotep and Amenhotep at Deir el-Bahari from the early third century BCE until its abrupt stop in 162 CE.[69] Scholars speculate that people practiced incubation at Deir el-Bahari based on an inscription from Polyaratos and one from Athenodoros, which indicates the specific location of the Bark Shrine as a site of healing. This is seen as comparable to practices at the temple of Imhotep in Memphis.[70] At the dual shrine, somatic practices were also used in conjunction with more ritualistic ones, such as the drinking of Syrian fig juice and consumption of the figs with bread while wearing an iron snake on the arm. Use of a snake charm has antecedents in both Asklepian medicine as well as in the worship of Theban goddess Meretseger, patron deity of the necropolis at Deir el-Medina.[71]

The island of Philae in the Nile at the first cataract has an extensive temple complex dedicated mostly to Isis. Its earliest construction dates to the reign of Taharqa (690–664 BCE), with building continuing until the reign of Emperor Diocletian (284–305 CE). Active worship of Isis at the site was eventually abandoned during the reign of Justinian (ca. 535 CE). Most of its buildings were created under the Ptolemies and then greatly embellished by Roman emperors. Although the original site is now flooded by the Aswan High Damn, the buildings were moved to Agilkia. Apart from Isis's connection to healing, there is also a shrine to Imhotep, built during the reign of Ptolemy V (204–180 BCE), and an earlier birth house for Ptolemy VI (180–145 BCE), with reliefs for Augustus (30 BCE–41 CE) and Tiberias (14–37 CE).

Various small shrines throughout Egypt can also provide valuable archaeological evidence for the history of medicine. Kanopos, just east of Al-

69. Lajtar, *Deir El-Bahari in the Hellenistic and Roman Periods*, 37.

70. Lajtar, *Deir El-Bahari in the Hellenistic and Roman Periods*, 53.

71. Lajtar, *Deir El-Bahari in the Hellenistic and Roman Periods*, 54.

exandria, had a significant healing shrine to Sarapis. To date, little excavation has been done in the area. Incubation may have been used at Kanopos[72] but possibly only in a later Roman period. Strabo reports that a stone stela with *iamata* attests to the power of the gods, while omitting the typical symptom description normally written with them.[73] If *iamata* were present at Kanopos, it is also likely that letters were deposited there, too.[74] The city of Ptolemais Hermeiou contained an asklepieion but followed the architectural layout of an Egyptian-style temple to Imhotep rather than the Greek form found at temples in Epidauros or Kos.[75]

One of the most important artifacts relating to the study of medicine is the cippus[76] statue, which depicts the child Horus standing on crocodiles and holding other dangerous, even poisonous animals. Texts accompanying the image recount the tale of Isis, hiding in the marshes from Seth, calling out to the Boat of Eternity on behalf of the sick. They include Horus and Thoth's spells for healing the child Horus, which end with the line "and the protection of the afflicted as well." This phrase extends the god's healing of Horus to any supplicant. The ritual with the *cippus* involved the afflicted person drinking or bathing in the water after it had been poured over the statue. This practice evolved from Egyptian religion during the Late period, since the *cippi* predate Ptolemaic control of Egypt; it does not seem to be connected to any form of Greek rituals involving water or incubations. Most famous is the Metternich Stela from the reign of Nectonebo II (360–342 BCE). Smaller *cippi* may have been used in a domestic setting rather than temple contexts.[77] Ideologically, it is easy to transfer concepts used with the *cippi*, plus long-standing tradition of dream interpretation, to the ritual of incubation associated with Asklepios. The inscriptions at Deir el-Bahari referring to both Amenhotep and Asklepios indicate just such a conflation of ideas.[78]

72. Lang, *Medicine and Society in Ptolemaic Egypt*, 67.

73. Strabo, *Geography* 17.1, 17.

74. Lajtar, *Deir El-Bahari in the Hellenistic and Roman Periods*, 56.

75. Lang, *Medicine and Society in Ptolemaic Egypt*, 57.

76. Pl. *cippi*.

77. Lang, *Medicine and Society in Ptolemaic Egypt*, 96.

78. J. Grafton Milne, "The Sanatorium of Dêr el-Baḥri," *Journal of Egyptian Archaeology* 1 (1914): 96–98.

## Cultural Concepts

### Anatomy and Physiology

There were no major shifts in anatomical and physiological concepts from those that dominated the Greek world of the fourth century but rather a refinement of some of the arguments based on more accurate anatomical knowledge.[79] Just as anatomy and physiology in ancient Greece could not be described with one dominant viewpoint, so too must the concepts in Ptolemaic medicine be understood by looking at seminal figures. Herophilus and Erasistratus are often credited as "fathers of anatomy" because of their reputations of human vivisection and dissection,[80] whereas previous and subsequent works depended on animal dissections as analogous to humans. Alexandria offered a unique opportunity to practice dissection and vivisection against the entrenched taboos found elsewhere in the Greek world. Similarly, the traditional Egyptian prohibitions on human dissection were initially suspended by the Ptolemies, and only with the increased power of the Egyptians did their taboos reassert themselves. It is not clear how the belief on the independence of organs or lack thereof impacted the practice of dissection. The *iatros* embracing a synonymous relationship between a person and his body may see dissection as a viable method of understanding that connection. But if the *iatros* does see body parts and the person as separate entities, then dissection could be excused on the grounds that it does not disturb the person/soul who no longer resides in the body. As for Egyptian cultural objections, the body will still function as a vessel for the person/soul after death, so it needs to remain intact to a certain extent. The rise of the Empiricist school additionally undercut the practice.[81] Thus, only a brief window of time in the third century BCE allowed for Herophilus and Erasistratus to practice dissection and vivisection on humans.

The organization of Herophilus's *On Anatomy* starts with the head; he believed that the brain is the governing principle of the body, which generated the nerves. From here, the digestive tract, reproductive organs, and fetus develop, followed by the vascular system. Herophilus added to the no-

79. Marganne, *La chirurgie dans l'Égypte Gréco-Romaine d'après les papyrus littéraires Grecs*, 158.

80. G. E. R. Lloyd, *Greek Science after Aristotle* (New York: W. W. Norton, 1973); and Porter, *Greatest Benefit to Mankind*.

81. Von Staden, *Herophilus*, 151.

menclature of the brain identifying the ventricles and their impact on limb movement. He likely understood the difference between motor and sensory nerves and correctly identified the optic nerve. While Herophilus wrote the most accurate physical description of the liver, Erasistratus correctly described its function in the creation of bile. Herophilus did not argue for the liver as the seat of the vascular system but assessed the absorption process of the hepatic portal vein.[82] This created a significant shift in the Greco-Roman understanding of the function of the liver. Herophilus, according to Galen, kept to the basic humoral theory espoused by Hippocrates and Praxagoras: "four faculties were said by Herophilus to govern living beings."[83] Yet the term "faculties" may also refer to types of pulses, as noted by von Staden.[84] Documents indicating that Herophilus rejected humoral theory appear to be forgeries dating to the Renaissance.[85]

Herophilus broke with the tradition of ascribing two chambers to the uterus; thus, gender was not determined by generation of the fetus in the right or left chamber. Herophilus kept to the idea that female anatomy was analogous to the male body, so the fallopian tubes were thought to have the same function as the sperm ducts. His description of these structures also argued against the ability of the womb to wander,[86] as in Hippocratic medicine. This undermines the older cultural idea of body parts as distinct entities with varying relationships between humans and gods. As we shall see, the development of the idea of involuntary movement starts to explain how organs behave mechanistically apart from relationships with humans and gods.

Hellenistic physicians debated the origins of the vascular system in either the brain or the heart. Herophilus maintained the theory of his teacher Praxagoras that vessels emerging from the right ventricle of the heart are veins, while those from the left ventricle are arteries, with the exception of the pulmonary artery situated on the right. This demonstrates the dominance of cultural values concerning left and right and the belief in the universe organized on the principle of opposites, even in the face of contradictory evidence. Erasistratus gave the most complete description of heart valves.

Based on anatomical structures of the brain, Herophilus ascribed bodily control to the hindbrain. This is in keeping with early theories of Alcmaeon

82. Von Staden, *Herophilus*, 181.

83. Galen, *De pulsuum dignotione* 2.3 (VIII, 870K); see von Staden, *Herophilus*, 311.

84. Von Staden, *Herophilus*, 243n4.

85. Von Staden, *Herophilus*, 244–45.

86. Von Staden, "Body and Machine," 87.

of Croton, as well as Egyptian medical texts, noting that head trauma can result in paralysis in limbs. He differs from these predecessors by more specifically locating areas of the brain connected to movement and sensory perception, as well as identifying the connection of nerves to the brain. This does stand in marked contrast to Aristotelian theory that the brain serves only a cooling function. He understood both motor and sensory nerves and described how the optic nerve worked by allowing pneuma to flow between the eyes and the brain, but he is not clear whether all sensory nerves functioned by flow of pneuma from the brain. There is no indication a similar form of pneuma allowed motor nerves to work. Giving a detailed physiology for perception seemed more important than motion. This would be in keeping with the Hellenistic cultural value toward the preeminence of the mind/philosophy as opposed to an idealized physicality. The mind perceiving the work of the gods has greater importance in the cultural sphere of the *iatros* than the body being in a physical state acceptable to the gods, as it would for a priest. Nerves, particularly motor nerves, caused voluntary motion and included muscles and ligaments, whereas involuntary movement was attributed to the arteries; observations of the pulse reinforced this position. None of the surviving fragments indicate how Herophilus reconciled the brain's prominence in pathophysiology with humoral theory.

Aristotle and Plato ascribed a vital role to the heart and its innate heat in the physiology of respiration, but Herophilus departed from this line of thought, disconnecting the movement of the heart and lungs. He understood the thorax and lungs as having their own natural, involuntary movement of expansion and contraction.[87] Dilation of the lungs sucks in outside air, or inhalation. The lungs then contract as the thorax dilates, which forces the pneuma into the thorax. It is at this point that pneuma can enter the arteries. The arteries seem to have their own cycle of expansion and contraction, which draws in the pneuma from the thorax. When the thorax is filled, the excess pneuma then flows back into the lungs. The lungs then contract, expelling the pneuma back outside as exhalation. With every breath, the lungs expand and contract twice, while the thorax only has one cycle of expansion and contraction. For this system to work, Herophilus suggests an imperceptible expansion and contraction of the lungs prior to the visible expansion of the thorax and another imperceptible expansion and contraction of the lungs just before the visible contraction of the thorax during exhalation. This derives from the theoretical position of involuntary movements rather

87. Aëtius Doxographus, *Placita* 4.22.3 (DG, 413–14); see von Staden, *Herophilus*, 320–21.

than being solely grounded in the observation of the body during breathing. It may impact ideas as to how body parts maintain relationships to each other by reducing it to a mechanistic process and in turn influence choice of healers.

Herophilus claimed that the arteries also contain blood, not exclusively pneuma. Blood carries nutrients, by the process of digestion, which both arteries and veins need, but the arteries have the capacity to expand and contract unlike veins; thus, the arteries will better absorb the blood/nutrients. Yet oddly, since the veins contain more blood, they actually better distribute nutrients to the body.[88] This theory seems to give a greater ideological value to things that can expand and contract rather than being passive. Yet taking certain agreed-upon facts to their logical conclusion creates a strange disconnect between veins and arteries in their role of delivering nutrients.

Herophilus coined the terms systole and diastole for the movements of the arteries, drawing indirectly from Aristoxenus's musical theory of time and meter.[89] Herophilus recognized the pulse as a constant function of the body, in agreement with Aristotle. Yet Aristotle linked the heart and lungs as the source of the pulse, with which Herophilus disagreed. This more neutral stance on pulsation differs from other Greek medical texts that see it as a sign of pathology, as Erasistratus did. Herophilus's theory linking the pulse with the heart contradicts Praxagoras, who thought the arteries had an innate pulsation. If the arteries had an innate pulse, then this would explain spasms and tremors and could be classified under the same physiological processes. The linking of the pulse to the heart then removed spasms and tremors from the vascular system and allowed Herophilus to categorize them with the physiology of nerves and muscles and then understand them as pathological involuntary movement of the voluntary motor nerves. Such an ideology pushes the role of the gods further into the background. Spasms and tremors become less likely a direct communication from the gods.

Herophilus's theory of spermatogenesis is in keeping with Aristotle's in that sperm derives from the blood. This is in contrast to other theories claiming generation from the brain or a constituent of all body parts. The anatomical justification for blood being the origin of sperm came from the observation that blood vessels contain a greater amount of blood further from the genitalia, but as they get closer, the blood changes to a milkier,

88. Anonymus Londinensis; see von Staden, *Herophilus*, 265.

89. Von Staden, *Herophilus*, 278–79.

seed-colored substance.[90] This differs from Aristotle in that the testes play a role in refining the sperm. Herophilus notes that the fetus has involuntary movements, especially a pulse, but that it is incapable of voluntary movement; hence, its nerves are not fully connected to the brain. This position is in contrast to the Aristotelian view that sentience is the contributing factor from the father and present in the fetus.

In contrast to many of the theories of Herophilus, the work of Erasistratus did not follow the dominant humoral theory. He had a mechanistic theory of physiology likely influenced by the work of Strato of Lampsakos, an Atomist, as reported by Diogenes Laertius.[91] This meant that his theories did not rely on invisible "faculties" as a driving force for physiological processes. Erasistratus worked with the understanding that all systems within the body are integrated, which is closer to the more traditional Egyptian physiological view.[92] He followed the Peripatetic/Aristotelian teleological idea of the body, holding that all organs serve a purpose. These ideas both allow room for illness as a form of communication from the gods and minimize the divine role in healing.

Erasistratus dismissed the idea of a single, continuous void (as advocated by Epicurus and contra Herophilus, who claimed there was no real void) and held rather that void was created by particles not fitting together, thus creating gaps, which is more akin to the theories of Strato of Lampsakos.[93] Matter will always fill the void. So within the body, its own fluids will fill the void.

He acknowledged the difference between sensory and motor nerves but refined its theory by demonstrating their connection to the brain and spinal cord. Erasistratus's overall physiology described the body as made up of a weave of veins, arteries, and nerves, with the heart working as a bellows pump.[94] This perspective was likely based upon the water pump of Ktesibios. Following Praxagoras, Erasistratus claimed that the left ventricle contains pneuma, passing it to arteries, while the right ventricle contained blood, thus connecting it to the veins. The bleeding of arteries came from the loss of pneuma, which attracts blood from the veins through capillary action.[95] Excess blood in the veins also leaks into arteries, which blocks the flow of the

90. Vindicianus, *Fragmentum Bruxellense de semine* I, e 6–16; see von Staden, *Herophilus*, 363–64.

91. Diogenes Laertius, *Lives of the Philosophers* 5.57–58.

92. Von Staden, "Body and Machine," 92.

93. Von Staden, "Body and Machine, 85–106.

94. Keyser and Irby-Massie, "Science, Medicine, and Technology," 252–53.

95. Keyser and Irby-Massie, "Science, Medicine, and Technology," 252–53.

pneuma causing disease. Erasistratus saw pulsation of the arteries as a sign of the disease process. Cutting an artery allows pneuma to escape, which draws blood from the veins, leading him to posit the existence of capillaries. He did keep to the idea of respiration as a cooling function connected to the heart, by outlining the trachea as drawing in air, passing it to the heart through bronchi (a form of arteries) and the pulmonary vein, then out from the left ventricle to the arteries throughout the body.[96] All pneuma throughout the body arises from the outside.[97]

## Disease Etiology

In keeping with classical Greek medicine, Ptolemaic physicians writing treatises moved away from the idea that diseases were a direct, personal message from supernatural entities. Instead, they saw the disease as a disruption in a regular, impersonal system established by the gods. How exactly this process worked was up for debate among the different philosophical schools. Some held to the humor theory, with the imbalance of substances causing disease. Others focused more on the movement of particular substances through the body, such as blood. This created a body of literature discussing the relationship between diagnostic signs and disease etiology. Specialists were needed to properly read and interpret these physical signs, but they did not need a special religious function or connection to the gods, like a priest or prophet, to give them authority. Precise observation and logic connected the *iatros* to the gods, while writing the treatises gave them authority.

Erasistratus thought that an excess of blood passing from the veins to the arteries disrupted the flow of other substances and thus caused diseases.[98] From this position, he maintained that the pulse itself was a sign of disease. Herophilus, though, espoused that the pulse was a natural movement and used variations in it as a diagnostic tool to discern an underlying disease process. The rapidity of the pulse in conjunction with the patient's internal temperature indicated fever.[99] He developed a portable water clock in order to accurately time the pulse. He could also adjust the timing of the clock to

96. Galen, *De usu respirationis* 2 (IV, 473–84K).

97. Galen, *De usu respirationis* 1 (IV, 471K).

98. Galen (V, 123K); see von Staden, *Herophilus*, 243.

99. Fever itself was a disease and not necessarily just a symptom, as modern medicine treats it.

match the age of the patient, since he held that the natural pulse rate varied between infants, children, adults, and geriatrics.[100]

But Herophilus did not rely on a purely mechanistic disease etiology. He identified a mental disorder, phrenitis, as caused by one of three types of dreams: (1) a dream sent by a god (contra Aristotle); (2) natural dreams, which are formed by the soul; and (3) the mixed dream, which has both external and internal stimuli, such as seeing something that then creates a desire in the soul.[101] There is no evidence that Herophilus went beyond just classifying dreams and used these etiologies in any type of therapeutic practices. But his outlining of such classifications shows that disease as direct communication from the divine still had a place in Hellenistic medical culture. By acknowledging that certain types of diseases arise from dreams, it gives space for particular healing strategies to also come directly from the gods through dreams. The *iatros* and the *asklepiad* could work in conjunction.

In contrast to the humoral theory, some Ptolemaic physicians understood diseases as stemming from food residues left in the body, a theory first developed among Knidian healers. The abundance of purgatives in Egyptian medical texts, coupled with a reference by Herodotus to such practices, makes it easy for later Ptolemaic Greeks and Roman-era writers, such as Diodorus Siculus and Anonymus Londinensis, to assume that Egyptian medicine worked on a similar principle to either residues or the humoral theory.

This brings up a debate among modern scholars about the relationship of the Egyptian substance *wḫdw* to Greek concepts of residues.[102] Lang criticizes modern scholars who see an Egyptian influence on classical Greek medicine via a Knidian school; she calls into question even the existence of such schools.[103] Although it is highly unlikely that Greek, especially Knidian medicine, directly borrowed Egyptian practices prior to the Ptolemaic period, it is not unreasonable to see, during and after the Ptolemaic period, a trafficking of disease concepts and therapies based on the similarity of Greek humoral theory or residues to the Egyptian idea of good health depending on the regular flow of substances through the *mtw* vessels. Likely, the similarity between the two cultures arose from a convergent evolution of ideas rather than a direct influence.

100. Marcellinus, *De pulsibus* 1; see von Staden, *Herophilus*, 353–54.

101. Von Staden, *Herophilus*, 306–7.

102. Lang, *Medicine and Society in Ptolemaic Egypt*, 115.

103. Lang, *Medicine and Society in Ptolemaic Egypt*, 117–19; contra Jacques Jouanna, *Greek Medicine from Hippocrates to Galen* (Boston: Brill, 2012) and Jacques Jouanna, *Hippocrates*, trans. M. B. DeBevoise (Baltimore: Johns Hopkins University Press, 1999); Nutton, *Ancient Medicine*, 74.

Lang compares the literary styling of disease coming like an arrow, citing references to both Sekhmet and Apollo, but sees the Egyptians as different, with an underlying concept of an outside active agent causing the disease, ranging from the mysterious semen of an incubus as the cause of the ʿ3ʿ disease to the more mundane infiltration of worms.[104] This is in contrast to the outside agent simply being the weather or foodstuffs, passive entities, which create an imbalance of humors in Greek medicine. Although classical-Greek disease etiology uses the idea of active external forces, it does appear in the texts that Ptolemaic medicine prefers a passive, predictable external force. This may be linked to the Ptolemaic dynasty separating themselves from the traditional Egyptian power structure grounded in the temples, governing on their own Greek authority. In turn, this created a culture for others, like the *iatros*, to also carve out a niche of authority divorced from religious power structures, even within the rest of Hellenistic society.

Lang's study points out the overlap in physical and metaphysical categories for Egyptian medicine, thus undermining the old science-magic dichotomy of earlier works on the history of medicine. Yet the distinction between active and passive agents as the difference between Egyptian and Greek medicine only shifts the emphasis while still depicting the Egyptians as engaging in magical thinking—the idea that disease vectors have volition. Scholars need to determine to what extent Greek medicine followed the same ideology. Passages about the wandering womb in the Hippocratic corpus indicate that organs can act of their own will but, even then, seem to be automatically responding to environmental conditions, such as dryness, within the body. The question then becomes to what extent the Egyptians similarly saw such active agents as ghosts and worms automatically responding to a situation compelled by their nature to attack rather than attacking from a conscious choice. We simply lack an Egyptian explanation for why the "active external agents" behave the way they do.

To follow Lang's distinction of active agents, then, a difference does exist. The Greeks understood that the gods manifested their work in a regular manner, perceived and affected by humans through natural philosophy, of which medicine is a subset, whereas the Egyptians did not explicitly claim the gods worked within a static, natural framework; rather, their ever-changing volition is the active agent. But still their actions and even motives can be perceived and influenced by the use of *heka* (access to power), which is its own predictable system. Despite the focus on active agents, Lang does

104. Lang, *Medicine and Society in Ptolemaic Egypt*, 108–10.

concede that Egyptian healers' "knowledge and authority is portrayed as dependent on consultations of eternally true and canonical texts."[105] Both Greek and Egyptian cultures held a middle course between what actions of the gods were knowable and not knowable; being able to distinguish the two categories and the work between them made healers unique personages in their respective societies.

## Restoration of Health

The more mechanistic the explanatory model of illness, the more available it becomes to the populace. Observation and logic can lead to democratization, even if that was not the intended outcome of the *iatros*, since for them only certain people, essentially blessed by the gods with the necessary mind, can undertake a proper study. Basic principles rather than specialized techniques allow almost anyone access to power in a new way. The complexity of the diagnosis and therapeutics in the treatises help to retard the tendency of democratization. Yet even the *iatros* at times would still embrace the more traditional reliance on communication with the gods.

Early Empiricists espoused a threefold view of signs for diagnosis: (1) Present symptoms allow the healer to understand the present condition. (2) Past symptoms indicate the patient's history and possible causes. (3) Future symptoms refer to the possible course of the disease and hopefully to the cure, indicated by treatment of previous patients. In contrast, later Empiricists depended on the study of symptoms to provide therapeutics.

Herophilus advocated treating both the symptoms and the cause, thus blurring the lines between etiology and therapeutics. His therapies included diet for both symptoms and preventative care, while exercise was just preventative medicine. He likely wrote a treatise titled *Therapeutics*, as reported by Caelius Aurelianus, espousing four general ideas: (1) remedies based on the position, color, and sensation of instrumental parts of the body, which are organs such as the heart, liver, eyes, or even a finger; (2) allopathy or treatment by opposites as a carryover of more traditional practices; (3) drug treatments that were acknowledged as "hands of gods"[106] rather than just purely the healer's skill or an inherent quality of the *materia medica*; and

105. Lang, *Medicine and Society in Ptolemaic Egypt*, 132.

106. Marcellus, "*Epistula Cornelii Celsi*" *De medicamentis* (*CML* 5.36); see von Staden, *Herophilus*, 417.

(4) venesection,[107] which had gained prominence since the fourth century BCE with healers such as Hippocrates and Praxagoras. The only evidences of Herophilus performing surgery, not counting dissection, are cases of tooth extractions and bloodletting, apart from a single abortion referred to by Tertullian.[108] Caelius Aurelianus reported that Erasistratus performed surgery to expose the liver and apply medication directly to it in order to relieve an illness.[109] This would have been highly unusual for the time and therefore a suspect account.

There is no indication that the somatic treatments in the older Egyptian medical texts, such as the Edwin Smith Papyrus, were abandoned. Thus, these therapies still conveyed obedience to the gods through physical rites and charged substances while maintaining cohesion among the human community. A significant cultural difference existed in that Egyptian medical practitioners did not use venesection, presumably because religious taboos about cutting into the body still held. Compound drugs, a feature of Pharaonic medicine, may have influenced Alexandrian physicians, because the advent of polypharmacy in Greek medicine occurred within the Ptolemaic period. Some attribute this to Herophilus and Mantias. Although Egyptian texts give a proportional relationship of ingredients, they do not precisely describe dosages. Greek texts prior to the advent of compound drugs lacked both ingredient measures and dosage. Although Ptolemaic medicine and later Hellenistic and Roman recipes adopted polypharmacy, hence measurements, the dosage amounts continued to be vague, since they would depend on other factors of the illness particular to each patient.

Both Greek and Egyptian therapies relied on a theory of similarity or homeopathy for the effectiveness of some drugs, such as the use of an ostrich shell mirroring the skull in a head wound.[110] Yet a system of allopathy or opposites was also applied when determining drug treatments, such as *materia medica* that cools the body in response to an illness caused by excess heat, as in *Regimen* in the Hippocratic corpus. Similarly, the Chester Beatty VI Papyrus includes prescriptions for cooling enemas.

Lang calls into question the accuracy of the ancient Greek perception that Egyptians relied on purgatives more than any other somatic treatment,

107. Galen, *De venae sectione adversus Erasistratum* 5 (XI, 162–3K); see von Staden, *Herophilus*, 412–13.

108. Von Staden, *Herophilus*, 403.

109. Caelius Aurelius, *Chronic Diseases* 3.4.65 (*CML* 6.1, 2.716.29–32 Bendz).

110. Edwin Smith Papyrus, case no. 9.

in contrast to Greek practices and its role in preventative medicine, which dovetails nicely with the Greek preconception of a healthy balance based on diet.[111] Yet without a comprehensive quantitative analysis of how often purgatives appear in both Greek and Egyptian medical texts, it is difficult to assess exactly how often one culture used purgatives over another, at least in a therapeutic context rather than a preventative one.[112] Even with such an analysis, there may be a disconnection between the frequency in written texts and in actual practice that our present historical evidence cannot illuminate. Modern scholarship is left with the ancient Greek view, though a pejorative one, that Egyptians employed purgatives more often than any other society with a significant medical culture.

Greek writers criticized the Egyptian use of dreckapothecary, although the Greeks themselves used it, mostly for gynecological matters. It is possible, though, that the Egyptians did not use real feces, but rather these are coded words within the recipes to prevent the average scribe from dubiously entering the ranks of more professional healers, such as the *swnw* or *wab* priest. Herophilus would use crocodile dung in some prescriptions,[113] likely a borrowing from Egyptian practices, even if a misunderstanding of coded texts. Dreckapothecary had an increase through the Roman period, including Galen, which indicates that it may have originally been misused at the folk level of healing but evolved into an accepted component of the professional healer's *materia medica*. Conversely, opium may have been introduced into Egyptian medical practices by the Greeks, since cultivated fields appeared in the Fayum starting in the third century BCE.[114]

Healing centers such as the asklepieion in Epidauros would see pilgrimages from the farthest cities in classical Greece. Yet, in Ptolemaic Egypt, places of healing such as Memphis would only serve a more local population. Most likely, this is due to the fact that the hellenized world still had the traditional Greek centers, in addition to the Egyptian ones now brought into the sphere of Greek influence. Non-Egyptians would more likely seek healing at a larger, more established asklepieion. The indigenous Egyptian population would either continue to use their traditional healing practices close to home or adopt Greek medicine that was brought into their area. For them, there

111. Lang, *Medicine and Society in Ptolemaic Egypt*, 161.

112. Lang is correct in pointing out that the Egyptian texts never prescribe a purgative to prevent illness, contrary to Herodotus's claim; see Lang, *Medicine and Society in Ptolemaic Egypt*, 162.

113. Lang, *Medicine and Society in Ptolemaic Egypt*, 167.

114. Lang, *Medicine and Society in Ptolemaic Egypt*, 170–71.

would not be a pressing need to travel great distances, unless they felt the local asklepieion was not effective and still wanted to pursue Greek medical help. Various reasons can explain the use of the asklepieia at Kos or Epidauros: (1) a dire, seemingly incurable illness; (2) a need to display a higher level of obedience to Asklepios; (3) the social need for an ostentatious display of wealth, inherent in long-distance travel; and (4) happening to be closer to one of these asklepieia because of travel for other reasons.

Lang divides healing strategies into two categories: (1) "healing procedures accessible at temples" and (2) "submission of oral and written prayers."[115] Although not explicitly stated, this seems to be addressing the strategies of Egyptians or Greeks on a comparable social level or those predisposed to a religious basis for their healing. It does not address the work of healers from the Greek medical tradition, such as Herophilus, other than to claim, "Wealthy protagonists of private letters preferred Greek pharmaceuticals, but the fact that temple libraries added or incorporated Greek medical materials within their own collections might imply an interest in Greek clients."[116] This indicates a colonial perspective that the Greeks, being the power elites, imparted knowledge only to the Egyptians rather than a recursive relationship. This may be accurate in a broad social setting, but among the healers themselves, there may have been a more fluid relationship of borrowing and adapting ideas. If the evidence from the Deir el-Bahari inscription is any indication, even for the layperson (nonmedical practitioner), therapeutic ideas from both cultures could be combined effectively.

Unlike Greek temples, especially the asklepieion, where purity could be achieved through ritual regardless of the afflicted's gender or social status, the Egyptian temples restricted personnel based on a priestly hierarchy. Commoners had no access to the interior spaces of a temple. This makes submitting a question or request for healing to cult officials a popular therapeutic tactic. Petitions for healing could be used even without consulting professional medical advice. It draws upon the traditional idea of gods sending a message through illness and demonstrates obedience with a physical and oral rite that could lead to physical healing as well as reestablish community cohesion.

Dream interpretation is another common therapeutic tactic continued from the Pharaonic period but not necessarily instigated by the sick.[117] A

115. Lang, *Medicine and Society in Ptolemaic Egypt*, 98.

116. Lang, *Medicine and Society in Ptolemaic Egypt*, 100.

117. Lang, *Medicine and Society in Ptolemaic Egypt*, 50n14.

god may initiate contact through dreams. During the Ptolemaic period, there is an upsurge in dream consultation that carries through the Roman period. From this period date a number of dream interpretation manuals that are typically considered separate from the standard medical texts.

Quite often the dream points to fulfilling cult obligations in order to effect healing. A commonly cited example is the third-century BCE case of Apollonios, an official of Ptolemy Philadelphos, who was told to build a sanctuary to Sarapis in a harbor town and who then became ill when he first refused this task. There is also the more Greek-styled practice of incubation, which would be carried out at the temple of Imhotep in Memphis. A second-century CE text reads much like the classical *iamata* from Greek asklepieia, in which the god must be memorialized.[118] Incubation can be thought of as a subset of dream therapeutics, since it specifically uses solicited dreams carried out in a sacred space.[119] The practice was not wholly borrowed from the Greeks, since Pharaonic dream oracles also made use of sleeping in the vicinity of a god, such as the court of a temple or otherwise "in the shadow of a god."[120]

Lang sees the use of dreams as de-institutionalizing, since it does not require an official intermediary. Traditionally, it was not a specialized skill, since many texts that could be consulted so readily would just be part of the overall scribal skill and thus likely carried out by lower-level temple personnel. This is in contrast to classical Greek practices in which specialized dream interpreters would work independently but near temples.

## Illness

### Disease

Given topographical variations in Egypt, the potential for diseases would vary according to the different environments. The marshes in Lower Egypt would be more disposed toward water-borne illness, such as malaria. Although malaria was not as problematic in Egypt as it was in Greece, the Hellenistic healers maintained the Greek culture of focusing on fevers in treatises dealing with diagnosis and explanations of the vascular system. The

118. Lang, *Medicine and Society in Ptolemaic Egypt*, 51.
119. Lang, *Medicine and Society in Ptolemaic Egypt*, 52.
120. Lang, *Medicine and Society in Ptolemaic Egypt*, 52.

deserts of Upper Egypt, especially away from the irrigation canals, would be less subject to such diseases, while snakes and scorpions would be more prevalent. Lang develops a picture of the overall pathogenic ecology of Ptolemaic Egypt extrapolating data from the Pharaonic period in comparison with similar data from archaic and classical Greece.[121]

Diarrhea in its own right was not considered a problem among the Egyptian population, since their regimen for health included regular purges, whereas they considered constipation a more serious concern in need of healing.[122] As in Pharaonic Egypt, typhoid may have been of particular concern especially in the Fayum, given the life cycle of *Salmonella typhi* and the dry climate of the area; the symptoms of typhoid also match the description of some fevers in the Hippocratic *Epidemics*.[123] It is possible that tuberculosis was a problem, yet the degree of prevalence cannot be determined with any exactitude. Evidence for it can be dubious since such a retrospective diagnosis relies on artistic renderings, as well as some skeletal remains. The depiction of a humpback in tomb paintings may indicate long-term exposure to tuberculosis, but the condition is exclusively rendered for servants, indicating a social marker rather than a clinical diagnosis.[124] The environmental conditions in Egypt made it predisposed to schistosomiasis, especially in comparison to Greece. Similarly, tapeworm and other parasites were endemic for Egypt.[125] The treatises of the Greek *iatroi* do not reflect a turn toward the types of diseases more prevalent in Egypt, as opposed to Magna Graecia.

### Trauma

Paleopathological studies have not yet revealed any unique pattern to trauma among Ptolemaic Egyptians. No particular community within Egypt has a higher incident of interpersonal violence or repetitive-use injuries based on gender or class. For now, it can be assumed that the normal frequency of these traumas found in other ancient societies likely was the same in Egypt. The relief at Kom Ombo gives us a unique glimpse at the type of work-related

121. Lang, *Medicine and Society in Ptolemaic Egypt*, 7.
122. Lang, *Medicine and Society in Ptolemaic Egypt*, 10–11.
123. Lang, *Medicine and Society in Ptolemaic Egypt*, 10.
124. Lang, *Medicine and Society in Ptolemaic Egypt*, 12.
125. Lang, *Medicine and Society in Ptolemaic Egypt*, 13.

injuries suffered during construction projects. Most likely, these work accidents spurred Herophilus to espouse the theory that certain types of wounds, such as round ones, take longer to heal based on the mathematical principles of surface area in relation to diameter and circumference.[126]

### Disability

As yet, there is no dedicated study on the issue of disability in Ptolemaic Egypt either from a cultural or paleopathological perspective. Lang's comprehensive study on medicine omits the category of disability. Most references in more general works assume that people who are blind, deaf, or the like were treated the same as they were in either Pharaonic Egypt or classical Greece, depending on their family's origins or social status within Ptolemaic Egypt.

### Conditional States

It is with the Ptolemaic physicians that the stages of life have a significant codified impact on medical culture in terms of diagnosis. Some of the Alexandrian physicians adopted Herophilus's idea of four phases to life: infancy, childhood, adulthood, and old age. Thus, many theories of health and disease, especially the significance of the pulse, revolved around the general age of the patient. Herophilus, in keeping with Aristotle, recognized a shift in the pulse over one's lifetime. Infants have a much faster rate that normalizes through childhood and into adulthood but then slows during old age.[127] With the exception of the pulse and outward signs of old age, such as greying/balding and increased muscular weakness, no specific disease process was identified as being unique to an age category, no common "childhood disease" as found in modern medicine. Instead, age played a significant role in reading symptoms and administering therapeutic measures.

Like all other ancient societies, puberty itself was not medicalized. An exception would be Herophilus's claim, in *Against Common Opinions*, that menstruation was both helpful and harmful, depending on the particular case of the woman rather than a blanket theoretical statement. Rites of ini-

126. Von Staden, "Body and Machine," 90.

127. Rufus Ephesius, *Synopsis de pulsibus* 4; see von Staden, *Herophilus*, 350–51.

tiation into adulthood would depend heavily on the socioeconomic status of the person, as well as one's claims to an ethnic identity. It would be interesting to note the frequency of hellenization of Egyptians trying to curry Ptolemaic favor, as well as adoption of Egyptian practices within the Greek royal court in order to bolster their legitimacy as rulers.

Khnum, one of the creator gods of Pharaonic Egypt, continued this role into the Greco-Roman period. Interestingly, a temple in Esna dedicated to the syncretized Khnum-Re gives details on the creation of humans, with the blood flowing and skin stretched over the bones; the respiratory, digestive, and reproductive organs were carefully put in place, and then finally life breathed into it. This attention to the formation of the body is not found in Pharaonic texts but may reflect an incorporation of the ongoing debates surrounding Alcmaeon's basic eight questions. The continued popularity of traditional creator and birth deities spoke to the common issue of infertility in the ancient world, especially given the high infant mortality rate.

The construction of birth houses became popular in the Ptolemaic period. This is a somewhat misleading fact in the history of Ptolemaic and ancient medicine. Typically, the birth house is a structure making up part of the temple complex, used in a ritual celebration of the birth of the child god Horus. One is attested at Philae in the temple to Isis.[128] Also, the shrine to Harpokrates inside the temple complex to Osiris at Alexandria may have served as a birth house. It is thought that these religious spaces developed from a Predynastic habit of women giving birth in special huts, although no evidence exists of such a practice. It is also suggested that some Ptolemaic family members were born in these temple birth houses, but that would go against the rules of purity for access to such sacred spaces.

Herophilus understood pregnancy as a normal or healthy occurrence and attributed pathology only to difficult cases of childbirth, which he addressed in his work *On Midwifery*. It does indicate that the female reproductive organs, such as the uterus, derive from the same tissue as the rest of the body and governed by the same faculties, namely, that an excess of humors can cause disease. Internal conditions interfering with childbirth include the position of the fetus and failure of the uterus to dilate properly. External conditions include diet, excessive heat or cold, as well as too much fat around the hips and upper abdomen. The humoral theory can be seen at work in notions like regulating heat and cold as well as dietetics. It is interesting to note that the distribution of body fat is an external condition rather

128. Lang, *Medicine and Society in Ptolemaic Egypt*, 63.

than an internal one, indicating that focus is on the fetus itself rather than the mother's body. Herophilus may have designated the normal duration of pregnancy at seven months.

## HEALERS

Pharaonic Egypt was famous for the many classifications of specialized healers focusing on organs such as the eyes, teeth, and even the anus. These, however, may be ranking titles denoting placement in a social hierarchy rather than indications of actual medical specialization on par with modern ophthalmology and proctology. In contrast, classical Greek medicine did not have designations for specialists based upon anatomy; all were simply either an *iatros* or physician. Ptolemaic government documents recording occupations simply gloss over the different Egyptian specialists, classifying most as *swnw* and using it as an equal translation to *iatros*. This speaks to the development of a professional healing class, in contrast to a folk or even popular one.

Yet medicine under Ptolemaic rule did have some overlap with the traditional Egyptian titles, such as an "enema specialist," thought to parallel the Pharaonic title "Shepherd of the Anus."[129] Classical Greece did recognize some healers as specializing in a particular therapeutic practice, such as bandaging or venesection. The enema specialist may then be part of this Greek tradition rather than a direct descendent of the Egyptian title Shepherd of the Anus. Some traditional Egyptian practices and their specialist titles could have survived under the Ptolemies, since their Greek counterparts could recognize a similarity and rename the Shepherd of the Anus as simply an "enema specialist" (*iatroklystes*), converting an anatomical focus to a therapeutic one.

Ptolemaic titles for Isis and Hathor included *rḫt*, meaning "knowledgeable woman."[130] This reiterates a title from the Pharaonic period used for women who could influence malevolent spirits, as well as poisonous animals. Although commonly seen as part of folk healing, Isis appears as this type of healer on the Metternich Stela, which indicates a rather high status even among the cultural elites. This argues against Kleinman's clear divisions of popular, folk, and professional healers. Certain titles for healers from the

129. Von Staden, *Herophilus*, 23.

130. Lang, *Medicine and Society in Ptolemaic Egypt*, 215.

Egyptian culture cannot be easily slotted into a social hierarchy. Lang sees it more as a private-versus-public-sphere division.[131] The "knowledgeable woman" does not appear in public in the capacity of an official religious office that practices healing, such as the priestess of Serket, yet in the Ramesside period, this "knowledgeable woman" healer still appears to have practiced outside her immediate domestic context, as dictated by the phrase "private sphere." To what extent this still held true during the Ptolemaic period is not clear. For ancient Greeks, women were more restricted to the home than their counterparts in Pharaonic Egypt. Coming out of traditional Egyptian medical culture, the Ptolemaic "knowledgeable woman" likely did not feel any restrictions practicing among the Egyptians. Her ability to extend her practice to the Greeks is not entirely clear.

Likely a separation existed between, on the one hand, the Alexandrian and other Greek-styled physicians and, on the other, the Egyptian healers, given the insularity of the two cultures, especially early in the Ptolemaic period. Wilcken provides German translation of a relevant but problematic papyrus attesting to an Egyptian healer who even had to make use of a Greek translator in order to service cross-cultural patients.[132] Greek medicine deriving from philosophy and not just religion focused on connections with other elements of natural philosophy, and its practitioners had to situate themselves within a community, competitively demonstrating knowledge with the precept: the wider ranging the knowledge, the better. Egyptian medicine, in contrast, did not follow a competitive theoretical model focused on demonstrating wider connections. For the Egyptians, competitive knowledge found its expression in the accrual of ranking titles. This would indicate, for those writing treatises, a shift away from healers separated by a focus on the human or divine community cohesion to a greater emphasis on just the human community.

Between 310 and 175 BCE, a medical tax was levied on local elites connected to military service in the less hellenized areas, as well as Ptolemaic-controlled cities outside Egypt, such as Halicarnassos. Perhaps this was a government supplemented form of health care, in that the physicians serviced the local elites paying the tax.[133] The work registers for places such as Deir el-Medina attest to a precedent within Egyptian Pharaonic culture. From Greek culture, Delphi had a similar arrangement to this tax to pay

131. Lang, *Medicine and Society in Ptolemaic Egypt*, 216.

132. Von Staden, *Herophilus*, 26.

133. Lang, *Medicine and Society in Ptolemaic Egypt*, 233.

for a public physician, and like in Delphi, the Ptolemaic tax only ensured the presence of *iatroi* in the area rather than in the modern sense of the government paying direct bills for services rendered for a particular patient.

Nothing within this tax system seems to have precluded the use of the Hellenistic *iatroi* by local Egyptians. This link between the *iatroi* and the government tax helped create a professional status for them apart from the authority they sought in writing. The Egyptian *swnw* were grouped together with the *iatroi* under this medical tax, which would further professionalize them in contrast to other Egyptian titles, such as the *sau* or *wab* priest. The taxes were paid monthly into a bank, and then eligible physicians could draw out the appropriate amount as needed. On some occasions, though, a soldier directly paid the healer as a form of paying the tax.[134]

In addition to the medical tax, there is also evidence that individual patients paid for services from a physician. Likely, Ptolemaic Egypt experienced a blend of different payment methods, with some healers employed by the city or royal court, whereas others worked more on private contracts. This is not too far removed from the typical remuneration practices of classical Greece and Pharaonic Egypt.

Only a few from the Empiricists or Herophilean school worked as physicians for the royal court. The Ptolemies did not seem to give any substantial patronage to physicians expressly for the purpose of research. How Herophilus and Erasistratus acquired bodies for dissection likely has more to do with the navigation of power structures than a Ptolemaic program of fostering medical research. Their patronage of the library and museum would itself provide an ideological impetus for research and breaking the taboos found in Greece proper, without the royal family having to designate specific funds for medicine. Yet the most prominent physicians of Alexandria, such as Herophilus, seem to have been independent and worked from within their houses, in rooms set up for treatment and dissection.

134. Papyri Hibeh 102 and 103; see Lang, *Medicine and Society in Ptolemaic Egypt*, 237.

# 9. Etruscan and Roman Medicine

## Location and History

The Italian peninsula during the first millennium BCE was home to two major ethnic groups, based on linguistics—an indigenous group, the Etruscans, as well as an Indo-European group, the Latins. During the first half of the millennium, the Etruscans formed a coalition under a titular king that dominated the northern portion of the peninsula, Etruria, and extended its power southward over some Latin tribes.

Rome itself lies on the Tiber River, the border between the Etruscan and Latin tribal territories in the sixth century BCE. This proximity not only put Rome under the political sphere of the Etruscan kings, as recounted by later Roman historians, such as Livy, Tacitus, and Pliny, but it also meant a cultural mixing between Latin Rome and the Etruscans. Slowly over the fifth and fourth centuries, the Etruscan tribal league lost power to Roman aristocrats, who formed a republic ruled by dual consuls and a Senate formed by the patricians. Internal strife created a shared governance with the lower-class plebeians as tribunes paralleling the consuls. During this time, the Gallic tribes of the north had been making their own incursions into Etruria, spreading as far south as the city of Rome. As the republic developed, the Romans expanded their military power to the north into Etruria and Cisalpine Gaul, as well as the northeast into the farmland of Sabinium and the hills of Umbria.[1]

The growing military prowess and expansion of Rome southward through the Italian peninsula into the territory of Greek colonies brought it into conflict with the trading empire of the Carthaginians,[2] who controlled

1. The Romans designated Gaul as the northern Italian peninsula along the Po River, eventually specifying this region as Cisalpine Gaul and the area of what is now southern France as Transalpine Gaul.

2. A group of Phoenicians from coastal Canaan on the eastern Mediterranean.

parts of Sicily in the third century BCE. The end result of these Punic Wars placed the islands of Sicily, Sardinia, and Corsica, as well as the Mediterranean coast of the Iberian Peninsula and parts of North Africa, under Roman domination.

More toward the eastern Mediterranean, the defeat of Philip V of Macedonia and later the Aetolians, along with the Seleucids, placed Rome in control of Greece and western Anatolia by the end of the second century BCE. Although the Roman senate and generals often found themselves allied with the Greek dynasty of Ptolemy in Egypt, the politico-military struggles between Octavian and Marc Antony, culminating in the battle of Actium in 31 BCE, brought an end not only to the Ptolemaic dynasty but the republican structure of Rome itself. Octavian assumed Egypt as an imperial province and took the title Augustus, finally transforming Rome into an empire. As early as the time of Etruscan domination, Greek culture permeated the Italian peninsula. This created a situation in which many of the underlying concepts important to the study of medicine are shared between the Greeks and the Romans, such as the ideas that all illness comes from the gods, who established a natural but understandable, predictable order to the universe. Consequently, many of the characterizations of the Greek gods regarding sickness and healing, can be transposed to their Roman counterparts.

## Religion and Culture

The interaction between humans and deities took on different forms as Roman culture expanded along the Italian peninsula and throughout the Mediterranean basin. A common way for modern scholars to analyze Roman religion is to divide it between public and private worship; this mode of thought parallels the supposed Greek system of state Olympian gods and the popular minor gods. Both forms of worship, though, accessed power or influence over the deities through ritual actions. Magistrates and priests oversaw the public rituals, such as sacrifices and care of temples, as "a pact freely concluded between the city's two partners, with a view to furthering the well-being of all."[3] In the sphere of private religion, families and individuals performed private banqueting rituals, as well as cared for domestic shrines with the same aim of mutual benefit. Sorcerers held a unique posi-

3. John Scheid, *An Introduction to Roman Religion* (Bloomington: Indiana University Press, 2003), 151.

tion, like their ancient Near Eastern counterparts, in that they could cause illness by a negative influence on the gods. Scholars slot them into the category of private religion, but similar actions, such as the cursing of enemies, could be found at the public, governmental level.[4]

The act of healing was not limited either to the public or private spheres. An important aspect of piety was consulting all the deities involved in a particular situation;[5] therefore, healing could take place among the public Capitoline deities[6] as well as the private ones if they were involved in someone's injury or illness. Most cases of healing that have come down to us do so in a private or personal context, but episodes of plague show that the public form of religion also plays a part in healing strategies. Whether public or private, a deity's role may have been to directly cause the health issue either as punishment or at the behest of a dubious magician, and therefore, the god is the one to heal it. Or the god may simply hear an appeal as a higher authority over those people and deities already involved. As we shall see, the direct and somewhat capricious actions of Etruscan and Roman deities in matters of health exist alongside a growing system of predictable divine systems that do not require religious forms of influence over them.

## Cosmology

Etruscans divided the sky into sixteen regions, with groups of deities residing in each of them. Etruscan gods often grouped together in councils, similar to the Mesopotamian and early Canaanite conceptions of gods working by a level of consensus. These divisions helped early augurs read and interpret messages from the gods. The first heavenly division, the abode of Veltune (Latin Jupiter) in the northeast, also contained Salus, a god of good health, while the personification of Wellness itself resided in the ninth section.[7] From this, we can see that the divine groupings were not simply by obvious subject categories, such as politics or health, but existed as mixed associations. Although there is a general sense of a "good to bad" spectrum moving

4. Scheid, *Introduction to Roman Religion*, 151

5. Scheid, *Introduction to Roman Religion*, 157.

6. A common phrase in Roman historical and cultural studies referring to those whose temples reside on the Capitoline Hill in Rome.

7. Martianus Capella relates the Etruscan cosmology in his fifth-century CE text *On the Marriage of Mercury and Philology*; see Nancy Thomson de Grummond, *Etruscan Myth, Sacred History, and Legend* (Philadelphia: University of Pennsylvania Museum, 2006), 45.

from east to west in the sky, the placement of Wellness shows that this is not a strict rule. Our surviving evidence of Etruscan religion does not shed enough light on the fairly nuanced relationships that the Etruscan deities had with each other as well as with humans.

The Piacenza Liver, dating from the third or second century BCE, attests to the continued practice of reading the celestial houses. This model of the liver has forty celestial houses mapped onto it and acts as an interpretive guide by which predictions could be made by haruspicy. Priests would interpret the physical condition of the sacrificed sheep's liver against the model. If abnormalities appeared in a particular section of the liver, it meant that a god residing in that particular celestial house was sending the message. By the end of the republic, the Romans reduced the heavens to just four sections, with negative readings coming from the left and positive from the right.

Some indication of the relationship between gods and humans for matters of health and medicine can normally be found in creation myths. Yet the peculiar character of the surviving myths makes it difficult to discern. The only known creation myth for the Etruscans comes from the third century BCE, with a Latin translation from the second century. It tells of the goddess Lasa Vecovia (Latin Vegoia) prophesying to Arruns Veltymnus about creation and warning of the consequences for those who do not follow the order of the cosmos.[8] The act of creation itself occurs with the separation of sea and sky, while Tinia/Jupiter sets boundaries, especially for Etruria. Storms, draught, and interestingly diseases stood as punishment for violating these boundaries. The aspects of proper order and physical separation of the world recall the role of Maat in the Egyptian cosmology as well as the power of the Israelite god. In the Etruscan story, though, the formation of human bodies is curiously absent. Although this myth explains one possible origin of disease for the Etruscans, it does not reveal much about a physical link, if any, between gods and humans.

Similarly, Roman myths focus on the foundation of the city of Rome and its acquisition of a population rather than human creation either *ex nihilo* or from earthly substances. Livy's account of the theft of the Sabine women highlights the hierarchical value of physical prowess and youthful beauty in the forms of the games for the gods, as well as the most attractive women being reserved for the senatorial class. It would be problematic to argue from silence that the absence of a specific human creation indicates that the Etruscans and Romans saw themselves as not intimately connected

8. De Grummond, *Etruscan Myth, Sacred History, and Legend*, 41.

to the divine or nature. Evidently, from Etruscan and Roman stories, the human body does exhibit a relationship, whether good or bad, between the people and the gods.

Sacrifices act as a main point of contact between the gods and humans, maintaining a positive relationship for the two groups. The Etruscans practiced three basic sacrificial rituals: (1) Celestial deities received a burnt offering on an altar decorated with wings. (2) Underworld deities received blood that flowed from the throat of the sacrificed animal, through a channel in the altar, and into a hollow in the earth. (3) Ancestors had libations and bloodless sacrifices.[9] Reserving blood for chthonic deities as opposed to celestial ones or ancestors indicates a belief about the relationship between living beings and the earth, but the exact nature of that relationship is not yet known. Although the Etruscans lacked (a surviving) tale of the gods' role in creating humans, there does appear to be a link through blood, given its role in sacrifices. Ritual sacrifices carried into Roman religious culture; these may have influenced later Roman concepts of blood's function in physiology. Roman medicine adheres to many theories originating in Greek medical culture, but the prominence of blood in a ritual/religious context could predispose Roman healers and patients to readily adopt and adapt medical teachings concerning blood. Patients may have accepted and rationalized bloodletting as a type of ritual sacrifice showing obedience to the gods in an expected exchange for healing.

Although Roman writers of the late republic and early empire, such as Cicero, Livy, and Seneca, pejoratively described Etruscan religion as overly superstitious, the Senate officially recognized the usefulness of the Etruscan rituals for taking omens in significant state matters and during times of crisis. Prior to this, a syncretization between Etruscan and Greek deities occurred around the sixth century BCE.[10] In conjunction, the growing power of Rome created a blend with the indigenous Roman gods. This resulted in multiple and sometimes linguistically related names for the same god. For example, the Etruscan Tinia/Veltune is Latin Jupiter, who equates with the Greek Zeus. The pantheon composed of Etruscan, Roman, and Greek deities possessed an overarching approach to issues of health and medicine. Every god had the ability to cause disease and injury as well as heal it, yet certain deities had a particularly close association with medical matters.

9. Sybille Haynes, *Etruscan Civilization: A Cultural History* (Los Angeles: J. Paul Getty Museum, 2000), 127.

10. Haynes, *Etruscan Civilization*, 268.

The following is a brief introduction to significant deities for the study of Roman medicine. As we shall see, some enjoyed a popularity throughout the territories governed by both republican and imperial Rome, while others had a significant role in healing for only particular communities or times.

## Etruscan Gods and Goddesses of Disease and Healing

### *Aesculapius*

One of the most obvious gods associated with medicine is Aesculapius, the Latinization of the Greek Asklepios. He retained much, if not all, of his characteristics as the physician par excellence, healing through dreams. His sanctuaries, the asklepieia, in the eastern territories continued to be popular pilgrimage sites for healing well into the late empire. According to Ovid and the *Anonymus Londinensis*, in the wake of a plague that struck Rome in 293 BCE, the senate consulted the Sibylline books for a solution. This resulted in the official importation of Aesculapius from his shrine at Epidaurus in 291 BCE. His Roman temple was built on the Tiber Island on top of a spring used in earlier healing practices. This particular shrine became a place of sanctuary for slaves rather than being frequented by patricians and plebeians.

### *Aplu*

Aplu is the Etruscan borrowing of Apollo, who had for the most part lost his healing role, except when the image was completely lifted from a Greek original, such as Aplu caring for an injured foot of Tinia. By the late republic and imperial periods, the Romans directly borrowed Apollo, including his healing aspects, with many of his shrines and temples to the east of the Italian peninsula still operational.

### *Diana*

An Etruscan healing shrine dedicated to Diana stood near Lake Nemi, just outside Rome, from the eighth to sixth centuries. In the fourth century BCE, as Diana became equated with the Greek virginal goddess Artemis, it converted to a more hellenized version of a temple.[11] Votives in and around the lake attest to Diana's role in childbirth and general healing, especially during the fourth century. It seems, though, that the process of hellenization forced Diana to lose her association with healing and protective childbirth for those living outside the immediate area around Rome. She became, like Artemis, a goddess with the ubiquitous general power to hurt and heal but no real specific medical function.

### *Herakles*

The Etruscans adopted the Greek Herakles as Hercle, which later became Hercules. Tribes in northern Etruria near Mount Falterona highlighted his healing abilities linked to his physical prowess. A shrine for Hercle might have stood on the shore of a mountain lake, or the lake itself served as a healing site, since archaeologists found in it bronze votives of body parts, as well as statuettes of Hercle and armed warriors.[12] Inscriptions and clothing motifs indicate cultural affinities between this population and Attic Greek. This Hercle also played a role with Menrva/Minerva in the birth of Epeur, a prophetic boy of Etruscan mythology.

### *Isis*

The Egyptian healing deity Isis began her integration into Roman medical culture during the late republic as the Ptolemaic Cleopatra joined alliances with the Roman triumvirates. The popularity of Isis gained ground under Caligula and the later Flavian dynasty. But she was never fully incorporated into the system of priestly colleges in Rome itself. For most of the Roman Empire, she was generally associated with health and safety, while in Egypt she retained a more prominent role in healing. Her healing shrine at Kanopos and Menouthis lasted until the late fifth century CE, when it was finally converted to a Christian church.

11. Audrey Cruse, *Roman Medicine* (Gloucestershire: Tempus, 2004), 117.
12. Haynes, *Etruscan Civilization*, 253.

### *Jupiter/Tinia*

The well-known Roman god Jupiter has several names stemming from his Etruscan origins as Tinia, which include Veltune, Voltumnus, and Vertumnus. Although head of the pantheon, he was one of several Etruscan gods that could throw lightning bolts. He possessed three types.[13] A benign one served as a warning, which Tinia could solely decide to use. Another one did both harm and good but needed approval of a divine group called the Consenting Gods. Finally, a destructive one needed permission from the Shrouded Gods. These latter types gave Jupiter the typical power of wounding and healing, but its requirement of consent from a divine council recalls the Mesopotamian story *Enuma Elish* and the Canaanite *Atra-ḫasis* that made disease a matter for the community of the gods rather than individual whim.

Jupiter was also associated with birth in several different contexts. Many mirrors show him with a baby, and one depicts him giving birth to Fufluns, a vegetation god, with the birth goddess Thalna and Aplu in attendance. In other images, Tinia gives birth to Athena/Menrva, with assistance from the birth goddesses Thanr, Ethausva, and Thalna.[14]

Jupiter is less important as a healing deity but extremely significant for understanding Etruscan and early Roman concepts of the body, gender, and its functionality. Jupiter/Voltumnus could also appear as the feminine Voltumna. This is not a separate god from Tinia but rather another incarnation. "Why do you marvel[15] that my one body should have so many shapes? . . . I am Etruscan, from Etruscans sprung. . . . My nature is suitable for all forms. Turn me into whatever you like, I'll still be handsome. Dress me in Coan silk, I'll become like a girl, and not rough. When I wear the toga, who will deny that I am a man?"[16] Interestingly, the physical expression of gender was not fixed for the Etruscan gods, but to what extent this was thought to apply to humans is not clear.

13. De Grummond, *Etruscan Myth, Sacred History, and Legend*, 53.

14. De Grummond, *Etruscan Myth, Sacred History, and Legend*, 58–61.

15. De Grummond, *Etruscan Myth, Sacred History, and Legend*, 67–69.

16. Propertius, *Elegies* 4.2; see de Grummond, *Etruscan Myth, Sacred History, and Legend*, 65–67.

### *Minerva*

The goddess Minerva formed one of the Capitoline triads with Jupiter and Juno. In her original Etruscan form of Menrva, she fulfilled a significant healing role, as evidenced by a sixth-century temple on the shores near Cerveteri, which contained terracotta models or votives of intestines, genitalia, arms, legs, and swaddled babies.[17] Once she became the equivalent to the Greek Athena, the Romans thought of her primarily as a goddess of wisdom and technology. Yet this association made her a patron deity for physicians, with many statues and coins depicting her with a coiled snake as the incarnation of Minerva Medica.

### *Salus*

The Roman god Salus, whose name means "health" or "safety," was associated with physical as well as moral welfare. Note the embodiment of these two concepts in one entity. The physical body is not distinct from the personality or behavior of the individual, which mirrors a Roman social value that the individual is not separate from the family or the public good (*res publica*). The Gauls called him Valetudo, with excavations at Glanum revealing that Agrippa in 27 BCE dedicated baths to Valetudo.

### *Birth Goddesses*

A number of goddesses could be involved with the protection of the mother and child during birth. Juno, a Capitoline deity and therefore linked to public worship, assisted with birth in all its forms, from humans to the birth of the new month with Janus. The Etruscan deities overseeing births were Thalna, who could change gender, Thanr, and Ethausva. Minor or private-sphere deities included Alemona, protector of the fetus, Partula, linked with delivery, and Vagitanus, associated with the initial cry of an infant. Cunina protected the cradle, and Rumina guarded breast feeding.

17. Haynes, *Etruscan Civilization*, 184.

### *Minor Deities*

Many minor or private-sphere deities could be invoked when health issues arose. A general healing deity was the goddess Bona Dea, but more often she was aligned with the cultic activity of married women. The personification of fever took the form of Dea Febris, who had three temples located in the city of Rome. Carna, likely an Etruscan goddess, protected the heart, stomach, and general well-being and also had a temple in Rome founded during the late sixth century BCE. Pales happened to be associated more with the health of flocks rather than people but could be called upon for either.

## Philosophy

In addition to healing practices growing out of the combined religious traditions of the Etruscans, Latins, and Greeks, a parallel medical culture developed based on the Hellenic natural philosophies. Yet, unlike scholarship on ancient Greek religion, there is no question whether the Romans believed in their gods. State-sponsored rituals to retain (or gain) citizenship was the norm, while these same learned men would argue theories of natural philosophy as the appropriate methods for practicing medicine. The unspoken assumption that the gods lie behind the ordered configuration of the natural world allowed some medical cultures, the treatise-writing *iatros* and *medicus*, to focus on the mechanistic aspects, giving the impression in surviving documents that the gods played no role. The teachings of Hippocrates, Epicurus, Plato, and Aristotle influenced these later Roman schools of thought, of which the three most prominent were the Methodists, Rationalists, and Empiricists. But even within this tripartite medical culture, certain men, such as Galen and Rufus of Ephesus, tried to stand apart. Galen gives an interesting outline of them in his work *On Sects for Beginners*, as does Celsus in his earlier encyclopedic work *De Medicina*.

The Roman Dogmatists, or Rationalists, continued much of their Greek predecessors' ideas. They relied on theoretical precepts for the development of their medical practices, instead of focusing on integrating clinical experience. They believed finding the "internal causal base of disease"[18] would lead to the proper treatments. Different theoretical branches developed among the

18. R. J. Hankinson, "The Man and His Work," in *The Cambridge Companion to Galen*, ed. R. J. Hankinson (Cambridge: Cambridge University Press, 2008), 26n12.

Dogmatists. Some scholars may slot Rufus of Ephesus into this category, since his writings were anti-Methodist and the Empiricists disavowed him, but he avoided being aligned with any particular school of thought, much like Galen.

Roman Empiricists developed from the Greek epistemological tradition that medical practices should be based on experiences and grounded in pragmatism. This contradicts the dogmatic search for "hidden causes," while sharing in Alcmaeon's idea that humans must interpret physical evidence, since they lack the divine ability to directly know things. Yet different stories circulate as to the origins of Empiricists, with some told as early as Pliny the Elder. Essentially, it formed as a reaction to Dogmatism by Philinos of Cos in 260 BCE, who rebelled against his teacher Herophilus. They espoused a tripartite system of personal observation, access to a wide body of knowledge, including the physician's own experiences, and recognizing the similarity of diseases, allowing for an overlap in treatment measures. Empiricists continued to flourish well past the second century CE.

Themison of Tralles (ca. 70 BCE), a student of Asklepiades of Bithynia (124–40 BCE), founded the Methodist approach to medicine, flourishing between the first century BCE and the second century CE. It runs a middle course between the extremes of the Dogmatists and the Empiricists. Methodists followed the theories of Democritus and Epicurus, positing that the body was composed of indivisible entities they called corpuscles and the space between them, pores. Diseases occurred because the movement of the corpuscles/atoms were either relaxed, constricted, or mixed. The Methodists did not strictly adhere to the Hippocratic idea of humors.

## Sources

Like the Greek ones, Roman texts often centered on arguments for epistemological authority rather than marketplace competition for patients. Thus, many of the medical texts come from this intellectual tradition, even if they were intended to be manuals for clinical use. To this end, Roman medicine saw little difference between theory and practice, even among the Empiricists. A good *medicus*, in this intellectual environment, knew the philosophical debates rather than just being trained in practical know-how through apprenticeship. This standard was a matter of pride in one's work rather than being regulated by any governing or licensing body. Unfortunately, our textual sources do not allow for a complete picture, especially the efficacy of the practicing *medicus* not caught up in theoretical debates.

## Texts

Even more so than ancient Greece, Rome provides us with a plethora of medical-related documents. In addition to the theoretical treatises are texts written for clinical reasons, usually associated with military outposts. Modern scholars try to collate and classify such varied sources in collections, such as the *Corpus Medicorum Latinorum*, a companion to the CMG stemming from the work of Herman Diels. The *CML* is an ongoing project[19] to collate all Latin texts relating to medicine, dating from the first to fifth century CE.

Another valuable resource for modern scholars is the *Corpus Papyrorum Latinarum*. It should be noted that any textual sources designated "papyrus" are coming from an Egyptian context. The $MP^3$ database, linked to CPL documents, reveals only one source[20] for the category "Medicine and Surgery," which lists the *materia medica* normally used for eye ailments in the Vindolanda tablets found in a first-century CE fort near Hadrian's Wall.[21] Other tablets from Vindolanda indicate medical activity, such as a list of ill and wounded soldiers.[22] Letters are also present, naming a *medicus*[23] and discussing the health of a prefect.[24]

Marganne has an interesting project, grouping together "iatromagical" papyri.[25] These documents reference protective charms and amulets from the first to seventh century CE. The majority of them are in Greek, only one in Latin, and three with intermixed Coptic. This collection has some crossover with the CPL, especially for the papyri from late antiquity, and interesting references to Jesus as a "heavenly *iatros*."[26] As Christianity grew in Egypt, only a few of the surviving Latin medical papyri directly reference Christ, yet an ample amount of Greek iatromagical texts from Egypt do make use of Psalm 90. Other studies look more closely at incantations within a

19. Housed at Berlin-brandenburgische Akademie der Wissenschaften and accessible at http://cmg.bbaw.de/publications/publikationen-cml.

20. $MP^3$ 3011.01.

21. T. Vindol 3.591; see Marie-Hélène Marganne and Magali de Haro Sanchez, "At the Crossroads of Greek and Roman Medicine: The Contribution of Latin Papyri 1. Medical Texts; 2. Iatromagical Papyri," in *"Greek" and "Roman" in Latin Medical Texts: Studies in Cultural Change and Exchange in Ancient Medicine*, ed. Brigitte Maire (Boston: Brill, 2014), 92–116.

22. T. Vindol. 2.154.

23. T. Vindol. 2.156.

24. T. Vindol. 2.344.

25. Marganne and de Haro Sanchez, "At the Crossroads of Greek and Roman Medicine," 92–116.

26. $MP^3$ 6101.

specific context, such as uterine amulets from Egypt.[27] Many of these texts classified under this type of heading, mixing the stereotyped categories of folk magic and rational use of drugs, have strong cultural similarities with the medical texts of Pharaonic Egypt. Some of the authors, such as Quintus Serenus Sammonicus (d. 211 CE), Oribasius (325–403 CE), and Marcellus Empiricus (ca. 399 CE), preserve remedies drawn from the lower classes of various territories, such as North Africa and Gaul, during the later empire.

An important linguistic division exists for Roman medical sources. Texts written in Latin tend to be documentary in nature, such as private letters, accounts, or lists, while medical treatises, especially by physicians, tend to be written in Greek.[28] Exceptions to this general rule of thumb are the encyclopedic works in Latin by men such as Pliny the Elder, expounding on the medicinal virtues of plants or other natural substances while denigrating Greek medicine. This reflects the cultural tensions within the greater Roman polity, despite a veneer of centrality.

Crateuas (ca. second century BCE) was most likely a root-cutter rather than a trained *iatros*. He wrote and illustrated an herbology, whose title has been lost. Codex Vindobonensis, from the early sixth century CE, may contain copies of his illustrations. A second work, *Root Cutting and Gathering*, is referenced by later writers, such as Dioscorides. Crateuas became the court physician for Mithridates VI (120–63 BCE), the king of Pontus with a reputation for paranoia. Mithridates tried to build up a tolerance for poison by regularly ingesting small doses of it, supposedly with the help of Crateuas.

Celsus (ca. 25 BCE–50 CE), who likely lived in Gaul, wrote or compiled *De Medicina*, which is one section of a larger work covering the topics of agriculture, warfare, rhetoric, philosophy, and law. It gives a history of medicine, mostly following a Hippocratic methodology stressing anatomy, diagnosis, and prognosis but with a greater reliance on the use of drugs and a preference for sporting activities rather than using a gymnasium. Originally thought to be a physician, modern scholarship now sees Celsus as "just an encyclopedist" rather than a practicing physician. This confusion highlights the issue of Greco-Roman physicians establishing their authority through epistemological debates rather than clinical practices.

*De Materia Medica*, written in 65 CE by Dioscorides of Anazarbus (40–90 CE), exemplifies the other end of the spectrum, targeting a more clinical

27. Katherine R. Marino, "Setting the Womb in Its Place: Toward a Contextual Archaeology of Graeco-Egyptian Uterine Amulets" (PhD diss., Brown University, 2010).

28. Marganne and de Haro Sanchez, "At the Crossroads of Greek and Roman Medicine."

audience. It focuses less on theoretically classifying ingredients and more on the consequences of different drugs when applied to particular cases of illness. Dioscorides envisioned the healer reaching for his manual and wanting a quick and clear answer to treat symptoms rather than an underlying pathology. He outlined approximately five thousand uses for one thousand drugs. His work is dedicated to Areios, with whom he studied at Tarsus, a known center for pharmacology. Interestingly, the introduction notes that he was a soldier and traveled extensively, which allowed him to gain knowledge of various plants and minerals in their native habitats, as well as to learn from people about their experiences with the drugs.

Rufus of Ephesus (ca. first century CE) studied in Alexandria and wrote *Quaestiones Medicinales*, urging physicians to take a detailed patient history, since diagnosis is more than analysis of the physical data presented by the body of the patient at the moment of consultation. Modern scholars have recently rediscovered the value of his work in light of the current patient-centered medical practices. Like Galen's writings, it stresses the uniqueness of each patient, but Galen does not reference *Quaestiones Medicinales*, despite referencing Rufus himself numerous times. Rufus's text is unique among ancient medical treatises in that it questions the patient, eliciting answers that the physician should incorporate into diagnosis and treatment.[29] Although no other Greco-Roman medical treatise uses the question tactic, this does not seem too far afield from the dialogue method of epistemology employed by philosophers such as Plato, the progenitors of the academic pursuit of medicine.

The physician Soranus, associated with the Methodists, trained in Alexandria and then worked in Rome approximately 98–138 CE under Trajan and Hadrian. He is reported to have written twenty treatises, of which only *Gynaecology* and a Latin translation of *On Acute and Chronic Diseases* survive mostly intact. Other texts, like *On Fractures*, are fragmentary or, such as *Pharmacology*, exist only as quotes by later writers. His teachings in *Gynaecology* survived in practice into the sixteenth century CE. He advocated a birthing chair and identified a disease in young children thought to be rickets. He gives directives to midwives for childbirth, which indicates that his treatise had a practical bent and was not intended just for academic argumentation. Unlike physicians of the nineteenth and twentieth centuries, in competition with midwives, Soranus's work demonstrates a more

29. Melinda Letts, "Rufus of Ephesus and the Patient's Perspective in Medicine," *British Journal for the History of Philosophy* 22 (2014): 996–1020.

cooperative nature across the different types of healers. The treatise, though, assumes they will listen to him as the authority based upon his experience, both educational and practical, across a wide variety of physical issues.

Galen, the most influential physician of the Roman Empire, was born in 129 CE in Pergamum. He originally studied philosophy but switched to medicine (ca. 145 CE) at the behest of his father, based on a dream. He began his medical training with Satyrus but left Pergamum in 149 CE for Smyrna to study with Pelops, a Dogmatist, and also associated with Albinus, a Neoplatonist. After a brief foray in Corinth, Galen ended up in Alexandria in 153 CE, working with the anatomist Numisianus. In 157 CE, he returned to Pergamum, taking up the position of physician for the gladiatorial school. In 161 CE, Galen traveled seeking herbal and mineral remedies in places such as the Dead Sea region, Cyprus, Thrace, and Macedonia, eventually moving to Rome by 162 CE.[30]

Galen cataloged his own copious amount of works in *On My Own Books* and *The Order of My Own Books*. The status of the physician was important to Galen. He did not want to be classified as a practitioner of magic or divination. Rather, he wanted to position the physician relative to the philosopher, one who arrives at diagnoses and prognoses by rational and empirical methods. He illustrates this with two autobiographical accounts in which his skills as a physician are put to the test by the philosopher Glaucon (*On Prognosis*), on the one hand, and the Herophilean physician Eudemus (*On Slander*), on the other.[31]

One often-cited reference for Galen is the twenty-volume[32] series by Kühn, published between 1821 and 1833.[33] The original Greek texts have a facing-page Latin translation. Volume twenty lists all Galen's treatises as well as a subject index. The important physiological text, *On the Usefulness of Parts*, is missing from Kühn, since its discovery in Arabic documents postdated his series. May provided an English translation in 1968.[34] A more recent edition of Galen's work appears in the series *Corpus Medicorum Latinarum*, which is making available previously unpublished treatises of Galen.

30. The most recent and definitive biography of Galen is by Susan Mattern, *The Prince of Medicine: Galen in the Roman Empire* (Oxford: Oxford University Press, 2013).

31. Hankinson, "The Man and His Work."

32. The series is numbered 1–20, but volumes 17 and 18 are subdivided into 17a, 17b, 18a, and 18b; this gives the count of twenty-two volumes cited in many overviews of Kühn.

33. Karl Gottlob Kühn, ed. and trans., *Opera Omnia* (Leipzig: C. Cnobloch, 1821–1833).

34. Margaret Tallmadge May, *Galen on the Usefulness of the Parts of the Body* (Ithaca, NY: Cornell University Press, 1968).

Of particular note are Galen's ideas on physiology, found in three major works: *On the Doctrines of Hippocrates and Plato* (*PHP*), *On the Natural Faculties* (*Nat. Fac.*), and *On the Utility of the Parts* (*UP*). This frequent crossover in various treatises for different aspects of physiology shows that Galen did not understand physiology as discrete systems but that all of them were interconnected. In some ways, the concern about community cohesion has shifted from the tripartite relations between humans, body parts, and the divine to one centered on humans and body parts; thus, cohesion is important for organ-organ rather than an organ-divine community.

Modern scholarship classifies the physiognomic texts as works of philosophy rather than medicine, but this was not so in the ancient world. They explain anatomy and physiology as signifying one's morals, thus demonstrating the ease with which Roman culture integrates its religious ideals with natural science. Marcus Antonius Polemon (90–144 CE) illustrates the use of physiognomy among the Second Sophists, although his work survives only in a medieval Arabic copy.

A wide variety of texts mention physicians, such as Martial's epigrams criticizing them as no different from gladiators and undertakers. Other literary works can provide valuable insight to the study of Roman medicine. Varro (116–27 BCE) and Cato (95–46 BCE) each wrote texts called *On Agriculture*, addressing the extensive use of plants in *materia medica* as well as the influence of weather on disease/health. *Natural History*, written by Pliny the Elder (23–79 CE), has significant sections addressing both formal healing by physicians and more traditional forms within the family structure.

Seneca's (4 BCE–65 CE) *Natural Questions* draws upon the Hippocratic texts to make comparisons for his ideas on ethics and epistemology.[35] He equates the Roman concept of *spiritus* with the Greek idea of *pneuma* as the universal agent causing unity, so the human body and the earth work on the same pneumatic principles.

> Our body is irrigated by blood; also by air, which runs along by its own routes. . . . In the same way this whole body of the entire earth is a passage way both for water, which takes the place of blood, and for winds, which you might call simply respiration . . . the movement of the veins also preserves its rhythm undisturbed while there is good health but when there

35. Frédéric Le Bay, "Pneumatism in Seneca: An Example of Interaction between Physics and Medicine," in *'Greek' and 'Roman' in Latin Medical Texts: Studies in Cultural Change and Exchange in Ancient Medicine*, ed. Brigitte Maire (Boston: Brill, 2014), 63–76.

> is something wrong the movement pulses more rapidly and inhaling and exhaling give signs of the effort and exhaustion. In the same way the earth remains unshaken as long as its condition is normal. When something is wrong, then there is motion just like that of a sick body, because the air which was flowing through it in an even pattern is struck violently and causes its veins to shake.[36]

Since air permeates everything, Seneca effectively denounces any use of the void, thus negating the Methodist sect of medicine.

Seneca's letters, *Moral Letters to Lucilius*, give another form of insight to medical practices. Personal letters found throughout the provinces provide details as to how people approached their health in a day-to-day context rather than the theoretical arguments of specific medical or other philosophical treatises. In particular, the papyri from Oxyrhynchus in Egypt illuminate the way in which people not only inquire about the health of a loved one but also trade medicants, recipes, and other healing advice between friends and family.[37]

An interesting glimpse into the patient's point of view, as well as the facile conjunction of religious and somatic medicine, comes from Aelius Aristides (117–181 CE), a highly acclaimed orator who wrote *Sacred Tales* in 170/171 CE. He intended this work to pay homage to Aesculapius. It integrates dreams given by the god with Aristides's life, describing his illness beginning in 141 CE and his problems seeking medical help from physicians, priests, and gymnastic trainers. His quest for healing takes him to Rome, Smyrna, and finally the asklepieion in Pergamum. The work contains references to his servant Zosimus as a healer, as well as the well-known physician Satyrus, but makes no real distinction in their healing abilities as one more skilled or professional than the other, negating a strict concept of a hierarchy of resort. It also attests to the Antonine Plague from which he suffered.

## Archaeology

Numerous archaeological sites supplement the textual sources to help develop an overall picture of Roman medicine. Some, such as the sanctuary at

36. Seneca, *Natural Questions* 6.14.1–2; see Le Bay, "Pneumatism in Seneca."

37. Jane Draycott, *Approaches to Healing in Roman Egypt*, BAR International Series (Oxford: Archaeopress, 2012), 15–16.

Marzabotto, in the foothills of the Apennines, speak to an early period when we have a paucity of written sources.[38] This Etruscan shrine built around a natural spring dates from the mid-sixth to mid-fourth century BCE. Bronze anatomical votives attest to its healing function. Similarly, bronze votives from Fiesole and Arezzo indicate an Etruscan shrine to Menrva along the Arno River, which date to 530–480 BCE.[39]

These early sites dedicated to Menrva are in contrast to the Minerva Medica, a popular tourist attraction near the central train station in Rome. These ruins, likely dating from late antiquity, were labeled the Minerva Medica, a temple dedicated to the healing aspect of the goddess Minerva, in the mid-sixteenth century CE by the artist Pirro Ligorio. He also claimed the Minerva Medica housed a Schola Medicorum, a type of medical training center. A temple for Minerva Medica did exist in the Esquiline district of Rome in the fourth century CE, but it cannot be identified with any structures still standing. By the late twentieth century, scholars identified the ruins by the train station as a type of garden pavilion rather than a temple or shrine. The *Turin Encyclopedia* claims that statues of Minerva, Aesculapius, Chiron, and Apollo that were found nearby were taken to the villa of Pope Julius III but have since been lost. This Minerva Medica exemplifies red herrings often created during the Renaissance and neoclassical periods that must be sorted through.

The Villa Vesuvio, a farmhouse outside Pompeii destroyed in 79 CE, contained a significant find for the history of medicine, a jar with remains of poppy seeds and the bones of reptiles and amphibians known for use in medical recipes, especially theriac. Fifty-eight percent of plant material retrieved from the jar matched known varieties used in both Pliny's *Natural History* and Dioscorides's *De Materia Medica*.[40] Additionally, excavators found a small cooker in one of the rooms, similar to ovens in workshop/houses within Pompeii. The presence of medical instruments identifies some of these structures as medical workshops. The same type of oven, though, as well as ingredients, can also be found in workshops involved in the production of dyes and soaps, which further complicates the picture with the possibility that dye makers could have engaged in healing.

38. Haynes, *Etruscan Civilization*, 192.

39. Haynes, *Etruscan Civilization*, 252.

40. Marina Ciaraldi, "Drug Preparation in Evidence? An Unusual Plant and Bone Assemblage from the Pompeian Countryside, Italy," *Vegetation History and Archaeobotany* 9 (2000): 91–98.

Sites outside the Italian peninsula are equally informative. A Roman-style garden at Fishbourne, near Chichester, contained a variety of plants common to a pharmacy garden. An upsurge in Mediterranean varieties of plants in Britain after the conquest in 43 CE acts as one of the indicators for the importation of medical practices. For paleopathology during the Roman period, the Dakhleh Oasis Project in Egypt has systematically recorded and analyzed human remains from the Roman cemetery at Kellis.

Medical kits from the ancient world are rare objects, since many overlap with cosmetic kits, but far more have come to light from ancient Rome than the earlier Hellenistic and classical Greek periods. In order for archaeologists to classify a find as medical, it must contain instruments used exclusively for medical purposes. These instruments tended to be practical, with many having a double purpose, such as hooks or spoons with one sharp end and one blunt end. Their functionality did not preclude decorative motifs, such as a mouse, which is normally associated with Apollo at Ephesus.[41] Similarly, knotty bark or a lion's head as a decoration links the surgical practices with Hercules. These decorative motifs likely had an apotropaic function, and they blended religion with somatic healing practices. Instruments made of wood, such as splints, textiles for bandages, and quills to administer powders, have not survived in these kits, though they are frequently mentioned in medical literature. The kits found in the Roman provinces of Germany, *Gallia Belgica* (northern France, Luxembourg, Netherlands, and the Rhineland), Hungary, and Britain are mostly in a grave context. Interestingly, a lesser amount of kits have been found around the Mediterranean basin, although the oldest visual reference to one comes from a wall relief in the Ptolemaic temple at Kom Ombo (180–47 BCE).

In 1968, the British Museum acquired an Italian kit, which dates to the early Roman Empire without further provenance.[42] This set of forty instruments includes catheters for both males and females, a speculum, bone chisels, a sharp spoon, a blunt hook, handled needles, a small tanged cautery, cylindrical medicine boxes, and a stone palette. Given the large number of instruments, objects such as a bleeding cup are oddly missing.

A Roman-style medical kit dating to the early empire was found in an Iron Age burial (ca. 50 CE) for a local tribal elite in Stanway, Essex.[43] The

41. Cruse, *Roman Medicine*, 151.

42. Ralph Jackson, "A Set of Roman Medical Instruments from Italy," *Britannia* 17 (1986): 119–67.

43. Ralph Jackson, "An Ancient British Medical Kit from Stanway, Essex," *The Lancet* 350 (1997): 1471–73.

kit most likely belonged to a Briton in service to a chieftain shortly after the conquest, which shows the rapidity of people adopting Roman medical practices. The materials for instruments vary between the Stanway kit and standard Roman ones. Roman instruments usually have bronze handles with iron blades, which allowed for either handle or blade to be replaced as needed. Hooks might have been tipped with silver as a way to prevent infection. The instruments in the Stanway kit are made from a single piece of iron, with the exception of the saw. Its spring forceps also had a loop, which is usually found on forceps in cosmetic kits, not medical ones. The presence of other, exclusive medical-use instruments, though, indicates that the kit is decidedly medical in nature. In addition to the kit found at Stanway, there were divination rods more typical of the religious and possibly medical practices of the indigenous Britons.[44] Although they were adopting Greco-Roman practices, they seemed to blend them with their own indigenous practices.

Baker's *The Archaeology of Medicine in the Greco-Roman World*[45] not only provides an introduction to the methods used in understanding traditional artifacts, human remains, and sites but also develops the concept of texts as a form of material cultural particularly important to the study of the history of medicine. This work centers on helping students and researchers formulate important questions to interpret medical data in the archaeological remains.

## Cultural Concepts

Like the other cultures of the ancient Near East and Mediterranean, an analysis of artistic representations can aid in understanding the development of the Roman explanatory model of illness from its Etruscan origins to its later blending with Hellenistic philosophical treatises.

44. Gillian Carr, "A Time to Live, a Time to Heal, and a Time to Die: Healing and Divination in Later Iron Age and Early Roman Britain," in *Practitioners, Practices and Patients: New Approaches to Medical Archaeology and Anthropology* (Oxford: Oxbow, 2002), 58–73.

45. Patricia A. Baker, *The Archaeology of the Medicine in the Greco-Roman World* (Cambridge: Cambridge University Press, 2013).

## Anatomy and Physiology

Villanovan civilization (1000–750 BCE) typifies the indigenous Etruscan culture of the Italian peninsula. They had trade connections with Sardinia that placed the Etruscans on the fringe of the greater commercial networks of the Mycenaeans. Not many artistic representations of the human body during this period survive, but some can be found on pottery urns in the shape of "matchstick figures" without any type of gender differentiation.[46] This is similar to the early representations of humans in Mesopotamia and Mycenae. This paucity of detail means we cannot discern the cultural values imparted to anatomy and physiology by the early Etruscans.

By the end of the eighth century BCE, an "orientalizing" process began as the Greeks and Phoenicians started colonies on Sicily, Sardinia, and the Italian peninsula. Human figures appeared more frequently on vases, following Greek artistic traditions,[47] but these still had a geometric shape, such as triangular chests for both males and females rather than a realistic expression. The males do have shoulders drawn with thicker lines than those for the females, but this may be a convention to depict gendered clothing, such as armor. Statuettes of mourners and the deceased have a formulaic appearance, yet they are identifiable as female by the presence of breasts. Some statues display a slightly more naturalistic appearance but are clearly linked to the Greek Daidalic artistic style.[48]

During this period, beards are used as a gender marker, as in Greece, but only for certain scenes in vase painting, such as from the *Iliad*. Some pottery had molded applications of human heads, which tended to a more naturalistic but still formulaic expression. Their youthful, clean-shaven appearance and lack of any hairstyle make gender identification impossible. This might be due to the molded faces having a relationship to certain Etruscan deities that could change gender, such as Thalna, Alpan, Leinth, and Lasa, as well as Artumes, the Etruscan styling of Artemis.[49] Monumental statues in tombs at Ceri have a block-like rendering of the body, similar to Hittite and north Syrian styles,[50] yet unlike these antecedents, the males are clean-shaven. It seems the presence of a beard is limited to those items directly lifted from Hellenic

46. Haynes, *Etruscan Civilization*, 7.
47. Haynes, *Etruscan Civilization*, 53.
48. Haynes, *Etruscan Civilization*, 83.
49. De Grummond, *Etruscan Myth, Sacred History, and Legend*, 21.
50. Haynes, *Etruscan Civilization*, 74.

representations, but when foreign artistic depictions of the body are applied to indigenous Etruscan contexts, the beard disappears. Other than culturally prescribed physical adornments to show social roles, the orientalized period of Etruscan history masks any indigenous ideology of anatomy and physiology.

The archaic period (575–480 BCE) saw an upsurge in the power of the local Etruscan cities forming a league.[51] Terracotta plaques from Acquarossa depict banquets and scenes from the story of Herakles.[52] These show people and animals with stout musculature but no indications of social rank by the size of the muscles and no striation to indicate a strain on the muscles in action. This is in contrast to the Mesopotamian depiction of musculature but in keeping with Greek artistic conventions. Statues of goddesses followed the Ionian model of depicting females, except in the Etruscan context they were nude, whereas Greek statuary depicted women always clothed.[53] Another feature of Etruscan statues of women is their stance with either a left hand supporting the right breast or the right hand extended downward covering the genitals. This positioning may have been borrowed from representations of the Phoenician-Canaanite goddess Astarte.[54] These are likely indications of fertility; thus, the statues are thought to be of fertility goddesses, such as Vei. Other statues of women show a combination of Daidalic and Attic artistic styles as well as the local Vulcian. One consistent Etruscan feature in reliefs and some statues is the prominence of the head in relation to the rest of the body. Additionally, many statues have large eyes to accommodate inlays. Possibly this indicates a value on the head and eyes, but no texts survive that reveal exactly what this value is. Like the schematic and geometric shapes of earlier periods, this blending of styles during the archaic period makes it difficult to understand how the Etruscans thought of the body, apart from a more liberal ideology about naked females than that of their Greek counterparts. This is not surprising given that their deities could easily change between male and female, indicating they do not have an entrenched notion of binary gender. The Etruscan ideology governing the relationship between gender and anatomy is still a mystery.

The depiction of deities underwent an interesting artistic development in Etruscan history. Throughout the Villanovan and most of the Oriental-

51. Many scholars see the formation of a twelve-city league as an imitation of the Ionian League or other amphictyonies of the eastern Mediterranean; see Haynes, *Etruscan Civilization*, 135.

52. An early Etruscan styling of the Greek Herakles and later Roman Hercules.

53. Haynes, *Etruscan Civilization*, 147.

54. Haynes, *Etruscan Civilization*, 129.

izing period, Etruscan religion was essentially aniconic. Rather than cult statues, natural objects like stones and wood represented the deities. The Etruscans also felt a divine presence in highly specialized fabrications such as swords.[55] Only around 600 BCE did the eastern Mediterranean practice of creating humanoid statues, reliefs, and paintings of the gods begin to develop around Etruria. The paucity of human figures prior to orientalizing and Hellenism may reflect an early Etruscan religious belief that placed the divine in a physical, natural world, while humans simply occupied a lower stratum than the gods in this cosmic hierarchy. The importation of anthropomorphic art indicates a changing perception of the place and power of humans in their cosmology. Although still weaker than the deities, humans increased in status vis-à-vis the natural world, which includes the field of medicine.

By the fifth and fourth centuries, the Etruscans were losing power to Rome. In turn, Roman expansion in the eastern Mediterranean during the third century BCE continued the importation of Hellenistic conventions for depicting the human body. To tease out the various strains of classical Greek, Hellenistic, and native regional Etruscan artistic styles, influence on nascent Roman Republican art would be a study in its own right and takes us too far afield from the history of medicine. Such a study, though, would be most welcome. The process by which the Romans adopted or adapted certain physical features could help us understand the late Etruscan and early Roman ideologies on anatomy and physiology.

In the late Republican period of Roman history, both statuary and paintings exhibited a strong adherence to realism, to the point of creating identifiable portraits. The underlying belief of this trend is that although general principles govern anatomy and physiology, one's body is also subject to individual contexts. This highlights an epistemological tension in the medical literature—the extent to which healers can rely on biological patterns and the rules developed from it.

Despite the growing realism in Roman art, they still held to a popular language of ideal body types. The depiction of youth and health reinforced the belief that these resulted from a well-balanced life not only for gods and heroes but prominent mortals as well.[56] Morals, social status, and health were intimately intertwined. Yet interpreting physiognomy did not always follow a simple one-to-one correspondence. There are numerous studies on

55. Haynes, *Etruscan Civilization*, 126.

56. Mark Bradley, "Obesity, Corpulence and Emaciation in Roman Art," *Papers of the British School at Rome* 79 (2011): 1–41.

the "other" in Roman art, which look at groups as varied as comedy actors, boxers,[57] hunchbacks,[58] and Africans.[59] Grotesque figurines provide a curious overlap between art and medicine. They blend realistic and caricatured depictions in one figure, which makes the tendency to diagnose from them both tempting and dangerously misleading. Many of them with holes for wearing as amulets have been found in Smyrna, a notable medical center in antiquity, which gives the possibility that these figurines were apotropaic or perhaps connected to medical training.[60]

Bradley has undertaken a study of physiological depictions throughout the Roman Republic and Empire, focusing on the popular tropes of obesity and emaciation.[61] The emaciated body conveyed a dual meaning representing, on the one hand, old age, sickness, or poverty. Yet, on the other hand, a thin or gaunt body signified an inner moral quality of stoicism and personal discipline.[62] The idealized form for many philosophers, including Hippocrates, was that of an old, emaciated man, highlighting their attention to the mind rather than the body.[63] Abundance of fat could signal the positive attributes of affluence and authority, as in the *obesus Etruscus*, from the fourth to first century BCE, and later coinage of the emperors, from Nero to Vespasian. But just as easily, it represented the negative traits of laziness and greed. The negative connotations do seem to be limited to male representations, while females and babies have a more positive association for fat in the highly popular forms of the Crouching Venus, with or without Cupid, as well as sculptures of the infant Hercules. Corpulent bodies could also represent those on the margins of society, such as boxers and wrestlers or foreigners, particularly from eastern kingdoms or Egypt. It is interesting to note that the Egyptian god Bes, imported into Roman culture through the cult of Isis, gained weight on his trip to Italy. A protective god for mothers

57. Alexander G. Mitchell, "Disparate Bodies in Ancient Artefacts: The Function of Caricature and Pathological Grotesques among Roman Terracotta Figurines," in *Disabilities in Roman Antiquity: Disparate Bodies* a Capite ad Calcem, ed. Christian Laes, C. F. Goodey, and M. Lynn Rose (Boston: Brill, 2013), 275–97.

58. Lisa Trentin, *The Hunchback in Hellenistic and Roman Art* (London: Bloomsbury Academic, 2013).

59. Frank M. Snowden Jr., *Blacks in Antiquity: Ethiopians in the Greco-Roman Experience* (Cambridge, MA: Belknap, 1970).

60. Mitchell, "Disparate Bodies in Ancient Artefacts."

61. Bradley, "Obesity, Corpulence and Emaciation in Roman Art."

62. Bradley, "Obesity, Corpulence and Emaciation in Roman Art," 20.

63. Bradley, "Obesity, Corpulence and Emaciation in Roman Art," 21–22.

and children, his physique of dwarfish proportions, with a protruding belly, became exaggerated in Roman art.

Roman medicine carried on the epistemological debates of its Greek predecessors; thus, no one theory of anatomy and physiology dominates the medical culture. At best, two general themes run through all the different viewpoints: (1) the body works on a balance of substances, usually described as humoral, and (2) there needs to be a regular flow or movement of substances through the body. Some might try to see this anatomically focused medicine as a break from the idea of body parts as unique entities capable of forming or maintaining independent relationships with the gods, but this would not be entirely accurate. Auspices, the common belief in the "wandering womb," and the use of votives all indicate that body parts could still be something distinct from the individual person's identity, but the concept was in flux in ancient Roman medicine.

Liver divination derived from Etruscan practices and was reinforced by later borrowings from the Mesopotamians, who maintained the idea that body parts are distinct, independent entities. The wandering womb would also indicate for some a fundamental difference between men and women, in that women have a body part that is not fully integrated with their identity as an adult human, whereas men do not suffer from something distinct attached to their bodies. This belief stands in contrast to the arguments of Asklepiades of Bithynia (124–40 BCE), who sees no difference between males and females, since the same atoms make up everyone. Yet Asklepiades's theory does not move Roman medicine away from the idea of distinct entities symbiotically sharing a person's identity, since these atoms exist completely independent from human identity and function without conscious knowledge. What makes his theory different from ancient Near Eastern conceptions of anatomy is that their relationship to the gods is fixed and therefore discernible and predictable. Independent parts are not sentient and do not have the potential to be made sentient through magical means.

Galen's theorizing on the capacity to attract, especially for the stomach's role in digestion, counteracts the nonsentient atom. "All of this shows that there exists in nearly every part of the animal a sort of impetus and as it were an appetite for its proper quality and an aversion from the alien quality."[64] Galen understands body parts as having a relationship with each other rather than with a god. It is assumed that God/Nature created the rules that govern

64. *Nat. Fac.* 2.159–60 = *SM* 3, 216, 17–22.

the anatomy's relationship with the world; therefore, the same type of rules would apply to the relationship between anatomical parts. This makes "magical" prescriptions unnecessary, since one cannot influence or manipulate the will of a god, body part, or other entity to effect healing. Manipulation could be done only by working within the cause-and-effect rules of Nature. In a way, this is rather mechanistic, although Galen seemingly disavowed a purely mechanistic approach to physiology.

The anatomical votive, as always, creates a separate entity acceptable to be in the presence of the divine. This aspect is less of a necessity in comparison to its Near Eastern counterparts, since the ailing person can be in the presence of the divine, as indicated by sick supplicants entering the asklepieion or having Aesculapius appear in their dreams. Yet the votive as a distinct entity reminds the god(s) of their relationship to the healed body part as well as the person. This dualistic function of representing separate as well as whole entities paves the way for a later conception of anatomy and physiology as integral to identity. The distinct body part does not lose its individual identity, capable of acting on its own, until the developing Christian communities incorporate Israelite/Jewish ideologies of monotheism and a soul infusing the whole body, blending them with Greco-Roman somatic medicine and physiognomic beliefs.

Although the medical treatises and some practices gave space for a shift in thinking about anatomy, the literature influencing nonphysicians still projected the idea of a symbiotic anatomy. For example, Lucan's account of the mutilation of Gratidianus describes "that man popped the eyeballs from their sockets; he dug out the eyes last, after they bore witness for the other parts of the body."[65] Like the votives, eyes bearing witness to the destruction of their own body hint at a conception of individual body parts having a degree of independence from the whole. In this case, Lucan's literary construction depends on the eyes having a relationship with the Roman citizenry also witnessing the destruction of the civil wars.

Many people held to physiognomic conceptions of the body, as expressed by Pliny the Elder, whose explanation of digestion noted that the longer the distance between the stomach and small intestine the more it made a person greedy, that an obese stomach indicates a less clever person, and that these conditions were associated with sterility.[66] These types of relationships between anatomy, physiology, and cosmology in the epistemo-

65. Lucan, *Pharsalia* 2.183–85.

66. Pliny, *Natural History* 11.200–213.

logical debates among Roman-era physicians centered on the two issues of animal dissection and teleology.

The Empiricists disavowed the practice of dissection, since the very act alters the circumstances under which the anatomical structures are observed. This would impede finding the hidden truths of the body and disease. Yet they would incorporate in their teachings the knowledge gained from dissections. The Methodists similarly eschewed the practice while using information gained from it.

In contrast, Galen claimed that animal dissection and vivisection were important for understanding anatomy, which was intimately bound with physiology.[67] Although certain functions can be posited only through rational methods, such as digestion or use of the liver, his aim was to demonstrate their functions through the anatomy. Galen used his ability to perform public demonstrations of dissections to win his positions, claiming that the wounded should be in the care of one with exceptional skills, as well as demonstrating his greater philosophical points, such as the seat of reason/soul.[68] In doing this, he moved his line of argumentation away from the theoretical to show its clinical value. Galen did not create demonstrations to pander to the masses with showmanship but drew upon rhetorical techniques of the philosophers, targeting the intellectual members of his audience.[69] Galen gave such primacy to anatomy, especially his abilities in dissection, that if others could not reproduce similar results, it was not the methodology in question but the skill of the other physician.[70]

Like Aristotle, Galen has a teleology for anatomy and physiology grounded in the belief that nothing is useless;[71] therefore, everything has a cause. Some are more immediate, such as an instrumental cause, but ultimately, there is a final cause, which he terms as a Demiurge, Nature, or God. This idea of a final cause is in contrast to the Methodists' more mechanistic view of systems at work rather than something that set it in motion. This point of motion or "faculties to act" underlies the variety of physiological theories in Roman medicine.

67. Armelle Debru, "Physiology," in *The Cambridge Companion to Galen*, ed. R. J. Hankinson (Cambridge: Cambridge University Press, 2008), 263–82.

68. Julius Rocca, "Anatomy," in *The Cambridge Companion to Galen*, ed. R. J. Hankinson (Cambridge: Cambridge University Press, 2008), 242–62.

69. Rocca, "Anatomy."

70. Rocca, "Anatomy.

71. *UP* III 268 = 196, 19–20 Helmreich.

Galen explained two broad categories for faculties or the capacity to act. One is the psychic faculty, which governs sensation and voluntary movements originating in the brain and carried out through the nerves. The other is the natural faculty, which governs generation, growth, and nutrition. Natural faculties depend on their tissues arising from elements and their mixtures, such as the hematopoietic faculty, which produces blood. The system at work: a combination of elements under the natural faculty creates an organ such as the liver, which can form other organs like the veins (generation) and create blood (growth), which is then spread throughout the body (nutrition). All the different faculties work together to maintain the body as a whole, a hierarchical yet cooperative system[72] creating equilibrium in the body. The entire system of faculties is governed by Nature or the Demiurge.

Galen adopted Erasistratus's theory about the role of voluntary muscles in respiration. Ultimately, this places Galen on the side of the brain rather than the heart as the source of speech and, most important, reasoning. One might assume then a hierarchy to the faculties, with the brain at the pinnacle of the natural faculties and the psychic faculty as the supreme one, since it allows humans—especially males, from an ancient Greco-Roman cultural perspective—to perceive and voluntarily act within the world. Yet Galen avoided any such hierarchy, adhering to Plato's tripartite division of the soul: brain for ruling, heart for emotion, and liver for vegetation or nutritional. Note that Galen focused on the organs in which these are situated rather than the use of the term "soul." Many organs and faculties work in cooperation, but the brain, heart, and liver are essentially independent from one another. This allows them to come into conflict, thus linking medicine with moral philosophy and the physiognomic texts. A healthy body has a functioning organ-organ relationship, whereas disease is a breakdown of this community cohesion.

The role of the kidneys and ureters in the production of urine provides a good case study for how competing physiological theories explained the same observable phenomenon.[73] Aristotle, Erasistratus, Asklepiades, and the Methodists all argued that urine resulted from the filtration of blood through the kidneys. Some, like Erasistratus, posited that the void was the attracting power and that things rushed into it to fill the void. Asklepiades differed by asserting that heat is what attracts corpuscles, not a simple void. Galen, who

72. *UP* III 18 = i 13, 7–9 Helmreich.

73. Rudolph E. Siegel, *Galen's System of Physiology and Medicine* (New York: S. Karger, 1968), 126–31.

claimed that parts of the body attract those things necessary for it (without fully explaining why), argued that the kidneys secrete water after separating it from the blood. The yellow color derives from the seepage of bile into the urine. Another competing but unattributed medical idea was that the bladder produces urine essentially through a process of condensation, but this then requires the urine to flow up into the ureters. Galen countered this with demonstrations of tying off the ureters at various points, showing urine collecting above the ligatures.

In addition to the attractive quality, Galen thought organs have the capacity to retain, alter, and expel. Blood flowing through the heart illustrates some of these principles. As the liver creates blood, building up pressure, the movement of the thorax during respiration forces the blood through the heart. Yet blood fills the ventricles because of their own attractive quality. Also, the heart itself can squeeze the blood between ventricles. According to Galen, the heart did not pump the blood through the body; this was the job of the thoracic muscles. Rather, the heart acted as a furnace, transferring its heat to the blood, while respiration itself provided air to cool the blood and heart, keeping the temperatures in balance.[74]

From this explanation of blood flow, we can see that Galen's physiology incorporated two popular medical beliefs: innate heat and pneuma. Innate heat, present at conception due to uterine blood, gives rise to all other organs. This innate heat wanes over time, also resulting in eventual death. Similarly, the thoracic muscles allow for breathing, an act integral to the pneuma, which is a primary instrument of the soul, governing sensation and voluntary movements. Asklepiades argued that the relaxed pores of the lungs drew in pneuma, which caused the pulsation in the arteries. Without pneuma, the person or animal ceases movement, that is, dies. Short of cessation, the functioning of pneuma and innate heat can be disturbed by an imbalance in the body, giving rise to diseases and illness.

## Disease Etiology

For many Romans, illness could have multiple causes. They could understand and accept a disease etiology explained by a physician from an Empiricist or Methodist school of thought but also adhere to the belief that a god like Aesculapius caused them to be ill. This apparent cognitive dissonance

74. Siegel, *Galen's System of Physiology and Medicine*, 83–87.

among patients was not problematic for the healers either, since they did not disavow the gods but only sought to understand the details of a natural, divinely created system. Although most medical sects operated with the same basic principles of balance, movement/faculties, innate heat, and pneuma, they differed on how they physiologically functioned and, in turn, caused diseases.

For the Dogmatists, the principles such as balance and movement that create a healthy body can change to cause a disease. Because diseases arise from any number of principles, they can have a single, independent cause; a simultaneous cause with each one creating different diseases but presenting symptoms all at the same time; or a concomitant cause with different principles working together to form one disease. Knowing these causes then determines which therapeutic option should be applied. The Dogmatists' disease etiology still rests upon navigating different relationships, but they are all centered within the natural world instead of incorporating the supernatural realm.

In contrast, Empiricists disavowed a theoretical analysis of disease etiology; one cannot know the hidden causes so should not waste time trying. Instead, they grouped and classified diseases by similar, observable symptoms. They worked with the idea that a successful treatment of a disease in one classification would then be successful treating all the diseases in that same group.

Methodists similarly rejected an in-depth causal analysis. They understood disease as arising from the movement of corpuscles, which are either obstructed/constricted or too relaxed, allowing an unhealthy amount of movement. Movement of corpuscles, not humors, would be out of balance. The constricted or relaxed conditions caused visible symptoms, and by addressing these symptoms, the disease is cured.

Galen, like the Dogmatists, was involved in causal analysis of disease. Interestingly, he effectively stamped out the competing theories of disease etiology by vehemently arguing against them, while simultaneously incorporating certain elements into his own form of Hippocratic medicine.[75]

He postulated two broad classifications for diseases, anatomical and humoral, though he referred to them as dissolution of the unity and disturbance of the balance.[76] We can see these at work in his description of fevers;

75. Alain Touwaide, "Disease, Conceptions of," in *The Encyclopedia of Ancient History*, ed. Roger S. Bagnall et al. (London: Blackwell, 2013).

76. *On the Difference of Disease* and *The Art of Healing*; see Siegel, *Galen's System of Physiology and Medicine*, 201.

some are due to lesions on anatomical structures, while other fevers arise from an imbalance of phlegm or bile. Although the lesions cause an imbalance, resulting in fever, Galen advises that it is difficult to locate the lesions. This is in contrast to the diagnosis of a general imbalance that is easier to treat, since the physician does not need to specifically locate the cause.[77]

In conjunction with the anatomical and humoral classifications, he described how disease moved through the body as part of understanding diagnosis. Bad humors could flow from the point of disease origin to remote organs, or a "primary irritation," something other than the humors, could move through the nerves to widely dispersed locations of the body. Galen explained five different types of movements, or sympathies, as he called them, adapting the Dogmatists' ideas of simultaneous or concomitant causes and applying them to the involvement of body parts.[78]

The disease classification and mode of sympathy leads one to follow a particular diagnostic chain for any illness, which consists of impairment, condition of impairment, cause of condition, and consequences. Diagnosis is the labeling of the condition of the impairment or, more specifically, the indications the body gives for the condition, and the condition is the target of therapeutic measures.[79] The conditions are an imbalance in the physiology. Interestingly, Galen does not assume a pure or perfect state of health in practice but only in theory. Anyone seeking a physician presents some type of imbalance, so a physician will never actually encounter true health. Additionally, even a "healthy" person has peculiarities that may not be the same as another's "health." Individual relationships, at least with the natural world, still have an impact. Within these parameters, Galen asserted that the best diagnostic indicators are urine and the pulse[80] and that moral upbringing can also have a positive or negative influence on health.

## Restoration of Health

The Dogmatist, Methodist, and Empiricist schools seemingly removed the aspect of obedience and consideration in the human-divine community

77. *On Crises*; see Siegel, *Galen's System of Physiology and Medicine*, 201.

78. Siegel, *Galen's System of Physiology and Medicine*, 361–62.

79. Philip J. van der Eijk, "Therapeutics," in *The Cambridge Companion to Galen*, ed. R. J. Hankinson (Cambridge: Cambridge University Press, 2008), 283–303.

80. Van der Eijk, "Therapeutics."

from their healing strategies, since there was no role for the gods to actively consider a patient's actions. A patient may still demonstrate obedience by engaging in somatic treatments, but this has two possible effects. It plays to the functioning of the human-human community. The wider human community considers the patient's obedience, whether submitting directly to the directives of the *medicus* or by demonstrating piety toward the gods by seeking a *medicus* or other healer when removing the sick role. This adherence to somatic treatments shows obedience to the gods and their natural order; thus, consideration becomes exemplified by the gods not disrupting the natural order and letting healing take place. Divine consideration becomes passive rather than active, in some circles of Roman medical culture. From an anthropological view, different types of somatic treatments are all naturally charged substances and rituals. The only difference is that how their power worked could now be explained and grasped by anyone blessed with the proper intellectual capacity.

Celsus divided therapies into the three categories of dietetics, pharmacology, and surgery. The detailed writings of Greco-Roman authors such as Galen indicate the vast amount of subdivisions these categories had, including venesection, plasters and bandaging, bathing, and purgatives, to name just a few. The Empiricists and Methodists focused especially on treating symptoms directly rather than discovering the cause of disease.

The Methodists approached therapies with the philosophy of opposites. If cold caused the restriction of pores and thus the movement of corpuscles, then heat would be applied to open them. They favored treatments based on massages, exercise, wine, and cold-water baths to maintain the proper movement of corpuscles. In their line of thinking, the use of *materia medica* worked because their atoms/corpuscles influenced the obstruction or flow of corpuscles in the body. Galenic medicine, following Hippocratic lines, did not explain the mechanism by which hot counterbalanced cold. These treatments focused only on the properties of substances being hot/cold and wet/dry to balance the humors, either through drugs or, more commonly, diet. Galen's overall approach to therapeutics can be outlined from the work *On the Therapeutic Method* and *Therapeutics to Glaucon*. The physician should be able to work within a general theoretical framework yet adjust therapies, depending on the specific conditions of each patient, an inherent tension in the field of medicine.[81] Influencing factors can be particular to the patient, such as age, gender, and lifestyle; environmental factors, such as seasonal

81. Van der Eijk, "Therapeutics."

shifts in temperature; or even the mode of therapy itself, such as internal or external application, raw or cooked *materia medica*. Healers must know the quality and quantity of relevant remedies, mode of their application, and ability to discern the right time for their application. Ultimately, the illness must be understood both on a level of general principle and on a specific level, with therapies targeting the different levels. To get a better understanding of Roman therapeutics, let us look at the healing techniques of surgery, pharmacology, amulets, and incantations as examples.

Surgeries tended to be limited to the surface of the body, such as the excising of cysts, the lancing of hemorrhoids, and eye surgery. Healers also commonly performed tonsillectomies,[82] since they can be accessed through the mouth. Another popular surgery was the partial removal of an uvula that had become swollen.[83] Roman era physicians did not strictly adhere to the general taboo of cutting into the body, as attested by the practice of cesarean sections as well as trephinations. Celsus also refers to the cauterization and excising of varicose veins.[84] Bloodletting, the most frequent type of surgery, had almost no variation in the style of cups used from as early as the sixth century BCE in Greece to the third century CE in Gaul.[85] The cupping instruments never appreciably changed, although the theoretical justification for the practice did. Galen touted venesection as a therapy, likely extending its popularity into the early modern period, while other prominent physicians of the ancient world, such as Erasistratus (304–250 BCE), had argued against it as useless and dangerous from an early period. Asklepiades of Bithynia, Themison of Tralles, and the later Methodists also disdained venesection.

Surgical instruments tended to have more than one use, such as needles for pricking as well as being heated for cauterizing, or the instrument itself was double sided. For example, a scalpel whose handle also had a blunt spatula could be used for multiple purposes during one surgical procedure. This type of instrument matches textual descriptions of surgery given by Celsus and later Byzantine physicians: "holding in the right hand a *polypus* scalpel, having its extremity shaped like a myrtle-leaf, we cut around the *polypus* or *sarcomatous* tumour. . . . Afterwards, turning round the instrument, we

82. Celsus, *De Medicina* 7.12.2.

83. R. P. J. Jackson, "Roman Medicine: The Practitioners and Their Practices," *ANRW* 37, no. 1 (1993): 79–101.

84. Celsus, *De Medicina* 7.31.2–3.

85. Jackson, "Roman Medicine," *ANRW* 79–101.

bring out the separated fleshy body with its concave part."[86] The dual nature of surgical instruments allowed the kit to be overall rather compact and portable, as Hippocrates advocated.[87] In this same work, Hippocrates urged the physician to keep the kit in a methodical order and, therefore, not to waste valuable time as the physician looked for a specific instrument.

Medical texts name different types of plants, but these can be problematic, since Roman references (like those from many ancient societies) are not always the same as those used in modern nomenclature. We can confirm the identity of some plants by correlating them with plant residues found in jars or remains from excavated gardens. Additionally, drawings of plants used in sources, such as Dioscorides's *De Materia Medica*, help identify them. Coins also bear images of important medicinal plants, such as *siliphium* from Cyrene.[88] This type of evidence attests to the increased variety of *materia medica*, due to the expansion of territory and trade during the republic. Pliny praises the peace brought during the Augustan period for its bountiful impact on the availability of drugs.[89]

There was no regulation of the pharmacopeia in the ancient world; thus, the potential for fatal doses was high if an inexperienced person handled the prescription or compounding of ingredients. This only added to the popular view that physicians were dangerous and could easily commit murder, as depicted in the rhetorical declamation exercises. Dioscorides, in describing the dosages of opium, took care to mention at what amount it can be fatal; this is in contrast to other, earlier medical texts, such as by Theophrastus (371–287 BCE), who simply states, "If he is to be killed," with the appropriate high dosage given.[90] The problem, though, with most recipes, including ones from Dioscorides, is that they did not have precise amounts. This is because the time of year, environment where harvested, size, age, and sex of patient could all impact the dosage.

Besides plants, other ingredients could make up the *materia medica*. Metals such as copper oxides were frequently employed in the preparation of eye salves, as Pliny references.[91] Images of Achilles binding the wound of Patroclus depict the use of filings from a spear tip. This type of image not only

86. Francis Adams, trans., *The Medical Works of Paulus Aegineta* (London: Sydenham Society, 1861), vi, xxv.

87. Hippocrates, *Decorum* 8.10–13.

88. Cruse, *Roman Medicine*, 63.

89. Pliny, *Natural History* 27.1.

90. Theophrastus, *Enquiry* 9.2.6.

91. Pliny, *Natural History* 33.28.

demonstrates the variety of ingredients but that the locus of healing is not always with a trained *medicus/iatros*. The soldier (figuratively represented by Achilles) would have some knowledge of the *materia medica* and how to use it. Ancient authors like Cicero, giving an account of Roman military medicine, claim that physicians were not assigned to legions until the Roman Empire, meaning that soldiers in the Roman Republic had to find treatment among themselves. Yet Cicero refers also to a military *medicus*.[92] A votive tablet from 82 CE mentions a *medicus* Sextus Titius Alexander, indicating they were in place during the empire.

The bones of animals such as reptiles and amphibians frequently appear in remedies for venom and poison, such as the famous cures mithridatium and theriac, perhaps based on theories of homeopathy. Curiously, though, snakes and lizards could not be used in the same recipe; we lack an explanation for why. These types of drugs could be highly complicated compounds, using up to forty-four ingredients for mithridatium and sixty-three for theriac.[93]

Yet these treatments presuppose only a somatic approach to medicine. Restoration of health includes the social aspect, especially reintegration with the community and a return to fulfilling obligations, including participation in communal worship. An argument can be made that patients using the somatic forms of healing are signaling to the divine as well as the human community their willingness to obey the natural laws set forth by the gods. This type of obedience, though, is more obvious when looking at therapies directly incorporating divine actions, such as amulets and incantations.

Throughout the Greco-Roman world, numerous amulets have been found for treating a variety of ailments, such as fevers, headache, and gout, with a large subsection of them devoted to controlling the wandering womb.[94] They usually depict a uterus, according to Galen's anatomy, surrounded by an Egyptian motif of a serpent devouring its tail. Others have the shape of an Egyptian scarab beetle. These ancient Near Eastern motifs can be found in sites as far away as Dicket Mead and the Rectory Farm in West Deeping in Britain.[95] The amulet from West Deeping contains the Greek name of its supplicant, Cleuomedes, with a Latin inscription making use of

92. Cicero, *Tusculan Disputations* 2.16.38.

93. Ciaraldi, "Drug Preparation in Evidence?" 91–98.

94. Elizabeth Ann Pollard, "Amulets, Greece and Rome," in *The Encyclopedia of Ancient History*, ed. Roger S. Bagnall et al. (London: Blackwell, 2013), 388–89.

95. Cruse, *Roman Medicine*, 55.

the names Yahweh, Sabaoth, and Adonai. Interestingly, these Hebrew names are written with the insertion of the Greek letter omega rather than the Latin "o." As Tomlin points out, this is not unusual for amulets.[96]

The precepts allowing amulets to work were not exclusive to one form of religion, such as sympathetic magic, which dictates the use of red hematite for issues with blood. Amulets acted as a conduit for human-divine communication. The belief in communicating through objects characterized all ancient religions. The choice to blend linguistics and artistic styles comes from what people thought the gods wanted rather than forcing a divine entity to communicate in a manner particular to one group of people. Even if the patient could not understand the specific symbols, especially true for writing, it was best to follow the gods' desires. The efficacy of certain styles proved which ones the gods preferred. The heyday for Greco-Roman amulets was the second through fourth century CE, which indicates that the somatic healing strategies espoused in the medical treatises did not dominate the healing options for many people.

Roman medical culture used incantations from an early period.[97] These often took a simple form directed at the disease and at times may have addressed a deity. In some cases, the incantation was needed to effect the power of a plant in a medical recipe blending magical and somatic therapies. This is much like the use of incantations in Egypt and Mesopotamia. Varro quotes an incantation and ritual for the curing of diseased feet from the older Saserna: "'I am thinking of you, cure my feet. The pain go in the ground, and may my feet be sound.' He bids you chant this thrice nine times, touch the ground, spit on it, and be fasting while you chant."[98] Similarly, Cato espouses the use of incantations with a ritual when treating dislocations.[99] This indicates that the magical properties of chants are not restricted to mysterious internal diseases but have an efficacy for traumas as well. Pliny the Elder, though, recognized within Roman culture a tension between, on the one hand, the magical thought processes of incantations and rituals and, on the other, the treatments grounded in the logical application of the rules of nature derived from philosophy.[100] This overlap in magic and somatic healing allowed the theories of Galen and other physicians to be adopted as

96. R. S. O. Tomlin, "'Sede in Tuo Loco': A Fourth-Century Uterine Phylactery in Latin from Roman Britain," *Zeitschrift für Papyrologie und Epigraphik* 115 (1997): 291–94.

97. Cruse, *Roman Medicine*, 52.

98. Varro, *On Agriculture* 1.2.27.

99. Cato, *On Agriculture* 160.1.

100. Pliny, *Natural History* 28.3.

Greco-Roman culture spread through ancient Europe and the Near East. For example, pre-Roman Britain and Gaul worked with the calendrical idea of auspicious and inauspicious times, which influenced decisions as to when one should or should not undergo medical treatments.[101] The use of augurs in Etruscan/Roman religion to determine appropriate times for action could readily be recognized by the newly conquered Britons. This, coupled with the timing for pharmacology in Greco-Roman medicine, would make it easier for the Britons to adopt the use of *materia medica* and their method of application from Roman *medici*.

## Illness

Knowing the types and prevalence of disease processes with which Romans contended would be helpful to the history of Roman medicine. To this end, paleopathology is a necessary complement. Such studies help determine the frequency of particular illnesses in contrast to a cultural emphasis in literary, religious, or even medical texts. Given the territorial vastness of the republic and the empire, it would be near impossible to characterize the paleopathology for all of Rome. This would then impact how a more universal medical culture applies locally.

### Disease

Gourevitch and Grmek assessed the classical period as a whole as suffering from a general decline in health.[102] As noted above, the environmental and cultural variations across Roman territory make this problematic. Etruscans practiced cremation and burial, but the soil acidity degraded the buried remains, making analysis difficult.[103] With a few usable samples, paleopathologists can identify different types of anemia. One is from nutritional deficit, as well as the genetic form thalassemia, which protects against malaria. The Etruscans also suffered from arthritis, spondylitis, osteoporosis, polio, and tuberculosis.[104] Later Roman burials, such as the one at Poundbury in Dor-

101. Carr, "Time to Live."
102. Bradley, "Obesity, Corpulence and Emaciation in Roman Art," 10.
103. Haynes, *Etruscan Civilization*, 8.
104. Haynes, *Etruscan Civilization*, 8–9.

set, England, give a slightly different picture of overall health, including periodontal disease, tuberculosis, and nutritional-based anemia. Demographic studies from Roman Egypt reveal not only a relatively younger population but that they were more likely to die during hotter months, due to a natural increase of infectious diseases during the summer.[105] An interesting cross-provenance study would look at the geographic dispersal of certain diseases, in comparison to isolated pockets of other diseases to help determine the contributing environmental factors. Even with regional variations in disease, certain illnesses had prominence in the medical literature, both ancient and modern, that can speak to the intersection of medicine and cultural values.

In 165/166 CE, the troops who fought the Parthians along the border region of Armenia brought a plague back to Rome. Over the next fifteen to twenty years, the plague swept across the empire and claimed the lives of the emperors Lucius Verus and Marcus Aurelius. Known as the Antonine Plague, it is considered the first recorded pandemic. Descriptions by Galen[106] indicate that it may have been a form of smallpox, but some scholars, reading the same account, think it was anthrax or measles. Problems diagnosing the type of plague stem from the fact that Galen did not focus on clear symptom descriptions and may have related them with borrowed rhetoric from Thucydides's description for the Plague of Athens. No sufficient paleopathological studies have been done to determine the exact disease agent. It is estimated that, in some areas, up to one-third of the population died from the plague, greatly altering the economic landscape as well as spurring a religious response that may have fostered the popularity of newer religious forms such as Mithraism and Christianity.

The marshy areas around Rome, especially between the seven hills in the city itself, made malaria a significant problem. In this regard, Romans took preventive measures by draining the marshes as well as building sewers and aqueducts. Unfortunately, the collection of water in cisterns exposed them to the rapid growth of bacteria and mosquito-borne malaria. The tertiary fevers of malaria may have influenced the medical texts' focus on fevers and theories of innate heat in the blood.

Although Gilfillan's theory of lead poisoning[107] is periodically revived and refuted, even the ancient Romans themselves realized the problematic

105. Draycott, *Approaches to Healing in Roman Egypt*, 8.

106. Galen, *Method of Medicine*.

107. S. C. Gilfillan, "Lead Poisoning and the Fall of Rome," *Journal of Occupational Medicine* 7 (1965): 53–60.

use of lead-lined pipes in their water-supply system and thus kept it to a minimum. Vitruvius warned, "Indeed that conveyed in lead must be injurious, because from it white lead is obtained, and this is said to be injurious to the human system. . . . This may be verified by observing the workers in lead, who are of a pallid colour."[108] He advocated the use of earthenware-lined pipes. This sentiment is echoed by Columella: "Rain-water is after all most suitable to the body's health, and is regarded as uncommonly good if it is conveyed through earthen pipes into a covered cistern."[109] The closer water is to the natural source, the better. Thus, Romans advocated using running spring water, but the urban reality made this nearly impossible for many.

Paleopathology cannot reveal the incidence of certain diseases, such as trachoma and cataracts. Based solely on the textual evidence, these were frequent eye diseases for the Romans.[110] Celsus describes surgeries for the conditions.[111] Trachoma needed removal of ingrown eyelashes. Cataracts were treated by inserting a thin bronze needle to push the cataract out of the way of the pupil or, if it floats back into view, cutting it up into smaller pieces to try to keep the cataract from blocking the vision.[112] *Collyria* are stamps to identify a medicant's maker, typically found on containers for eye salves. Although used throughout the empire and usually associated with bath houses, the majority come from Gaul and Britain, while none have been found in the Levant or Egypt.[113] This attests to a localized bias in their use, perhaps linked to certain guilds of healers or other cultural contexts. For example, the Egyptians since the Pharaonic period used kohl around the eyes as a preventative measure from insect-borne diseases and thus did not need *collyria*.

## Trauma

All societies must contend with the typical industrial accidents, war wounds, and animal bites. Rome additionally had traumas from its gladiatorial games. Galen provides a good source for investigating these injuries, which would

108. Vitruvius, *On Architecture* 8.6.10–11.

109. Columella, *Agriculture* 1.5.2.

110. Debate surrounds the frequency of eye diseases and blindness in the ancient world, given the ubiquitousness of it as a literary trope, especially in religious or other moralizing texts.

111. Celsus, *De Medicina* 7.7.8.

112. Celsus, *De Medicina* 7.7.14e.

113. Cruse, *Roman Medicine*, 166.

be the same as those acquired in battle. Two areas of particular importance, though, for ancient Rome are eye injuries and bites from snakes and crocodiles. Given the importance of the gaze in Roman culture,[114] it is not unusual that the nonmedical documents tend to focus on the loss of an eye. An eye injury, especially from battle, serves as a badge of honor and courage. Sallust describes Sertorius's wounded eye: "for it showed how gloriously he had preserved the rest of his body."[115] In this context, the eye symbolizes the sacrifice that one is willing to make not just for personal well-being but for the republic. Similarly, the eye is seen as sacrificing itself for the whole of the body. Once again, this reinforces the idea of organ-organ relationships or communities.

More particular to Egyptian documentation are snake and crocodile bites. This is due to the traditional religious significance of these animals in the Predynastic and Pharaonic periods. Because Roman domination did not significantly disrupt traditional religious practices, crocodiles were still seen as agents of the god Sobek. Bites from them held religious connotations beyond just an animal attack. As the healing aspect of Isis increased in Greco-Roman culture, snakes, although not part of her original iconography, became associated with the goddess. This is due in part to the presence of snakes with Isis in the ancient Egyptian story *The Contendings of Horus and Seth*, which is then coupled with the association of snakes with Aesculapius. When suffering from these animal bites, patients had to account for their religious significance, if they decided to seek treatment.

## Disability

Romans, much like the Greeks, culturally valued the perfected physical form and therefore provide little documentation directly addressing disability. In fact, Greco-Roman census data from Egypt shows that females and disabled children were not counted.[116] This in itself speaks to the ideal of the Roman body at least in relation to the government. Unlike the modern world that

114. David Fredrick, ed., *The Roman Gaze: Vision, Power, and the Body* (Baltimore: Johns Hopkins University Press, 2002).

115. Sallust, *Historiae* 1.88; see Lisa Trentin, "Exploring Visual Impairment in Ancient Rome," in *Disabilities in Roman Antiquity: Disparate Bodies* a Capite ad Calcem, ed. Christian Laes, C. F. Goodey, and M. Lynn Rose (Boston: Brill, 2013), 100.

116. Christian Laes, "Silent Witnesses: Deaf-Mutes in Graeco-Roman Antiquity," *Classical World* 104, no.4 (2011): 453n8.

categorizes mental and physical as separate issues requiring specialists, the Roman world saw them as integral to one another. An ancient mental deficit, such as melancholy, resulted from a physical problem of the brain, heart, or stomach, so that writers like Galen expound on what today would be in the discipline of psychiatry. The Roman view that an underlying physical condition results in "intellectual" problems does not necessarily equate to the classification of learning disabilities in the modern sense, such as Down syndrome. This disconnect comes from the modern approach to "medicalize" disability rather than seeing the term, like the Romans did, as a social label intertwined with issues of status and power relations.

Gellius, addressing the legal definition and use of terms pertaining to the sale of slaves, comes closest to outlining a Roman concept of disability, distinguishing between disease and defect, with the difference being whether someone can work; the defect prevents work and might be analogous to the modern term "disability."[117] Gellius, though, goes on to outline legal cases where opposite verdicts have been given with regard to the same disease/defect, such as being a eunuch, barren women, nearsightedness, and even missing a tooth.[118]

At the heart of the matter is how the Romans defined disability. It cannot simply be deviation from the norm, whether ideal or standard, because then all humans present some sort of disability by Galen's theory that no one actually embodies the ideal and even the standard is difficult to come by. This idea of deviation from a norm is exactly how Gellius defines disease, not defect/disability: "Disease is an unnatural condition of any body, which impairs its usefulness."[119] So, by definition, all diseases are defects, but not all defects are diseases. "However, the converse is not also true; for one may have defects and yet not be diseased."[120] But it is in this separate notion of defect, free from disease, that one may find a Roman definition of disability.

If they defined disability by social function, then the extent to which physical impairments do actually hinder someone can vary from place to place. Typically, it is assumed that caring for the disabled would have been a heavy burden for many citizens and subjects of Rome, given their precarious

117. Gellius, *Attic Nights* 4.2; see Christian Laes, C. F. Goodey, and M. Lynn Rose, "Approaching Disabilities *a Capite ad Calcem*: Hidden Themes in Roman Antiquity," in *Disabilities in Roman Antiquity: Disparate Bodies* a Capite ad Calcem, ed. Christian Laes, C. F. Goodey, and M. Lynn Rose (Boston: Brill, 2013), 1–15.

118. Gellius, *Attic Nights* 4.6–12.

119. Gellius, *Attic Nights* 4.3.

120. Gellius, *Attic Nights* 4.5.

subsistence level of living; only the well-to-do would have the resources to provide for those unable to work.[121] Garland, asserting that only the economic elites had access to physicians, claimed that even simple traumas such as a broken leg would result in permanent disability.[122] This assumes that only the philosophically trained physician could properly set a limb when, in fact, even those healers trained through a basic apprenticeship would have the skills necessary from years of practical experiences. Yet it is just as likely that failure to seek treatment stems from patient reluctance, for a variety of cultural reasons, rather than a simple economic inability to pay for a healer.[123]

Many with disabilities could still find an occupational niche within Roman society. Blindness may not be as problematic for someone in an urban environment as in a rural one, or vice versa. Their integration within the family and larger community is also key. The economic burden of caring for a blind person may be spread out among the community rather than fall to just the individual or his immediate family. The presence and strength of many religious and occupational fraternities in Roman society could have easily absorbed the supposed economic burden of the disabled.

Visual impairment could interfere with full cultural participation, since the Romans highly valued the use of spectacle. Yet Roman society did provide avenues by which some could still participate.[124] War veterans suffering from a damaged or missing eye could receive financial benefits from the state as well as some degree of legal immunity.[125] Analysis of Latin terms shows that the culture did distinguish between degrees of partial blindness and total loss of vision due to various causes. The frequency of vision impairment would necessitate a variety of strategies to compensate, depending on socioeconomic factors. Unlike the priesthood in Israel, physical imperfections such as blindness did not exclude anyone from priestly offices. Augustus did not have to give up the office of Pontifex Maximus in light of his blind left eye. Suetonius exemplifies the cultural implications of blindness when he notes the morally degenerate emperors Nero and Domitian as causing blindness, contrasting them with the exemplary emperors Vespasian and Hadrian miraculously healing blindness. Interestingly, the miracles follow

121. Robert Garland, "Disability," in *The Encyclopedia of Ancient History*, ed. Roger S. Bagnall et al. (London: Blackwell, 2013), 2156–57.

122. Garland, "Disability."

123. Trentin, "Exploring Visual Impairment in Ancient Rome," 89–114.

124. Trentin, "Exploring Visual Impairment in Ancient Rome."

125. Trentin, "Exploring Visual Impairment in Ancient Rome."

similar plotlines as healing dreams attributed to Aesculapius, as well as Jesus's power of touch.

Applying modern demographic studies, one can reconstruct that approximately one out of one thousand people experienced congenital deafness in antiquity; isolated populations may have experienced a higher frequency based on their genetic pooling. Galen mentions that the Greeks, in particular Hippocrates, linked deafness and muteness. Some ancient healers theorized that the linkage is due to the nerves for the tongue and ears being connected and that sometimes they are damaged in unison (congenital defect) or injured separately (acquired deafness or muteness), especially by external trauma. Other ancient scholars simply assert that the inability to hear from birth meant that one cannot learn speech, hence muteness. Celsus claimed that cutting of the lingual frenulum should cure the mute, but in actuality, it rarely does.[126]

Roman law viewed both the deaf and the mute as mentally deficient and suffering from an illness. If the condition was present at birth, they would not be able to make wills or be a witness to them; they were excluded from holding public office or acting as judges. Note that this disability makes one unacceptable to public life (i.e., government) as opposed to the divine. Many of the legal restrictions on children were applied to the deaf-mute. Both Greek and Latin texts distinguish between deaf and mute, but the Greek in Matthew 9:33 and 15:31 uses the typical term for deaf to indicate muteness.

Greco-Romans privileged mutes over the deaf, as exemplified in the story of Croesus's son.[127] Although first identified in Herodotus as a deaf-mute, later writers such as Nicolaus of Damascus (first century BCE) focus on the boy's recovery of speech. Similarly, Cornelius Gellius (125–180 CE) reports on muteness only in his *Attic Nights*. These stories follow the medical theory that an obstructed tongue caused the muteness and that learning to speak frequently involved the procedures of learning literacy. Laes suggests that the culture's emphasis on rhetorical skill causes this valuation of muteness over deafness. The inability to hear or speak excluded the deaf-mute from the oral-based education system; thus, society viewed him or her as also being mentally deficient. This would then be a serious functional disability among the upper classes, whereas deaf-mutes among the agricultural laborers may still work, developing an individualistic communication system for their immediate friends and family. Ample evidence exists of deaf and

126. Celsus, *De Medicina* 7.12.4.
127. Laes, "Silent Witness."

mute slaves, especially within the royal household, whose condition did not interfere with their social roles.

Estimates for the modern world is that 3 percent of births have a congenital defect, with that figure rising to roughly 8 percent by the time the child is five years of age; it would be reasonable to assume similar statistics for ancient Rome.[128] Roman Egypt up through the third century CE had a prevalence of brother-sister marriages not seen in other Roman provinces at roughly 15–20 percent.[129] Likely, this is in imitation of the earlier Ptolemaic practice being continued, since it is mostly found among the Greek elites within the urban areas. It is unclear to what extent and percentage of the population of children from such a union had congenital defects, either in infancy or surviving into adulthood. Approximately 40 percent of Roman cognomens do refer to some sort of physical abnormality, such as the name Strabo, meaning "cross-eyed."[130]

The phrase "monstrous births" referred to any abnormality, from the mythic Minotaur to the perceived dangers of moral degenerates, such as Caligula, to the physical impairments of the Emperor Claudius, who stuttered and limped. Upper-class/wealthy Romans would keep slaves with deformities as a type of pet, especially dwarfs; Plutarch writes about the "monster market" for acquiring them.

The Roman notion of a monstrous birth included the modern category of intersexed people, which in Latin had a variety of terms, the most frequent being the Greek loan words *androgynus* and *hermaphroditus*.[131] During the Republic, those with indeterminate gender were viewed as a bad omen, precipitating wars or other disasters. In order to assuage the anger of the gods, these individuals would be sacrificed, particularly by drowning. This practice seems to be a carryover from Etruscan rituals. Yet by the time of the Roman Empire, Roman culture viewed the hermaphrodite as an erotic entertainment. It is unclear what caused this shift in perception of intersexed people.[132] Interestingly, the positive shift continued into the early Christian period when Augustine declared them descendants of Adam

128. Luts Alexander Graumann, "Monstrous Births and Retrospective Diagnosis: The Case of the Hermaphrodites in Antiquity," in *Disabilities in Roman Antiquity: Disparate Bodies* a Capite ad Calcem, ed. Christian Laes, C. F. Goodey, and M. Lynn Rose (Boston: Brill, 2013), 181–209.

129. Draycott, *Approaches to Healing in Roman Egypt*, 8–9.

130. Trentin, "Exploring Visual Impairment in Ancient Rome."

131. Graumann, "Monstrous Births and Retrospective Diagnosis."

132. Graumann, "Monstrous Births and Retrospective Diagnosis."

and therefore part of God's design, which humans not fully understanding should not disparage.[133]

## Conditional States

Modern somatic medicine subdivides life stages into the specializations of pediatrics, obstetrics, and geriatrics, whereas Roman medicine only tangentially touches upon these categories. Medically, little was made of children apart from their tendency to be hotter and therefore more problematic when determining treatments like venesection. This was a continuation of the Greek medical perspective.

Most likely, the onset of puberty for both males and females occurred at about fourteen years of age, due to nutrition. Although they had no legal age of majority, it seems to have happened around the age of seventeen, especially for males. A common rite among the upper classes was to sell a son into slavery, with his immediate manumission as a way of separating from the *paterfamilias*, thus marking him as an independent adult. Roman culture, much like Greek, saw teenage boys as an avenue for elite families to make political alliances by offering their sexual favors to older men with established careers. Some of the medical literature reports recipes for hair removal in order to make these young men more attractive. Pliny mentions midwives such as Salpe as providing effective depilatories. This shows midwives more in a role of overall family care rather than in just issues of pregnancy and childbirth.

For women, the ideal passage into adulthood comes with marriage, shortly after the onset of puberty. In practice, marriage was often delayed until the age of seventeen or eighteen for women, especially from the wealthier families. Physicians such as Soranus focused on the physiology of proper maturation resulting in fertility. He went so far as to advise men not to look at a woman's lineage or wealth, the culturally prescribed requirements for a "good marriage," but at her ability to reproduce as the primary consideration. Many Romans considered menstrual blood to have powerful properties, including physicians who noted midwives using it in therapies to cause abortions.

Most of our information on practices associated with pregnancy and childbirth comes from Soranus's *Gynaecology*. Some of the more striking

133. Augustine, *City of God* 16.8.

innovations come from his advice to use a birthing stool over a reclining position, as well as the disposition of the midwife to ease the anxieties of the mother. Apart from medical treatises, calendars provide divinations pertaining to pregnancy: "June 2nd. If in any way it should thunder, women in labor will have an easy delivery, but there will be an abortion of cattle, yet there will be an abundance of fish."[134]

As early as the sixth century, terracotta votives depict mothers holding infants, with a popularity that extended into the first century BCE.[135] Similarly, statues from the fifth century show nursing mothers with the child being larger, almost toddler sized; this imagery owes to Etruscan culture, whereas Greek culture never depicted nursing mothers until the Hellenistic period. A common votive motif was the swaddled baby with only its face and toes showing, wearing an amulet around its neck. These votives asked for protection of the child from the deity of a particular sanctuary.

The elderly comprised roughly 6–8 percent of the total population of ancient Rome,[136] which is dramatically lower than the modern world, with an elderly population closer to 18 percent. This is due not just to a shorter life expectancy in the ancient world but to the rather unique baby boom of the late 1940s to early 1950s, which is now an aging population. Romans took different approaches to defining old age, either by degradation of physiology or by a change in cultural expectations, which differed by gender.[137] Ovid and Galen mark "old age" around sixty to sixty-five years of age. Culturally, for men, the age of sixty-five exempted one from public duties such as serving on a jury, while military requirements were waived for those as young as fifty. Ultimately, though, appearance and ability, such as balding and graying hair, failing eyesight and hearing, or faulty memory, garnered the label "old." Women entering menopause in their forties or fifties signaled a new geriatric status.

Physiological explanations for graying, balding, and wrinkling of the skin rested on the humoral theory; as one ages, one naturally depletes internal heat, thus causing a drying out that results in changes to the hair as well as other aspects of the body. This implies a finite amount of heat in the body present at birth. Diet may supplement and replenish some of the heat, but the body overall loses more than it can take in over one's lifetime. Although Seneca

134. De Grummond, *Etruscan Myth, Sacred History, and Legend*, 43.

135. Haynes, *Etruscan Civilization*, 361–62.

136. Trentin, "Exploring Visual Impairment in Ancient Rome."

137. Karen Cokayne, *Experiencing Old Age in Ancient Rome* (New York: Routledge, 2013), 1.

labeled old age as a disease,[138] Galen saw it as a part of nature and therefore did not count it as a disease but as a stage midway between health and illness.[139] Medical writers discussing old age tend to focus on symptoms rather than diagnosing any specific disease as being more prevalent in the elderly. Yet they acknowledge that the overall frail health of the elderly made them more susceptible to common illnesses such as colds and bronchitis.[140] Some prescriptions for staving off the effects of old age, rather than its symptoms, aimed at restoring the body's heat (e.g., wine), while they advocated dry foods that would not overly tax the digestive system as well as regular exercise.

Physiognomies lack any direct reference to the appearances of old age, but many literary texts reference the stigma of old age. Since physiologies espoused that hair and semen have the same origins, lack of one would lead people to assume lack of the other, concluding that bald men suffered from impotency; premature baldness such as that of Caligula indicated moral degeneration.[141] These attitudes, beyond simple vanity, would explain the abundance of therapeutic recipes designed to restore or prevent hair loss, even though the physicians note it is inevitable. Conversely, portraiture and busts as early as the first century BCE, with the realism of baldness, wrinkles, and sunken cheeks, were viewed positively by the Romans. Such appearances of old age signified dignity, wisdom, and authority.[142]

## Healers

Modern scholars debate using the distinctions high/low, rational/supernatural, and science/magic, especially in relation to the different types of healers.[143] Nutton is correct in that medicine in the ancient world "was open to influences of all kinds and could be studied, and indeed practiced, by many who did not think of themselves as doctors."[144] This leaves us with the problem of how to translate, if at all, the Latin and Greek terms for healers popular in ancient Rome without obliterating the access to cultural power inherent in their plurality of titles.

138. Seneca, *Moral Letters to Lucilius* 108.28.

139. Galen, *On Hygiene* 1.5 and 5.4.

140. Cokayne, *Experiencing Old Age in Ancient Rome*, 39.

141. Cokayne, *Experiencing Old Age in Ancient Rome*, 14.

142. Cokayne, *Experiencing Old Age in Ancient Rome*, 20–21.

143. Draycott, *Approaches to Healing in Roman Egypt*, 2.

144. Nutton, *Ancient Medicine*, 313.

There is most definitely a power struggle playing out, but not between science and religion, as commonly assumed in the modern world. Ancient healers fought over authority within the human community based on their particular epistemological strategies. Terms for healers, such as the Greek *iatros* and Latin *medicus*, were meant to reflect their position within the educated society's power structure. Similarly, the distinction between types of medicine is to capture where it is concentrated within a socioeconomic cultural spectrum. The fact remains, though, that patients, regardless of their education or wealth, could easily move between these categories as their particular situations warranted, hence a hierarchy of resort. It should be remembered that the medical-anthropology phrase "hierarchy of resort" functioned more as a heterarchy.

According to Galen, patients should assess a physician (*iatros/medicus*) based on his knowledge of anatomy; the greater the breadth and depth, the better the physician.[145] Methodists taught that medical knowledge can be observed by any thinking person and therefore needs only about six months of study. This is in great contrast to Galen's years of study. Rome had no system or regulation for being an *iatros* or *medicus*. Many of the authors, such as Galen, used the term *iatros* because they came out of the Greek-speaking part of Roman territories and saw themselves as heirs of Hippocratic or other Greek physicians. But anyone with some amount of learning/training could use the terms *medicus* or *iatros*.

We can categorize healers as official in the sense that they occupied a government post or had a tax exemption. For Roman Egypt, the traditional title *swnw* is absent by the first century CE, and no specialist titles appear,[146] like the *medicus ocularius* seen in Gaul and Britain. Interestingly, during the reign of Tiberius (14–27 CE), the Roman senate outlawed for Britons not just Druids and diviners but also healers.[147] Specialized titles in Roman Egypt were connected to the administration, such as *archiatros*, which started out as a physician for the royal court but eventually became a public physician paid by the state; this type of title can be seen throughout the empire, especially the western provinces. Designated public physicians do not provide indigent care, or any care at all. Their function was to certify death or to document injuries and illnesses for legal proceedings.[148] As the Roman gov-

145. *On Examinations by Which the Best Physicians are Recognized* (*Opt. Med. Cogn.*) CMG Suppl. Or. IV, 115, 24–25.

146. Draycott, *Approaches to Healing in Roman Egypt*, 21.

147. Pliny, *Natural History* 30.13; see Carr, "Time to Live."

148. Draycott, *Approaches to Healing in Roman Egypt*, 24.

ernment oversaw the Egyptian temples, healers normally attached to them also became *de facto* functionaries of the state. Other frequent specialized titles include the *medicus ordinarius* to indicate a physician in the army.

The status of physicians is not clear-cut. We have more evidence from the eastern part of the empire, where an *iatros* is likely to have a high-status government position. Status seems to be based upon association with a patient's class, especially in the western half of the empire. At the college of physicians in Tibur, one *medicus* had a low status since he cared for slaves. Another *medicus* in Aix-en-Provence had an extravagant lifestyle on par with his wealthy patients.[149] A problem affecting the status of a *medicus*/*iatros* is the classification of healer as craftsman in the minds of many people. The itinerant nature of many physicians reinforces this perception. Like other craftsmen, families of doctors passed on knowledge to the next generation (i.e., Asklepiads). There were also husband-and-wife teams of physicians, such as Glycon and Pantheia in Pergamum or Aurelius Gallus and Auguste in Pisidia.[150]

It is not clear to what extent being a *medica* differed from a *medicus* or that such a title conferred any greater status to them over midwives (*obstetrices*). No theoretical treatises from female physicians survive, but ancient authors do mention their written works. The more common term for female healers was *obstetrix* or midwife, denoting their primary role in childbirth. Yet therapeutic recipes attributed to the midwife Salpe indicate a much wider range of medical issues under their care, such as numbness, sunburn, eye ailments, and fevers.[151] Given the typical physician's tendency to situate himself as an authority, it is not surprising that their references to midwives would place them in a subordinate position. At the same time, these references show the midwife not as a simple "old woman with experience in childbirth" but as a fairly erudite practitioner engaging in epistemological debates. Soranus's outline of requirements for a good midwife included being a Methodist rather than Empiricist or Dogmatist.[152]

Augurs may have worked as the earliest healers, providing diagnoses and prognoses based on reading signs from the god(s) behind the illness. Varro and Cato praised traditional rural Romans as strong and healthy, not

149. Vivian Nutton, "The Medical Meeting Place," in *Ancient Medicine in Its Socio-Cultural Context*, ed. Philip J. van der Eijk, H. F. J. Horstmanshoff, and P. H. Schrijvers (Atlanta: Rodopi, 1995), 11.

150. *GV* 2040; *MAMA* VII 566 and *IGR* III 376; see Nutton, "Medical Meeting Place," 18.

151. Pliny, *Natural History* 28.38, 66, 82.

152. Soranus, *Gynaecology* 1.3.1–5 and 1.4.1–5.

needing urban Greek medicine. This traditional stance on medicine dovetailed with the Roman conception of the *paterfamilias* as the ultimate authority looking after the well-being of all members of his household. Therefore, the traditional Roman healer was ideally the *paterfamilias* dispensing herbal remedies.[153] Ironically, the herbal/diet-based cures espoused by Cato and Varro recall the Hippocratic advice in *On Regimen* and likely spurred Romans to adopt Greek medical practices.

Looking at the development of the Roman *medicus*/*iatros*, Nijhuis posits an interesting scenario of a Roman patient going to a Greek doctor for healing a dislocated shoulder joint.[154] The scene plays out with the patient expecting a ritual splinting, incantation, and dietary supplement along the lines of Cato's description.[155] But the Greek physician would manipulate the joint and perhaps insert a cautery based on humoral theory. This situation highlights the differences between traditional Roman and theoretical Greek medicine. The blending of the two is highlighted in Pliny's dislike of Greek medicine but also in his praise of Hippocrates's pharmacology. Pliny focuses on the role of nature and therefore distrusts Greek methods of compounding and changing ratios of things found in nature.

The eventual integration of Roman and Greek medicine occurred as a multivariate process resting on patient needs, perceived ineffectualness of traditional Roman medicine, and the Greek doctor's ability to present treatment in a manner that the Roman patient recognized as an acceptable variation. The Greek doctor in Nijhuis's scenario could have presented manipulation and bandaging as a type of ritual akin to the one described in Cato. The imperial household used mostly Greek physicians during the first and second centuries CE, which probably helped foster their acceptance among the upper classes, who also began to use slave physicians of Greek origin in imitation. Such practices would eventually filter down through democratization and elite emulation.

The first recognized Greek medical practitioner in Rome was Archagathus of Sparta, who was invited as an official of the state in 219 BCE. Others likely came to Rome before him but not by invitation of the state. Pliny describes him as a heavy-handed butcher. It was not until the arrival

153. Cruse, *Roman Medicine*, 57.

154. Karin Nijhuis, "Greek Doctors and Roman Patients: A Medical Anthropological Approach," in *Ancient Medicine in Its Socio-Cultural Context*, ed. Philip van der Eijk, H. F. J. Horstmanshoff, and P. H. Schrijvers (Atlanta: Rodopi, 1995), 49–67.

155. Cato, *On Agriculture* 160.

of Asklepiades of Bithynia in 120 BCE that Romans began to outwardly accept Greek medical practices. Asklepiades had the reputation of not relying on surgery, which likely made him more acceptable than Archagathus. Under Julius Caesar, the state gave tax-free status to physicians practicing in Rome, perhaps to address the paucity of certain types of healers in the city. Augustus, Vespasian, and Hadrian all continued granting privileges to physicians.[156] The state eventually funded medical teaching in Rome itself during the reign of Severus Alexander (222–235 CE), but it provided for only a lecture room; any type of physicians overseeing the selection and appointments of new physicians did not occur until 368 CE.[157]

A knowledge network of physicians developed,[158] particularly among anatomists, starting with Quintus, who trained Satyrus, Lycus of Macedonia, and Numisianus. The latter two wrote anatomy books; Lycus's enjoyed popularity at the time, while Numisianus's did not. Numisianus went on to teach Pelops, whose writings have not survived. Pelops then taught Galen, who began his medical career under Satyrus and later studied with Numisianus.

The process started under the Presocratics, such as Thales, and was continued by Hippocrates, to assume that the gods are behind everything and therefore that physicians should focus on understanding the greater cosmological rules by which the body operates. They carried this almost to a logical conclusion of never mentioning the gods directly. As we move into later Roman periods, medical treatises do not mention the relationship of specific gods as a cause for either health or disease but only vaguely reference a more powerful entity, such as Demiurge or Nature, as the ultimate source of health and illness. Interestingly, though, none of the medical treatises actively dissuade anyone from believing that the gods exist. Rather, they concern themselves with charlatans who, while healing, do not employ philosophy, logic, and rigorous methods determined by the rules of nature. On the surface, this may appear as a science-religion dichotomy, but in actuality, Roman physicians such as Galen attacked bad practitioners and not religious ones *per se*. Rhetorical exercises strengthen the cultural association between the moral character and technical expertise of the physician; if one makes poor diagnoses or prognoses, then they also lack sufficient moral character.[159]

156. Jackson, "Roman Medicine," 79–101.

157. Jackson, "Roman Medicine," 79–101.

158. Rocca, "Anatomy."

159. Craig A. Gibson, "Doctors in Ancient Greek and Roman Rhetorical Education," *Journal of the History of Medicine and Allied Sciences* 68 (2013): 529–50.

This underpins much of Galen's charge against other physicians that they lack expertise; failing to learn and understand is a type of laziness, immoral in its own right, but then leads to further immoral behavior by harming a patient. Galen thought that simply listening to a patient made it too easy; even someone not trained as a physician could then diagnose.

One can contrast the tactics used by Galen and Rufus. Galen asserted that the good physician should demonstrate his knowledge by diagnosing from physical signs, minimally speaking with the patient to the point of almost seeming magical. This is not a matter of ego; Galen and Hippocrates both advocated giving a strong impression to the patient through leading questions in order to ensure obedience. Notice that the object of obedience has shifted from the gods to the healer; the human-human community is emphasized. They feared that patient noncompliance would result in further harm or death.

Rufus employed a more free-form conversation, focusing on areas of discussion rather than predictable, almost scripted questions. He understood that there are physical signs evident to the patient since symptoms are deviations from normal behavior, but these are not always directly observable by the physician. These "hidden signs" may be the key to an accurate diagnosis and proper treatment. To ignore the patient's observed signs could lead to the wrong diagnosis, making proper treatment impossible. Rufus's use of questioning would eliminate the role of an intermediary, since the third party cannot accurately answer these more open-ended questions. These intermediaries on behalf of the sick person were a common sight at the asklepieia. Although Rufus's method pit him against Hippocrates and later Galen, his highly individualistic approach was meant as a rejection of Methodist teachings. Rufus's perspective drew the ire of the Empiricists, who disavowed hidden causes.

When looking at the history of medicine from the patient's perspective, a frequent question is where the common person went for healing. People most likely went to the home of the healer if they were not attached to the imperial household or the military. Excavations at Pompeii and Rimini have revealed specialized rooms or medical workshops attached to private homes.

Some histories of Roman medicine discuss hospitals, but this is a bit of a misnomer, since nonreligious institutions dedicated to healing, like our modern hospitals, really did not exist in the ancient world. The closest institution to the modern concept of the hospital comes from a military context, not a civilian one. The Roman army maintained in encampments a dedicated space called the *valetudinarium* (place of health), which many translate simply as "hospital." Although the writers Vegetius[160] and Pseudo-Hyginus[161] claim that every fort had a substantial *valetudinarium*, archaeology cannot support such ubiquitousness; structures with a medical function tended to be on a much smaller scale, as found in places like Hadrian's Wall. Surviving examples of large scale *valetudinaria* for a legion include one at Novae/ Bulgaria, built under the reign of Trajan during the wars with the Dacians in the early second century CE. A *valetudinarium* contained not only rooms for patients but offices for personnel, storerooms, kitchens, and temples dedicated to Aesculapius and Hygea with votive inscriptions.[162] Studies of settlements along the lower Danube show that there seems to be a blurry line between soldier-physicians and civilian ones, especially on frontiers where many healers were hired by the state.[163] The largest and most extensively excavated *valetudinarium* is at Xanten, Germany (Vetera I), built during the first century CE.[164]

160. *Epitome of Military Matters.*

161. *De Munitionibus Castorum.*

162. E. Künzl, "Aesculapius in the Valetudinarium, or: The Hitherto Existing Interpretation of Roman Military Hospital Is Furthermore Valid," *Würzburger Medizinhistoriche Mitteilungen* 24 (2005): 99–109.

163. Dan Aparaschivei, "Healthcare in the Roman Province of Moesia Inferior," *Mankind Quarterly* 53 (2012): 110–29.

164. Cruse, *Roman Medicine*, 99.

# 10. Second Temple and Early Rabbinic Medicine

## Location and History

The phrase "Second Temple" is commonly used when referring to the history of the Levant, but its exact time frame can be a little unclear without context. The Babylonians destroyed the temple in Jerusalem in 586 BCE, exiling the elite population. In 539/8 BCE, the Persian king Cyrus II allowed the exiled population to return to Jerusalem and rebuild the temple. Already, a dispute arose as to who could assert an authoritative claim of inheriting the covenants and mantle of God's chosen from the Israelite and Judahite kingdoms. The biblical books of Ezra and Nehemiah describe the struggles between the returning exiles and those who had remained in the land. This rebuilt temple stood until its destruction in 70 CE by General Titus, which essentially ended the Great Revolt against Rome. But during those intervening six hundred years, the political and cultural landscape of what became known as Syria-Palestine dramatically shifted. The phrase "Second Temple" can thus apply to more specific times within that 539 BCE–70 CE date range.

Some will mark the beginning of the Second Temple period with the Hasmonean[1] Dynasty (142–63 BCE). After the death of Alexander the Great, the general Seleucus established his kingdom in Syria, extending it down the eastern coast of the Mediterranean. This put the areas of Israel and Judah at the center of conflict with the Greek Ptolemaic family, who ruled from Egypt and tried to incorporate the Levant. While under Seleucid domination, the priest Mattathias began a rebellion in 165 BCE. His son Judas the Hammer (Maccabee)[2] carried on the fight. His brother Simon finally established

1. The family name Hasmonean likely developed from the town Heshmon associated with the family of Mattathias, although he lived in Modein. In traditional Canaanite/Israelite culture, families did not carry last names; this practice was adopted from Greek culture.

2. The Hebrew word for hammer became a name for the family but usually only applied

himself as an independent king in 142 BCE with Roman backing. By 140 BCE, Simon was also anointed as the high priest in the temple in Jerusalem. Although the Hasmonean Revolt began as a retaliation against Seleucid control and hellenization of the culture, the dynasty by the first century BCE became itself hellenized and intertwined with growing Roman power. Other scholars focus on the expansion of the temple complex under Herod in 20 BCE as the Second Temple period. Although these starting dates for the Second Temple vary, the destruction in 70 CE usually marks the end. One exception is the Bar Kokhba Revolt (132–135 CE), which for some scholars may serve as an ideological end point rather than a physical one for the end of the Second Temple.

However one marks the beginning and end of the Second Temple, a significant development in the religious culture occurred during this period. Judaism as distinct from the ancient Israelite religion begins with the return of the Babylonian exiles in 538 BCE. It was not a uniform practice but had sectarian variations across the ancient Near East and Mediterranean. Josephus describes four major sects of Judaism within Palestine[3] by the late first century CE. They are the Sadducees, Pharisees, Essenes, and the Fourth Philosophy, sometimes referred to as the Zealots. These are by no means the only sects but are representative of the plethora of variations, many of which can no longer be accounted. Given the paucity of textual information on the various sects, it is nearly impossible to reconstruct the practice of medicine for each one. Instead, we must investigate the medical culture, acknowledging that it is weighted toward the forms of Judaism that have survived, namely, rabbinic Judaism.[4]

The tendency, especially for those not practicing Judaism, is to think of rabbinic Judaism as essentially the same ancient Israelite religion that once prevailed in the area. Given the political and religious climate since the reign of the Seleucids and Ptolemies, it is easy to overlook the influence of hellenization, as well as Persia, specifically the Sasanian Dynasty, on the development of Talmud and the practice of medicine in keeping with it. Apart

---

to Judas and his brothers rather than the dynastic line as a whole. This name also became the title of the books in the Apocrypha describing the revolt and the time period.

3. Flavius Josephus, *Jewish War* and *Antiquities of the Jews*. Use of the term Palestine reflects the contemporary Roman designation of the area; Josephus targeted a Roman audience with his writings.

4. Early Christianity can also be slotted into this category as a form of Judaism, but its development into its own various sects makes it too large of a topic for this study. See the introduction.

from the Pharisees and rabbis, other sects of Judaism concerned themselves with medical matters, such as the Essenes and the scholar Yeshua ben Sira (ca. 150 BCE). Both Josephus and Philo of Alexandria refer to the Essene's medical practices.

## Religion and Culture

In order to understand the development of medical culture through the Second Temple period into the early rabbinic movement, let us look at some of the more well-known sects of Judaism from the Roman province of Syria-Palestine, as well as the diasporic community in Babylon, that have had an impact on the study of medical practices. To date, there is no in-depth study of the impact the Alexandrian Jewish community had on the development of rabbinic/talmudic medical culture. For the most part, these early sects of Judaism adhered to the same cosmology of covenantal monotheism as found in the Hebrew Bible, but the exact interpretation of specific passages varied depending on the sect's political fortunes and relationship to hellenization.

### Cosmology

The Essenes are one of the larger sects within Second Temple Judaism and appear in the writings of Josephus, Philo, and Pliny the Elder. They likely originated in the wake of the problematic Hasmonean succession in 63 BCE,[5] or possibly earlier in defiance of the Hasmonean assumption of the high priesthood. Scholarly consensus attributes the Dead Sea Scrolls (DSS) to the Essenes, but this association is increasingly questioned, thus making the documents as a source of Essene culture problematic. Striking a middle ground between the DSS and Josephus's assertions of extreme but admirable piety, we can describe the Essenes as a hierarchical group focused on brotherhood, communal life and property, and strict maintenance of purity, while adamantly refusing hellenization. There is no surviving evidence attesting to the sect after the first century CE, especially in wake of the destruction of the

5. The brothers Hyrcanus and Aristobulus vied for the throne, involving the Romans, who eventually established their political dominance in the area and left Hyrcanus in place as the high priest.

temple. This reinforces the idea that a fundamental ideology of the Essenes related to issues with the temple.

There are several theories on the meaning behind the name Essene. Most understand it as derived from *hasidim* (saints) or words for "pious" or "secret." Yet another theory, espoused by Vermes, holds that the name came from a Greek corruption of the Aramaic term *assaia*, meaning "healer." In keeping with this, Philo describes a sect as *therapeutai theou* (servants of God). He also goes on to describe the name "in the sense of '*cure*' because they profess an art of healing better than that current in the cities which cures only the bodies, while theirs treats also souls oppressed with grievous and well-nigh incurable diseases."[6] If the Qumran Scrolls were produced by the Essenes, there is a curious incongruity between their writings and the descriptions of Essenes by Philo and Josephus with regard to healing practices. These ancient writers depict the Essene community as one that collectively pays for the healing, whether a physician or the medicants, for its members. Yet modern scholars understand the Qumran community of Essenes as having "war-camp-like conditions" where "there was no place for handicapped 'soldiers,'" citing 1 QM VII: 4–5, which claims that anyone with a limp, blindness, or permanent blemish cannot go to war.[7] This underscores the uncertainty of linking Qumran with the Essenes. But it also creates an ideological parallel between warfare and being in the presence of God, since the Qumran community used the same purity requirements.

Josephus counts about six thousand Pharisees, including himself, during the first century CE. The New Testament makes frequent mention of them in opposition to Jesus and states that Paul originally belonged to this sect. They believed in maintaining Levitical piety, an eternal soul that could be punished, cultivating harmonious relationships within the community, both among the Jews and with the ruling powers, and following a "tradition of the fathers" not found in the Torah. Some argue that the valuing of these traditions led directly to the development of the Talmud; thus, the Pharisees were the forefathers of the rabbis. Their ideology attained some popularity with the general population, even if many did not directly align themselves with the Pharisees. Although the Pharisees were not a ruling class, they often worked with different factions of the Hasmoneans, they took part in

6. Philo, *Contemplative Life* 1.2.

7. Samuel Kottek, "Hygiene and Healing among the Jews in the Post-Biblical Period: A Partial Reconstruction," *ANRW* 37.3:2862.

the Great Revolt (66–70 CE) against Rome, and they would work with the Romans, as Josephus later exemplifies.

Although rabbinic Judaism did not directly develop from the Pharisees, there is considerable overlap between the two groups, especially when looking at the Pharisaic "tradition of the fathers" and the rabbinic oral traditions that developed into the Talmud. Josephus does not mention rabbis. Only Simeon ben Gamaliel is noted as a rabbi before the destruction of the temple in 70 CE. Vespasian allowed Rabbi Yohanan ben Zakkai to escape from Jerusalem and set up a high court in Yavneh on the coast; this area and the students of R. Yohanan become the core of rabbinic Judaism. Yet the rabbis in Palestine after the Bar Kokhba Revolt in 135 CE had little ability to wield any considerable power, due to Roman rule. During the third century CE, rabbinic centers appeared in Tiberias, Sepphoris, and Caesarea. Through the third and fourth centuries, Roman authority retracted in the area, allowing for growing rabbinic power.[8]

Meanwhile, the Babylonian Jews tended to isolate themselves from other Jewish groups, based on a perceived hierarchy. This is in keeping with Persian cultural practices of no movement between the classes, in contrast to Roman culture that did allow for a relatively greater degree of interaction between *plebeians* and *patricians*.[9] Yet the rabbis in Palestine derided Babylon, saying, "He who eats earth of Babylon is as though he ate the flesh of his ancestors; some say, it is as though he ate of abominations and creeping things, because it is written."[10] Talmud conveys the belief that residence in Palestine itself acts as a preventative to disease; the holiness of the land and its ability to heal draws upon biblical precedent.

The cultural environment of the rabbis played an important part in the adaptation of Greco-Roman medical practices. Living in a hellenized world created conflicts among the Jewish communities. Talmud assesses the infighting of the Hasmoneans, stating, "Cursed be the man who would teach his son Grecian Wisdom,"[11] blaming their hellenization for the strife. Newmyer points out, though, that allowances could be made for learning Greek, not for its own sake but to advance one's career.[12] Pragmatism would

8. Seth Schwartz, "The Political Geography of Rabbinic Texts," in *The Cambridge Companion to the Talmud and Rabbinic Literature*, ed. Charlotte Elisheva Fonrobert and Martin S. Jaffee (Cambridge: Cambridge University Press, 2007), 75–96.

9. Richard Kalmin, *Jewish Babylonia between Persia and Roman Palestine: Decoding the Literary Record* (Oxford: Oxford University Press, 2006), 1.

10. Shabbat 113b.

11. Bava Qamma 82b.

12. Newmyer, "Talmudic Medicine and Greco-Roman Science," *ANRW* 37.3:2895–911.

dictate for healers, at least in the Alexandrian and Palestinian communities, to learn the basics of Greco-Roman medicine. Rabbinic sages concerned with anatomical manifestations of purity and impurity likewise could find Greco-Roman anatomy invaluable for their "profession of Torah." While they can accept the anatomical knowledge, they would reject the physiological theories tied to it. In turn, as these ideas become a part of the Palestinian Talmud, they would then find their way into the Babylonian Talmud, especially among the *tannaim*[13] like Simeon ben Gamaliel, whose education and subsequent teaching espoused an all-inclusive, lenient ethos.

Boyarin claims that Babylonian Judaism is, essentially, an act of Hellenism itself rather than an incorporation of Hellenistic tendencies or a subjugation to hellenization. He argues that the Babylonian Talmud inserts itself into the tradition of Greek dialectic by creating a third option for answering dilemmas.[14] Especially with regard to medical problems, it depicts both sides of an issue, thus allowing it to exhibit both an acceptance of Galenic medicine as well as a rejection of it. This makes it stand apart from the Palestinian Talmud, which seeks either to accept or reject an answer. For the Babylonian Talmud, the dialectical act becomes the devotional act rather than an adherence to the correct answer.

Just as Galen argued against the use of pure rationalism and pure empiricism in medicine, talmudic rabbis such as Simeon ben Gamaliel found themselves arguing against religious dogmatists. Talmud preserves the contention within the rabbinic community over the different approaches to learning. The subcategories of purity and impurity came to symbolize a difficult, technical study of terminology that easily succumbed to manipulation.[15] Numerous passages[16] depict sages committing a sin by publicly revealing someone failing to adhere to the letter of the law. One in particular relates the story of Rabbis Meir and Nathan trying to humiliate Simeon ben Gamaliel by displaying his assumed lack of knowledge of *uqtsin*.[17] It is inter-

13. Aramaic word meaning "teachers," referring to specific rabbis during the period 10–220 CE.

14. Daniel Boyarin, "Hellenism in Jewish Babylonia," in *The Cambridge Companion to the Talmud and Rabbinic Literature*, ed. Charlotte Elisheva Fonrobert and Martin S. Jaffee (Cambridge: Cambridge University Press, 2007), 336–64.

15. Mira Balberg and Moulie Vidas, "Impure Scholasticism: The Study of Purity Laws and Rabbinic Self," *Prooftexts* 32 (2012): 312–56.

16. Hagigah 14a; Sanhedrin 38b, 67b, 107a; Bava Metzi'a 59a.

17. Horayot 13b. The word *uqtsin* means "stalk," which designates one of these subcategories concerning purity.

esting to note that the incident centers on Simeon ben Gamaliel, one of the rabbis that advocated following human consensus in non-biblical matters. This is the very charge laid against the study of *halakhah* (law) in comparison to *haggadah* (exegesis)—it espouses the human majority more so than divine intervention.[18] The self-reflection and self-criticism exhibited in the use of terminology for purity and impurity exemplify the inherent Hellenism in the Babylonian Talmud.

## Sources

There are no known texts dedicated solely to the study of medicine from the Jewish communities during the Second Temple period. It should be noted that the texts addressing medical issues do not come from practicing physicians, as far as we can tell, but from the rabbis, essentially theorists of religious law. This is important because there are references to healers, the *rophe'im*, as part of the Jewish communities, yet unlike their Greco-Roman contemporaries, they did not engage in a literary discourse on their profession. In contrast to the variety of textual sources is a dearth in archaeological ones.

### Texts

The Talmud is a collection of sayings from rabbinic sages dating from the first century CE to the closing of the canon in roughly 770 CE. Sages or rabbis from the first and second centuries CE, referred to as the *tannaim*, were located in Palestine. The sages from the third and fourth centuries in Palestine and the fifth century in Babylonia are called the *amoraim*. The Talmud is divided into the Midrash, Mishnah, Gemara, and Tosefta. Midrash is an exegesis of the Hebrew Bible mostly derived from the teachings of Rabbi Akiva (50–137 CE) and Rabbi Ishmael (90–135 CE). Mishnah is a collection of legal rulings (*halakhot*), mostly centered on Rabbi Judah ha-Nasi (135–219 CE) and organized into six orders, while the Gemara are the interpretations of the Mishnah. The Tosefta contains variations of the Mishnaic *halakhot*, with additional explanations and scriptural references.

The codified oral traditions of the earliest sages provide insight on the Jewish communities' medical practices during the first and second centuries

18. Bava Metzi'a 59b.

CE as well as later antiquity and even the early medieval periods. Ironically, common use of the term Talmud in the modern era refers to the Babylonian Talmud (*Bavli*), yet in antiquity, the Jerusalem Talmud (*Yerushalmi*) also influenced Jewish practices. Therefore, rabbinic teachings on medicine are located in two geographical areas, Roman Palestine and Persian Babylonia. Tradition holds that there were four generations of sages living in cities such as Sepphoris and Bosra in the Roman province of Syria-Palestine; these are referred to as the sages of Eretz-Israel. During the fourth century CE, the *amoraim* settled in Babylonia, ushering in the next seven generations of sages, thus creating the Babylonian Talmud. Some view this migration as Jews fleeing Christian persecution, while others see it as part of the more complex problem of the deportations of Romans from conquered territories in Syria, Anatolia, and Armenia by the Persian king Shapur I (239–272 CE). Most writings pertaining to medical ideas and practices are in the Babylonian rather than the Jerusalem Talmud.

The Babylonian Talmud was written after the fifth century, with its final redaction around 770 CE. Halivni sees two layers to the Babylonian Talmud. The first consists of the legal rulings and their terse explanations from the *amoraim*. The second layer consists of in-depth explanations, often in dialectic form, by anonymous writers more than a generation after the *amoraim*.[19] Throughout the texts, various interpretations and explanations of biblical passages relate concepts of healing that were popular among the rabbinic community. Talmud also mentions a Book of Medicine written by King Solomon. Interestingly, "Pesaqim 56a and Berakhot 10a states that King Hezekiah was instrumental in causing this Book of Medicine to disappear, and the Sages praised him for that action."[20] Although Solomon's Book of Medicine seems like a fictional creation of the talmudic sages, Josephus, in *Antiquities of the Jews*,[21] also refers to Solomon composing medical incantations, making it likely that at least during the Second Temple such a medical treatise focusing on ritualistic therapies did exist, even though it was probably of contemporary authorship. It was common practice in the ancient Near East to have an older, respected name attached to writings, such as the name Solomon, in order to give them legitimacy and authority.

19. David Weiss Halivni, *The Formation of the Babylonian Talmud*, trans. Jeffrey L. Rubenstein (Oxford: Oxford University Press, 2013), xxi.

20. Samuel Kottek, "The Essenes and Medicine: A Comparative Study of Medical and Para-Medical Items with Reference to Ancient Jewish Lore," *Clio Medica* 18 (1983): 81–99.

21. Josephus, *Antiquities of the Jews* 8.2.5, 45.

This is in contrast to the contemporary practice of the Greeks and Romans attaching their own names, such as Herophilus or Galen, to their works. Yet even within Greco-Roman culture, false attribution for claims of authority were common, especially for the names Hippocrates and Galen.

Slightly predating the Babylonian Talmud is the Jerusalem Talmud, which was redacted around 400–420 CE by Rabbi Yochanan in Tiberias. This is overall a shorter work. Its narrative portions are in a much simpler form of Hebrew. Scholars think it underwent less editing and redaction than the Babylonian Talmud; therefore, Jerusalem gives a clearer picture of the original oral teachings. This can be helpful in understanding which medical practices may have been earlier or unique to Palestine.

Scholars for the history and anthropology of medicine use rabbinic sources apart from Talmud, such as Piyyut and Hekhalot, but their composition after the third century CE, mostly dating to the medieval period, make them too late for the scope of this study. A significant source, though, relating to the Second Temple period may be found in the *targumim*.

*Targum*[22] means a translation of the Hebrew Bible into Aramaic, but the word is reserved for those translations made within the rabbinic culture rather than just any translation. The *targumim* started toward the end of the Second Temple period and stretched into the end of the tenth century CE. The *targumim* are divided into Babylonian and Palestinian recensions. The most noted Babylonian *targumim* are Onqelos, a translation of the Torah, and Jonathan ben Uzziel, which translates the Prophets. Neofiti is the surviving Palestinian *targum* for the Pentateuch. Both the Babylonian and Palestinian *targumim* were written in Roman Palestine, but the versions brought into Babylonia became codified earlier, while the Palestinian translations were allowed more fluidity for a longer period. Talmud references certain *targumim*, such as Onqelos, which may shed light on late Second Temple medical practices, depending on the translation choices for medical passages in the Bible.

As we have already seen, the writings of Flavius Josephus (37 to ca. 100 CE) shed considerable light on the Second Temple period. Josephus was an aristocratic Judean who originally fought against Rome as a general in the Galilee during the Great Revolt. After surrendering to Vespasian's army in the siege of Jotapata, he traveled to Alexandria and Rome under the protection of Vespasian. He wrote four works that can be used to glean information about medicine in first-century Judea and Rome: *Jewish War*, *Antiquities of*

22. *Targum* is the singular form; *targumim* is plural.

*the Jews*, *The Life*, and *Against Apion*. These texts can be problematic, though, especially in light of later Christian corruptions of the texts.

Many of his references to medicine are elaborations on biblical passages, such as Saul's melancholy in 1 Samuel 16:15–16. The biblical text simply has the servants declare an evil spirit has descended and that a harp player should be used. Yet Josephus adds, "Physicians[23] could devise no other remedy save to order search to be made for one with power to charm away spirits and to play upon the harp."[24] Whereas the original Israelite cultural context of 1 Samuel uses appeasement of spirits without recourse to a physician, the Greco-Roman milieu of first-century Judea necessitates some reference to the ubiquitousness of the *iatros* or *medicus*. Although some form of healer attending Saul is an anachronism on Josephus's part, he still maintains the gist of the medical culture of Iron Age Israel when retelling the story.

When describing the illness of Herod the Great, Josephus indicates a more popular Greco-Roman view of medicine, especially with the negative portrayal of physicians participating in assassination conspiracies.[25] In addition to this, he describes how some Jewish sects approach medicine, such as the Essenes: "They display an extraordinary interest in the writings of the ancients, singling out in particular those which make for the welfare of soul and body. With the help of these, and with a view to the treatment of diseases, they make investigations into medicinal roots and the properties of stones."[26] Such passages indicate that Jews likely experienced to some degree an incorporation of Greco-Roman medicine, regardless of the particular sect of Judaism they followed.

A collection of scrolls found in caves along the Dead Sea near Qumran have proved significant for the study of the Hebrew Bible as well as the Second Temple period. They are commonly known as the Dead Sea Scrolls, but some scholars refer to them as the Qumran Scrolls. Each scroll is designated by its cave number, the letter Q, and the title of the document. Additionally, a superscript letter designates a particular version. As an example, $4QExod^c$ refers to a scroll from cave number 4 at Qumran, containing the text of Exodus, designated c (as opposed to others called a and b). Qumran contained not only books of the Hebrew Bible, with the exception of Ruth, but also texts that outline the rules and belief system of the community that created them.

23. Writing in Greek, Josephus used the term *iatros* rather than the Hebrew *rophe*.

24. Josephus, *Antiquities of the Jews* 6.166.

25. Josephus, *Antiquities of the Jews* 14 and *Jewish War* 1.

26. Josephus, *Jewish War* 2.8, 6, 136.

In particular, the Damascus Document depicts the contemporary political-religious culture of Judea. Like Josephus and the Talmud, these documents make reference to issues that are of a concern to the history of medicine, although none of them are specifically medical treatises. A problem exists in that scholarly consensus sees Qumran as a community of Essenes, but there is a growing debate about this association. The medical information in the Qumran Scrolls may be compared to Josephus's description of the Essenes' interest in medicine.

Another valuable source is the Septuagint (LXX), a Greek translation of the books of the Hebrew Bible, but it is a recension different from the Masoretic Text (MT). The MT and LXX recensions reflect a cultural difference between the Israelites of the Bronze/Iron Age and the Jews of the Hellenistic period. The LXX is not a single translation either, but a series of translations spanning centuries and then collated together. The diasporic community in Alexandria seems to have started a Greek translation of the Pentateuch in the early third century BCE, with the other books of the Bible being translated in Palestine into the late second century BCE; later revisions were done into the second century CE. Of particular interest for the study of medicine, the LXX uses anatomical parts different from those in the MT of Lamentations, such as "heart" for "bowels." The LXX also uses euphemisms like "my honor" instead of "my liver."[27] Such shifts indicate a hellenization of cultural ideas about anatomy and physiology.

The Apocrypha is a collection of religious texts not included in the Hebrew Bible/Old Testament canon but still recognized as authoritative. Since 1546, Catholic Bibles contain the Apocrypha, but Protestant Bibles do not. These texts were composed mostly in Palestine between 300 BCE and 70 CE and can give information concerning healing during the Second Temple period, especially among Jewish groups that played a role in the development of early Christianity.

1 Enoch 7:1 mentions the angels who took human women as wives and taught them the magical properties of roots and stones to ward off evil spells. Jubilees 10:11–17 describes not only that the good angels taught Noah about the medical properties of plants to cure diseases but that Noah actually wrote them down in a medical treatise intended for his son Shem. Although no dedicated medical treatises survive among the writings from the biblical period, it is interesting that these Jewish religious texts of the Second Temple incorporate the ubiquitous Greco-Roman epistemological practice of

27. Thomas, *Anatomical Idiom and Emotional Expression*, 1.

recording medical knowledge in focused treatises. Additionally, the specific naming of Shem reinforces the growing reputation of Jewish healers/physicians (and later Arabic ones in the Middle Ages). During this period, there is a divide between the good angels who bring cures and bad angels or demons who send the disease. This seems to be an adaptation in light of the growing dualistic ideologies, such as in Zoroastrianism from the east and Neoplatonism from the west, yet it stands in tension with the avowed monotheism of Judaism and early Christianity.

The Wisdom of Ben Sira contains a poem linking the physician's skill with wisdom and beneficence of God.[28] This passage seems to be a reconciliation between the Second Temple interpretation of biblical teachings, eschewing physicians and the use of the growing practice of using physicians, especially from a Greco-Roman medical milieu. Similarly, good health is connected to fear of the Lord[29] and to one's emotions.[30] In keeping with idea that disease is a form of direct communication (and sometimes a punishment) from God, healing is then accomplished through God. Ben Sira advises that one must forgive others if expecting God to forgive and heal, maintaining in equal importance community cohesion for both human-human and human-divine relationships.

In 1911, Julius Preuss published the comprehensive study *Biblisch-Talmudische Medizin*, which Fred Rosner originally translated into English in 1977.[31] This still stands as the most complete collation of medical material in the Talmud, covering anatomy, physiology, pathologies, *materia medica*, and physicians. Preuss sets the Jewish *rophe* in a hellenized cultural context, drawing comparisons with the Greco-Roman practitioners. The only drawback to his study is the collapsing of biblical with talmudic medicine, giving a false impression that the practices and ideology of the Second Temple also apply to the Bronze and Iron Ages. Given that the rabbis drew upon the Hebrew Bible for justification of their medical concepts, it is hard to avoid such conflation but not impossible. It is important for those studying medicine in both the biblical and Second Temple contexts to keep in mind that they are closely related but not synonymous practices.

28. Sir 38:1–15.

29. Sir 34:17–20.

30. Sir 30:14–20.

31. Preuss, *Biblical and Talmudic Medicine*.

### Archaeology

Although many archaeological sites relating to the Second Temple are being excavated across Israel, nothing has been published on finds specifically relating to the practice of medicine in a purely Jewish context. The closest artifacts would be the *mikvot*,[32] ritual baths used in purification rituals, such as after menstruation. The most readily identifiable sites and artifacts stem from Greco-Roman culture, such as asklepieia found in Kedesh and Jerusalem. It is unclear to what extent Jews participated in this aspect of Greco-Roman medical culture, although it seems reasonable to assume some use. On the hierarchy of resort, the asklepieion could have been a first recourse or as a last resort, depending on the personal ideology of the afflicted.

## Cultural Concepts

Although there are writings apart from Talmud that attest to different sectarian views that could influence multiple medical cultures during the Second Temple, it is difficult to place them in their appropriate social contexts to draw an accurate picture of them individually. These texts come to us from a later collation, which makes them better suited for understanding early Christianity. This study will then focus on the explanatory model of illness expressed in the talmudic uses of anatomy, physiology, disease etiology, and restoration of health during the shift from Second Temple to rabbinic Judaism.

### Anatomy and Physiology

Talmud's emphasis on the breath of life in the Hebrew Bible reinforces the monotheism of rabbinic Judaism. The Hebrew Bible depicts a life force that enters the body as a breath through the mouth or nose.[33] Unlike the Greco-Roman medical texts, though, the Bible omits any explanation of how that breath moves through the body or the mechanism by which body and soul interact. For Judaism, there is no mechanistic explanation for the linkage between body and soul. It is simply God acting through the body.

32. Singular form *mikvah*.

33. Gen 2:7; 7:22; Isa 42:5; 57:16; Job 27:3.

God, and only God, gives a soul to humans. This undercuts attributing any aspect of humanness to other gods. Yet this monotheism also created a parallel ideology with Galen's teleology of Nature/Soul. Additionally, God is equally present in all body parts due to the breath of life.[34] Talmud came to reject a symbiotic anatomy as a continuation of biblical monotheism. There simply are no other gods with which the body parts can form relationships. So this means that the anatomy itself is not independent of the human. God created humans and their body as one single entity, so what was a three-way relationship for the Egyptians, Mesopotamians, and Canaanites became a two-way relationship in Judaism, the relationship between humans and God.

In turn, monotheism and the two-way relationship meant that Jewish healers did not need complex explanations of the link between anatomy and physiology or even disease etiology. This obviated a need for the Greco-Roman organ-organ relationship. God was at the root of all disease and trauma as well as the proper functioning of the body. Yet this also meant they could use a mechanistic explanation of physiology as long as they recognized God as the ultimate source of that mechanism, much like Galen's teleology of Nature/Soul. This duality explains the lack of physiological analyses in Talmud but also their ability to adapt Greco-Roman practices without compromising theology.

Talmud focuses on anatomical descriptions in order to identify that which is acceptable by purity standards. Through this, an ideal body type can be reconstructed. It does not seem to be used as a clinical baseline for determining illness in an academic/epistemological sense. The rabbis did not diagnose illness in the way the biblical prophets and even the Levitical priests had done. No sacrifices necessary for the removal of the sick role could be done since the temple was gone, thus influencing the relationship of the rabbis to the issues of purity and illness.

Preuss claims that Talmud expressly forbids the use of comparative anatomy in the *tosefot*[35] for Hullin 42b and Zevahim 116a.[36] The reasoning of the medieval commentaries points to the obvious differences between Adam (humans) and animals. Yet the late date of these prohibitions makes them a moot point for determining the ideological stance of rabbis in late antiquity. It would be hard to imagine, as Preuss also points out, that the practice of inspecting animals for sacrifice and food preparation did not

34. Gen 2:7.

35. Commentaries on the texts written in the medieval period.

36. Preuss, *Biblical and Talmudic Medicine*, 41.

create some tendency to compare the anatomy of humans and cattle. Perhaps this tendency prompted the medieval *tosefot* to stress the uniqueness imparted to Adam by his soul, expressed through his anatomy. But it seems that, unlike their Greco-Roman counterparts, the Jewish healer idealized in Talmud refrained from dissecting even animals for the express purpose of learning anatomy and physiology.

Although Talmud does prohibit the desecration of a corpse[37] based on Deuteronomy 21:22–23, interestingly, it does not unilaterally forbid the dissection of human corpses. It tries to limit the practice to cases of absolute necessity, such as saving the life of a child or making certain determinations. Three passages discuss human dissection. Hullin 11b preserves an autopsy request in order to assist a murder case; the rabbis rejected the request on the grounds it would not influence the outcome of the case and therefore not be of benefit. A second request for an autopsy to determine someone's age in a legal case surrounding the validity of a sale contract was also rejected on similar grounds.

The disciples of Rabbi Ishmael ben Elisha (90–135 CE) boiling the corpse of a female prostitute to count the bones stands out as an exception.[38] The act is partly forgiven since her count of 252 bones exceeded the normal attribution of 248 bones, which made it a case of pure versus impure and allowed R. Ishmael to then expound on the intricacies of female anatomy, in that God allows women to have "two extra hinges." Mundane legal cases concerning contracts and even murder do not justify the need for human dissection. Judging purity or impurity, though, does present a pressing need that allows for human dissection, working around the prohibition in Deuteronomy 21:22–23. Further excusing the dissection is the idea that Ishmael ben Elisha, a Palestinian from the upper Galilee, was not a Babylonian rabbi and therefore more likely to act in accord with the nearby "Alexandrian physicians," whose practices seemed mysterious to the Babylonian rabbis.[39] These Alexandrian physicians, renowned for dissections in late antiquity, included Herophilus, Erasistratus, and Galen.

This underscores the understanding that Greco-Roman medical practices most likely infiltrated the Babylonian Talmud via rabbis closely connected to the Palestinian/Greco-Roman cultural milieu. At no point does

37. Hullin 11b.

38. Bekhorot 45a.

39. Although Rabbi Ishmael did not partake in the dissection, he is not depicted as taking issue with it; see Preuss, *Biblical and Talmudic Medicine*, 44.

Talmud validate dissection purely for empirical knowledge. But it also does not forbid anatomical knowledge gained from dissections, so the works of Greco-Roman physicians such as Herophilus, Erasistratus, and Galen may be employed by the talmudic rabbis.

Unlike Galen, the rabbis did not explicitly outline the physiological rationale behind bloodletting, and Talmud provides insufficient information to fully reconstruct rabbinical understanding of the physiology underlying the practice. Possibly, rabbinic Judaism merely picked up the practice of venesection from its Hellenistic neighbors without further theoretical knowledge. This seems especially true if one focuses on Abaye's (280–340 CE) reference to his mother as a form of justification. Yet the link between bloodletting and the pulmonary disease of *askara*[40] made by Rabbi Ishmael ben Jose (early third century) indicates some understanding of Galen's theory that breathing has a direct relationship with the blood and that he was not just applying folk traditions. In fact, he argues against the folk remedy of bloodletting to cure fevers, which contradicts a fundamental aspect of Galen's physiology, that blood carries an innate heat.

Three possibilities exist for why Rabbi Ishmael ben Jose argued against bloodletting for fevers. One, the observation of bloodletting amply demonstrated its dangers, an unnecessary risk for the relief of fevers. But warnings about where and when to let blood and making allowances for patients to eat and avoid chills after the bloodletting show that these risks were known and, for some, adequately managed, regardless of one's knowledge of Galen's physiology. Two, he simply wanted to undermine the increasingly widespread Hellenistic folk practice without knowing Galenic theories. Both of these answers, though, beg the question: why undermine bloodletting for a broad category of ailments such as fever but advocate it for a specific illness like *askara*? Three, he knew both theoretical precepts that the blood carries innate heat and that breathing influences it, but he only partially accepted them. Prescribing bloodletting for *askara* incorporates the Hellenistic (if not specifically Galenic) link between breathing and blood while also maintaining the biblical idea of God infusing humans with the breath of life.

Since the link between breathing and the soul is never explicit, it leads to contradictions within rabbinic Judaism. A folk tradition in the third century CE warns that sneezing can endanger one's life, while Tosefta Shabbat

40. Symptoms are described as affecting the throat, and the Aramaic term comes from the root *sakar*, meaning "to close, shut," in reference to the breathing difficulties. Modern scholars have tried to identify the disease as croup or diphtheria.

prohibits such beliefs.[41] The association of the soul with the breath of life through the nose makes sneezing a positive omen and a good prognosis in the ill.[42] This idea is continued in Talmud with the assertion that odors can affect the soul but not the body; one's sense of smell directly links to the soul because of the "breath of life."[43] Yet this argues against the idea of the body and the soul being a singular entity in relationship with God. More in keeping with the symbiotic anatomy of the surrounding ancient Near East and Mediterranean is the talmudic claim that although the parents contribute the physical matter that makes up the human body, the ability to see, hear, speak, walk, and, most important, understand comes from God.[44] This does maintain the sense of anatomy and physiology found in the Hebrew Bible.

As for the linkage of blood and breathing, according to Galen, the blood's innate heat arises from the semen that initially formed the body. This heat not only provides the mechanistic link between body and soul, but it also forms the physiological explanation for fevers. An excess of the blood or a problem with one's breathing that normally cools the blood allows for a buildup of the heat, resulting in a fever. Since the Bible does not address the mechanics of the breath of life once it enters the body, this allows for rabbis either to accept or reject various parts of Galen's theory of blood, innate heat, and respiratory problems causing fevers. It appears Ishmael ben Jose accepted the understanding that blood and breathing are related, hence the recommendation of venesection for *askara*, but he ultimately rejected the belief in blood's innate heat and therefore dismissed its use in reducing fevers. It is possible Ishmael ben Jose's rejection of innate heat derived from its use in explaining how the soul interacted with the body.

Mar Samuel[45] (165–257 CE) recommended fasting before bloodletting, which directly refutes Galen's admonitions to never combine the two practices. Galen's treatise against the Erasistrateans[46] explains the danger of overly weakening the patient by combining fasting and bloodletting and that

41. t. Shabbat 7:5.

42. Berakhot 57b.

43. Berakhot 43b.

44. Berakhot 43b.

45. Samuel bar Abba, a first generation *amora*, not to be confused with the twentieth-century Metropolitan Athanasius Yeshue Samuel, also known as Mar Samuel.

46. Peter Brain, *Galen on Bloodletting: A Study of the Origins, Development, and Validity of His Opinions, with a Translation of the Three Works* (Cambridge: Cambridge University Press, 1986).

fasting is the slower, less efficient of the two methods to eradicate *plethora*.[47] The Erasistrateans, originally opposed to bloodletting, finally adopted the practice during Galen's lifetime, partly in response to the increasing popularity of Galenic medicine in Greco-Roman culture.[48] Given that Mar Samuel, roughly a contemporary of Galen, studied under Rabbi Hanina bar Hama (d. 250 CE) in Sepphoris, he was most likely aware of the debates surrounding the issue of fasting and bloodletting. Mar Samuel reasons that if one eats beforehand, then the only thing leaving the body with the blood is what you just ate. By fasting, one is getting straight to the matter, essentially bad blood, causing the problem. Despite contradicting Galen in terms of practice, this actually incorporates Galenic theories—the efficiency of bloodletting and "bad" blood. This creates a physiology in which the "good" parts of the body are synonymous with the soul, while the "bad" parts are separate from the human-divine community. As we see from these examples, rabbinic medical culture was in flux, much like Greco-Roman medical culture, on how exactly the human, body parts, and the divine formed relationships.

Many talmudic authors adopted the notion of *plethora* as a reason for bloodletting,[49] but Mar Samuel's explanation for fasting also indicates use of the "intrinsically bad blood" ideology. Galen argues that two types of blood exist, the intrinsically bad due to infection and blood that is bad for the body because it is in excess, or *plethora*. Even he acknowledged, though, the difficulty in visually recognizing infected "bad" blood from normal blood and cautions against trying to excise only the bad blood, since the digestive and cardiovascular systems transformed food and air into the vital *pneuma* carried in the blood. Both Jewish and Greco-Roman healers attest to the obvious change in blood's color, becoming darker as the letting progresses, but the color changes signaling infected/bad blood are much more difficult to discern.

Mar Samuel deviates from Galenic physiology, though, as a way to determine bad blood. In keeping with the biblical notion of a breath of life infusing the whole body, Mar Samuel's physiology sees food as infusing the entire body through the bloodstream. The observable change in the color and character of blood during the course of a letting only reinforces the idea that the food temporarily infuses the body. It essentially "rides" through the

47. A disease state marked by the physical characteristics of redness, tension, and pulsation.

48. Brain, *Galen on Bloodletting*.

49. Fred Rosner, *Medicine in the Bible and Talmud: Selections from Classical Jewish Sources* (Hoboken: Yeshiva University Press, 1995), 150.

bloodstream but does not necessarily transform the body, let alone directly link one to God. Galen's transformative process of *pneuma* directly links the body to the soul. It would not be surprising for Mar Samuel to reject this particular aspect of Galenic medicine, as one's soul is not created by food and air. Since the transformative process is no longer necessary and food infuses the entire body, like the breath, then fasting becomes an important component to successful venesection. Once the patient has fasted, then bloodletting becomes, as Galen claimed, the most efficient process for clearing the body of "bad blood" and ultimately disease.

Hullin 56b gives an overall assessment of human anatomy and physiology. Mar Samuel, drawing upon Deuteronomy 32:6, declares that God had made "in man every organ on its foundation, so that if any one organ is twisted man cannot live." Hullin has various sections describing the anatomy, especially of the thorax and respiratory system, in some cases more accurate than Galen's description, but the passages lack any explanation of how breathing worked or its function in relation to the rest of the body and its processes, such as digestion. One's anatomy comes from specific contributions from each parent; the father's semen forms the "child's bones, sinews, nails, the brain in his head and the white in his eye," while the mother's seed, denoted as red, gives the child "his skin, flesh, hair, blood and the black of his eye."[50] This explanation likely comes from the rabbis' exposure to and adaptation of Greco-Roman understanding of fetal development. Yet the rabbis understand a third contributor to the formation of a child: "And the Holy One, blessed be He, gives him the spirit and the breath, beauty of features, eyesight, the power of hearing and the ability to speak and to walk, understanding and discernment." The talmudic rabbis also debated fetal development; some argue that it begins with the head, while Rabbi Saul claimed that it was the naval.[51]

Berakhot 61b claims that the lungs absorb all liquids; this seems to be in keeping with the description in Plato's *Timaeus* and works with the Hippocratic idea that the heart absorbs fluid from the lungs. It is not clear whether this was borrowed from Greek physiology or simply an indigenous assumption, given the sponge-like appearance of the lungs, which would have been known from butchering and sacrificial practices.

Isaiah 6:10 gives the idea that the eye itself does not see, but the faculty of perception depends on the mind. Rabbi Judah (230–270 CE) attributed

50. Niddah 31a.

51. Newmyer, "Talmudic Medicine and Greco-Roman Science," *ANRW* 37.3:2895–911.

logic and reasoning to the brain in Yevamot 60a, but the passage Avodah Zarah 28b explains perception by connecting the eye to the heart, which seems to be a borrowing from Aristotle.[52] This indicates an attempt to reconcile the popularity of Greco-Roman medicine with adherence to biblical understanding of how the universe works, including human physiology. A similar process of reconciliation appears when investigating digestion. Talmud depicts digestion as taking place in the stomach, which not only grinds up food but causes sleep; this is counteracted by the nose, which helps wake up a person. When the function of the two organs is reversed, death ensues. How these are connected is not clear; Preuss assumes that it is the same mechanism in Aristotle by which the vapors of digestion rise to the head, inducing sleep. The rabbis debated how the stomach ground food; some sages describe it as mechanical, in keeping with Erasistratus and Alexandrian medicine, while others see it as a process of putrefaction, as advocated by the Dogmatists. It is clear that Greco-Roman medicine, if not directly used by Jews during the Second Temple and early rabbinic period, still influenced their approach to anatomy and physiology.

## Disease Etiology

Like other ancient Near Eastern and Mediterranean cultures, a disruption to the cohesiveness of the human community causes diseases. But rather than God making an individual decision to send a disease, communicating displeasure for a specific incident, etiology in Talmud follows a more mechanistic process in keeping with the surrounding Greco-Roman culture. According to Rabbi Jose, the painful skin condition *ra'athan*, which necessitates divorce, is thought to arise from both a man and a woman having intercourse after being bled but without first eating; for some, it is the subsequent child that will actually suffer *ra'athan*.[53]

As the etiology of the skin condition indicates, Talmud reinforces the biblical idea that a community suffers due to the transgression of a leader. Since a Jewish king is no longer present during the early rabbinic period, this responsibility for community health falls to the parents. Ketubbot 60b–61a outlines the causes of eye ailments in children by the types of foodstuffs consumed by the mother. Hullin 69a recognizes, though, that a blind father

52. Preuss, *Biblical and Talmudic Medicine*, 72.

53. Ketubbot 77b.

does not necessarily produce a blind child. Individuality is not totally absent from talmudic disease etiology.

Apart from the Talmud, Josephus maintains the biblical belief that all illness comes from God for some form of transgression. When the high priest Alcimus suffered a stroke, Josephus attributes this to Alcimus's opposition to Judas Maccabee.[54] Additionally, disease etiologies linked to transgressions are applied to the royal family for Aristobulus, Queen Alexandra, and Agrippa. Curiously, though, Alexander Jannaeus's illness was accredited to heavy drinking and exhaustive military campaigns rather than a direct punishment by the hand of God for moral failings. This incorporates the Hellenistic form of disease etiology reliant on a mechanistic interaction with the environment. Ketubbot 111a and Berakhot 43b note that either an excess or paucity of exercise can be detrimental to health, indicating that the talmudic rabbis picked up similar mechanistic ideas. Since the natural world is a manifestation of God, people failing to obey the rules of a natural order essentially cause a disruption in the human-divine community.

When investigating diseases, rather than looking at specific or even categories of disease etiologies and their relationship to physiology, the rabbis classified disease based more on linguistic similarities. The Hebrew terms for "bitter" and "sickness" are cognate to the term for "gall." Thus, gall and the gall bladder are responsible for a number of diseases that affect the entire body; this number is noted as eighty-three, since the Hebrew cognates have that value in numerology.[55] Such classification reflects the rabbinic value of closely studying the wording of authoritative texts.

## Restoration of Health

For all the sects of Judaism, the restoration of health ultimately resides with God, since disease and trauma stem from transgressions or at least a separation from the proper community with God. According to their cosmologies, disruptions among the human communities also create disruption in their community cohesion with God. The avenues by which one heals the relationship with God also heal the body, although these avenues do vary by communities.

54. Josephus, *Antiquities of the Jews* 12.413.

55. Rosner, *Medicine in the Bible and Talmud*, 108.

The underlying ideology for Essene therapeutics was to perfect the soul, therefore making it receptive to God.[56] This is a slight ideological shift from being acceptable in the presence of God, likely a response to the loss of the temple, so God must now reside among people rather than in a specific physical location. The Essenes mostly used herbal remedies, amulets, and prayer/incantations, but the exact process for them is not known. We can tell that they essentially satisfied the requirements of charged substances in oral and physical healing rites in the Essenes' attempt to perfect the soul and reestablish community cohesion both among themselves and with God.

Similarly, Talmud itself requires one to recognize that illness and thus healing are in the hands of God. "Man must ever pray not to become ill for if he becomes so, it is demanded of him to show merit in order to be healed."[57] In order to "show merit," the afflicted in rabbinic Judaism uses various *materia medica*. This allows for a combination of biblical medical ideology with hellenized therapeutic practices. Drawing upon a passage in Ezekiel, "along the river will grow every kind of fruit tree with leaves. . . . And their fruit will be good to eat and the leaves medicinal,"[58] the talmudic rabbis often resorted to diet or compounds to treat many ailments. They give little explanation for why certain foods are curative, so medical historians have difficulty pinpointing an underlying humoral or other physiological theory at work. In broad terms, these foods and compounds are the charged substances in a ritual of obedience directed toward both God and the sectarian communities.

A system of homeopathy seems to be the basis for several treatments, such as using a poultice of squashed flies to counteract a hornet sting.[59] Also, a particular medicinal substance may have multiple uses, such as rosewater for both eye ailments and headaches.[60] Josephus makes reference to the use of the natural hot springs around Tiberias as well as to various plants. Of note are the use of bitumen, honey, and oil during the Second Temple period, not only among Jews but for the Greco-Romans as well.

It is highly doubtful that the practice of venesection originated on its own within Judaism, given that Leviticus 19:28 prohibits the piercing of the skin, a passage cited in Talmud as preventing bloodletting.[61] Yet multiple

56. Rosner, *Medicine in the Bible and Talmud*, 13.
57. Shabbat 32a.
58. Ezek 47:12.
59. Shabbat 77b.
60. Gittin 68b.
61. Makkot 20b and 21a.

passages in Talmud attest to its widespread use among Jewish communities. One in particular remarks on the difficulty of finding someone who does not have the puncture wounds of bloodletting.[62] The ubiquitousness of the practice found its way into legal matters. One case of assault has the injured person pay the offender the price of bloodletting, since it saved him the trouble of having to visit a venesectionist.[63] Such frequency of bloodletting among the Jewish population may indicate that it was a rite of obedience directed at maintaining cohesion with the surrounding Greco-Roman communities.

Mar Samuel recommended regular bloodletting preceded by fasting, as a measure of maintaining good health, but its frequency should be determined by age.[64] This incorporates Galen's dictum to follow an age guide when cupping, although he warned not to let blood those under the age of fourteen. In contrast, Talmud indicates that bloodletting was done at much younger ages throughout the Jewish communities, a common occurrence among the non-Galenic practitioners of Greco-Roman medicine. The advice not to let blood in children depends on the physiological belief that blood has an innate heat and that children have more blood, therefore making them more susceptible to fevers.[65] Bloodletting upsets their natural balance of humors, designed to compensate for the heat of the extra blood. This physiological basis for bloodletting is only partially accepted by the rabbis. Although noted as useful, Talmud cautions that excessive bloodletting does considerable harm.[66] Such a basic position derives from experience more so than reactions to Greek philosophical reasons for physiology.

Such habitual bloodletting indicates that the practice derived from the Greco-Roman culture, which understood the balance of humors as its theoretical basis. Geller asserts that the talmudic writers did not know the ideology behind bloodletting and, especially, did not adopt the technique from Galen.[67] This is in contrast to Newmyer's claim that the rabbis were well aware of Hippocrates's humoral theory.[68] Given the Hellenistic slant to the education of Simeon ben Gamaliel and Mar Samuel, it would seem

62. Sanhedrin 93b.

63. Sanhedrin 109a.

64. Shabbat 129b.

65. Rosner, *Medicine in the Bible and Talmud.*

66. Gittin 70a.

67. Markham J. Geller, "Bloodletting in Babylonia," in *Magic and Rationality in Ancient Near Eastern and Greco-Roman Medicine*, ed. John Scarborough et al. (Boston: Brill, 2004), 305–24.

68. Stephen Newmyer, "Talmudic Medicine and Greek Sources," *Ḳorot* 9 (1985): 34–57.

likely that at least some rabbis knew about the theories of Hippocrates and Galen, even though we cannot prove a direct borrowing from their writings. Culturally, the bloodletter or *gara* held a low position in society and was not considered on par with the physician or scholar.[69] This is in contrast to the high esteem given to physicians in Greco-Roman culture, whose practice included bloodletting. An exception to this rule is the great reputation of the bloodletter Abba, mentioned in Talmud.[70]

Although venesection became a typical practice, Talmud indicates that even its proponents could not agree on when to do it. Rabbi Ishmael ben Jose advocated bloodletting for treating the *askara* disease but not for other ailments, including fevers.[71] Abaye, though, advised bloodletting on the second day of a fever, which was the custom of his mother,[72] while others warned never to let blood during the height of a fever or for eye ailments.[73] Additionally, one should not consume small fish, cress, and vinegar or bathe immediately following a bloodletting.[74] Timing was also an important factor, with prohibitions on cloudy days or while a south wind blew.[75] This last directive incorporates traditional Mesopotamian medical beliefs about wind-borne illness.

Modern studies on talmudic medicine note the references to amputation[76] and a splenectomy.[77] The splenectomy, though, is not a cure for an illness but rather a form of literary hyperbole about making one run faster. This results in a later medieval commentary from Rashi, who connects the heaviness of the spleen with slowing down one's running. Apart from cesarean sections, there are no known practices of such an invasive abdominal surgery in the ancient world, especially an elective one.

Biblical prohibitions on cutting into the body make surgery a rare therapeutic form in the Talmud. Yet Ketubbot 77b gives direction for removing some sort of organism from the brain to treat a painful skin condition. Oddly, the presence of the organism is not the etiology of the disease but only mentioned in its cure. Surgery *per se* is not performed, in that nothing

69. Qiddushin 82a, Kelim 12:4, and Derekh Eretz Zuta 10:2.
70. Ta'anit 21b.
71. Yoma 84a.
72. Gittin 76b.
73. Avodah Zarah 29a.
74. Avodah Zarah 28b.
75. Yevamot 72a.
76. Gittin 56a.
77. Sanhedrin 21b.

pierces the skin. A prescription attributed to Abaye has a compound mixture applied to the head, which softens the skin enough to peel it back, exposing the organism, which many translations render as "insect," and then removing it with tweezers. When analyzing the parts of the body that can cause defilement, though, even a small portion of the skull as removed from a surgeon's drill can transmit uncleanliness,[78] thus indicating that some form of trephination may have been practiced.

Shabbat 53a–b refers to amulets to prevent suffering in both humans and animals, though it is acknowledged that only amulets proven successful are actually acceptable. The issue for the talmudic sages is whether something is working through the power of God, hence proven acceptable, or is operating with a different "power source," thus not acceptable and not likely to work. Josephus refers to the use of stones by the Essenes, most likely meaning amulets made of stone, but it is not clear whether they derived this practice from Egyptian or Pythagorean use of amulets[79] or directly from the biblical antecedents of the precious stones representing the twelve tribes of Israel on the breastplate of the high priest's clothing.[80] This overlap of three medical cultures would increase the likeliness. If the Qumran Scrolls are Essene writings, it is curious, though, that they do not mention such knowledge and medicinal use of stones.

For much of the ancient world, illness signifies a disruption in community cohesion, which finds expression in the Hebrew Bible by physically removing the afflicted from the human community. In contrast to this, Talmud calls for the practice of *bikkur ḥolim* (visiting the sick) as one of the holy duties in Judaism.[81] Rabbi Huna (216–296 CE) thought that visits reduced the illness by one-sixtieth; therefore, sixty visits would cure the patient.[82] During the visitation, one must cook, clean, and generally make the patient comfortable, but also, importantly, pray for the person. Even without being in the presence of the sick person, one is supposed to pray as a fulfillment of *bikkur ḥolim*. Interestingly, there is a requirement to pray only in Hebrew if the patient is not present, because the ministering angels understand only Hebrew. But if one is in the patient's presence, one can use any language, since God is then ministering to the patient directly.[83] *Bikkur*

78. Ohalot 2:3.
79. Kottek, "Essenes and Medicine," 81–99.
80. Exod 28:17.
81. Sotah 14a and Bava Qamma 100a.
82. Leviticus Rabbah 34:1.
83. Rosner, *Medicine in the Bible and Talmud*, 178.

*ḥolim* demonstrates the human community's obedience to God instead of just the patient's. The instructions for appropriate language choice indicate God's consideration in the process. Certain types of ailments are exempt from such visits, such as diarrhea and diseases thought to be contagious.

The laying on of hands is a practice seen in many of the pre-Hellenistic cultures and especially tied to the healing powers of a king. *Genesis Apocryphon* from the Qumran Scrolls relates a story of the Egyptians suffering from plagues and of the pharaoh asking Abraham to pray and lay hands on him to effect a cure. In Talmud, Berakhot 5b describes how Rabbi Yohanan (180–279 CE), in fulfilling *bikkur ḥolim*, raised up Rabbi Hiyya as well as Rabbi Eleazar, which is interpreted by some as not simply helping the sick to physically move but as the laying on of hands and healing them.[84] Christian writings also make use of this practice quite frequently.

The principle of like curing like, homeopathy or sympathetic magic, can be found throughout the ancient world. Sanhedrin 7:4 prohibits the use of magic, but positive references to it do occur in Talmud. Rabbi Matthia (135–170 CE) advised that "one whom a mad dog has bitten may be given to eat the lobe of its liver," while subsequent sages did not consider this particular practice a cure.[85] Part of the controversy over whether this is an effective cure is the reputation of Rabbi Matthia, who is said to have had a conversation with the angel Raphael,[86] as well as the traditional cultural importance of the liver over other organs, especially in the Hebrew Bible.

Sympathetic magic is not just the pairing of a dog bite with the liver of a dog but that the etiology of the madness lies in the liver; therefore, eating specifically liver will cure it. In this, though, there is a blending of Greco-Roman medical ideology. Deuteronomy 12:23 declares that blood is life, so the anatomical understanding that the liver contains a great amount of blood makes such sympathetic magic work within the mandates of Judaism. Yet the anatomical knowledge of the importance of blood and the liver is reinforced by the Galenic explanations of anatomy and physiology. Although this particular instance of sympathetic magic with the dog's liver is not derived or dependent upon Greco-Roman medicine, it does signify an ideological overlap that would allow for a trafficking of therapies between the two medical cultures.

84. Kottek, "Essenes and Medicine," 81–99.

85. Yoma 84a.

86. Raphael means "healer of god."

## Illness

### Disease

Currently, there are no publications on the paleopathology of Jewish bodies[87] from the Levant during the Second Temple period in order to determine prevalent diseases and types of traumas. Legal prohibitions in modern Israel on the handling of Jewish bodies make an in-depth paleopathology difficult. But one can reconstruct the environmental conditions of Jewish groups in the diaspora, such as at Rome, based on studies of both Jewish and non-Jewish remains in those areas. Given the extent of the diaspora through the Mediterranean to the west and the Iranian Plateau to the east, an investigation of the paleopathology of these diasporic communities reaches beyond the scope of this present study.

In the absence of significant paleopathology, we must rely on textual sources to understand the types of illnesses Jewish communities encountered in the Second Temple and early rabbinic periods. Diseases of particular concern in the textual sources tend to be eyesight, which often carries a theological message rather than a purely clinical one. This may be a reflection of the valuation on eyes and the gaze in Roman culture. In keeping with biblical antecedents, skin disorders figure prominently as well in the texts of many Jewish sects. Besides the theological focus, the Talmud also describes diseases through a legal lens. This is most clear in a discussion concerning death resulting from circumcision. Rabbi Judah declares that, after the death of a second son, the third does not have to be circumcised. Yet Rabbi Simeon ben Gamliel claims that it is only after the death of the third son that the fourth shall be exempt from circumcision.[88] Other than the slight recognition that a disease process is at work,[89] no attempt is made to understand the underlying physical condition, likely hemophilia.

Hellenism, additionally, influenced the presentation of diseases. The talmudic writers often adopted the Greek terms for diseases, such as *podagra* for gout. Gout is not a communicable disease arising in a particular population and then spreading, like Hansen's disease; it results from di-

87. In this study, the designation of a body as Jewish is wholly dependent on its cultural context, determined by the site and associated artifacts of the body.

88. Yevamot 64b.

89. Maimonides (1138–1204 CE) is a late talmudist noting that the disease seems to be inherited from the mother.

etary deficiencies and excesses. Therefore, it can arise in any population and likely existed in the earlier Israelite community. The rabbis' borrowing of *podagra* is not due to the disease suddenly appearing after contact with the Greeks. The adoption of a Greek term indicates a cultural exchange of medical knowledge. For all their disavowal of Greek learning, the talmudic sages and likely the larger Jewish population had recognized some level of expertise in diagnosing and treating the disease within Hellenistic medicine, thus spurring the incorporation of a Greek word.

### Trauma

The Talmud does not go into detail on injuries, except some notable remarks on dog bites, in particular that the bite of a mad dog is always fatal.[90] Josephus relates many non-biblical episodes of trauma, either from accidents, battle, or torture, but gives little in the way of clinical descriptions of the wounds and almost nothing of their treatments; he mostly states whether they lived or died and whether an attempt at healing was made in the most general of terms. The lack of paleopathological studies means we cannot tell whether there is a disproportionate amount of injuries due to interpersonal conflict or the types of daily labor, based on gender lines, that leave marks on the skeletons.

### Disability

There are recent studies by Julia Watts Belser on disability in early rabbinic literature, but most scholarship has centered on the work of medieval rabbis or the developing Christian perspective during the Second Temple period. Talmud outlines the categories of deaf-mute, mentally disabled, and even youth as stigmatized. This conception parallels the same attitude seen in Roman medicine. It is highly unlikely that the rabbis adopted these ideas through hellenization. Rather, the rabbis experienced a similar ideological development given that both cultures valued an educational system based upon a dialectic form of argumentation. Rabbinic texts depict physical disabilities as a result of the body's interaction with its environment, especially its social context, such as slavery.

90. Yoma 8:5.

The lived experience of those with disabilities was in tension with the rabbinic ideals of a perfected body. Belser argues that in the process of eschatological healing, disability acts as a temporary marker of individuality.[91] This indicates a shift in the ancient Near Eastern concept of a three-way relationship between the person, body parts, and the gods. Anatomy is not so much a distinct entity but a bridge between humans and God. During a mortal life, body parts are more closely associated with the person, but upon resurrection, the body becomes more distinct and useless as the person now joins his or her identity with the afterlife and God.

## Conditional States

Talmud addressed puberty and its physical changes as a legal and socio-religious issue rather medicalizing it. The rabbis noted that in both males and females, there are upper and lower signs of the body, with ultimate determination by the upper signs, since these develop later than the lower signs. For males, beard growth is the determining factor in reaching an age of majority in relation to fulfilling the obligations of the Torah. Mar Samuel asserted that for legal-scientific purposes he made observations of his female maidservant's pubescent development.[92] Talmud contains some discussion on whether the left or right breast develops first in women due to their socioeconomic status. Poor women have the left develop first due to carrying things like water jugs, while upper-class women have the right breast develop because of the rubbing against head scarves that hang down on the right side. Some thought that the lower classes developed the upper signs earlier, since the arm muscles are worked more from grinding.[93]

The legality of menstruating women participating in temple sacrifices is of particular concern; talmudic consensus is that she cannot participate in a state of impurity caused by menstruation. With regard to legal purity, the sages try to determine whether a bloody discharge is something other than menstruation. It is interesting to note that repeated uterine bleeding after intercourse, although a cause of ritual impurity and grounds for divorce, does not preclude the woman from remarrying. There is the idea that the cause

91. Julia Watts Belser, "Disability, Animality, and Enslavement in Rabbinic Narratives of Bodily Restoration and Resurrection," *Journal of Late Antiquity* 8 (2015): 288–305.

92. Preuss, *Biblical and Talmudic Medicine*, 13.

93. Preuss, *Biblical and Talmudic Medicine*, 129.

of the bleeding is due to the husband, and therefore changing husbands may in fact resolve the condition. Before the second marriage, the woman had to undergo an examination by an approved physician, which gives textual evidence of the first vaginal speculum.[94]

Cases of menorrhagia or metrorrhagia have appeared in Matthew 9:20, in which the woman unsuccessfully sought healing from physicians. This indicates that women were not limited to consulting only midwives for such gynecological issues, but there is no evidence that the male physician would have physically examined her. The miraculous healing stories of the gospels indicate one strategy in the hierarchy of resort not unlike those seen in the rabbinic texts or the Greco-Roman asklepieion.

The use of midwives for issues of fertility, pregnancy, and likely all gynecological matters means the topic of pregnancy would be limited in Talmud. Some folkloric advice on choosing the sex of a child does appear, but for the most part the rabbinic sages admonished the belief that one can do something to determine the gender of offspring. They claim that God decides a child's gender, based on Ecclesiastes 11:5. Talmud noted a variation in the length of pregnancy; God determined some fetuses to gestate for seven months while others for nine. If a seventh-month fetus stayed in the womb until the eighth month, it would be fine. Yet the Hippocratic idea that an eighth-month fetus is not viable seems to have crept into the *tosefta* in Shabbat 15:5. The talmudic tractate Hullin 58a claims that the fetus is an appendage of the mother.

Geriatric issues do not appear as a medical condition in texts from the Second Temple and early rabbinic periods apart from a recognition of the effects of aging on anatomy and physiology. In particular, the physiological process of grinding food was thought to slow down as one ages.[95] The more autobiographical passages in Talmud mention a reduction of visual acuity for some of the sages.

## Healers

The rabbis, while outlining the minimum number of people needed in a city to have a Sanhedrin, advised that scholars should reside only in cities with

94. Niddah 66a; see Newmyer, "Talmudic Medicine and Greco-Roman Science," *ANRW* 37.3:2895–911.

95. Shabbat 15a.

certain features such as a synagogue, public bath, circumciser, and notably a surgeon/physician.[96] The Wisdom of Ben Sira also indicates a shift toward a positive attitude for physicians in the Second Temple period. "Honor physicians for their services, for the Lord created them; for their gift of healing comes from the Most High."[97] These passages come from a cultural context in which many Jews saw secular healers as idol worshipers or magicians. There is a change in the use of terms during this period. In Talmud, the Hebrew word for physician, *rophe*, biblically associated with God, gives way to the Aramaic *assaia*. A more thorough analysis of various Aramaic terms for healers appears in Preuss, with the conclusion that in the rabbinic communities, there is no real presence of specialists.[98] One might think the *mohel* (circumciser) is an exception, but he was not considered part of the medical community. Either a *mohel* or a physician can act as a stand-in for the father, who is the one obligated to circumcise his son. Harris's *Popular Medicine in Graeco-Roman Antiquity* includes a more recent study of rabbinic attitudes toward the prevalent *iatros/medicus* in ancient Palestine.[99]

It is not entirely clear whether the rabbis acted as practicing healers or whether their advice is confined to the academic world of talmudic study. Mar Samuel is the only one of the *tannaim* accredited as a physician, and he is noted for even preparing an eye salve for Rabbi Judah Hanasi.[100] Abaye, who wrote on medical topics, accredited much of his expertise to his stepmother, whom he references frequently.[101] Although Rabbi Yohanan would make certain pronouncements touching upon medical issues, his knowledge comes from literary study rather than clinical experience. It is quite possible that their position in society as men of learning would lead people to seek them out as healers, perhaps on the upper end of the hierarchy of resort, a common occurrence in the ancient world. In this respect, they are on par with the Greek *iatros* and Roman *medicus*, although the rabbis did not specifically study medicine or apprentice themselves to noted healers.

Talmud identifies a few non-rabbinic physicians, although with not enough detail to give a clear picture of their practices. Tobiya appears by

96. Sanhedrin 17b.

97. Sir 38:1–2.

98. Preuss, *Biblical and Talmudic Medicine*, 14–15.

99. Catherine Hezser, "Representations of the Physician in Jewish Literature from Hellenistic and Roman Times," in *Popular Medicine in Graeco-Roman Antiquity*, ed. William V. Harris (Leiden: Brill, 2016), 173–97.

100. Bava Metzi'a 85b.

101. Some accounts describe her relationship as more akin to a foster parent.

name in Rosh Hashanah 1:7, and Bar Girute (ca. 200 CE) is mentioned in Betzah 1:60c. According to Avodah Zarah 28b, a physician called Benjamin (ca. 280 CE) proclaimed that only fluid from the kidney is beneficial to the ear; several texts indicate that the disciples/apprentices of Benjamin conflicted with the rabbinic sages.[102] Non-Jewish sources such as Galen and Celsus refer to Jewish physicians. Galen mentions a Theodas, who may be the same Theodoros of Alexandria appearing in Bekhorot.[103] The Galenic treatise *Epidemics* also notes that Rufus Samaritanus worked in Rome around 100 CE.

The most noted female healer in Talmud is the stepmother of Abaye. Like her Roman counterparts, she was not simply a midwife restricted to the care of pregnant and parturient women and infants. She had cures for ear infections, heart problems, fevers, and scorpion bites.[104] Beruriah, the wife of Rabbi Meir and daughter of Rabbi Hanina, although likely a fictional construct or conflation of different women, is noted as a scholar, which brings up the issue as to the extent women could indulge in Greco-Roman learning, which was otherwise prohibited for Jewish men. This also raises the question of where exactly did Abaye's stepmother acquire her knowledge of medicine. Yaltha, the wife of Rabbi Nahman, is noted as a healer in the passage Gittin 67b. Rabbi Yohanan is said to have sought out healing from a Roman woman when suffering from a disease of bleeding gums,[105] now equated with modern scurvy.

Unlike the itinerant physician, common in Greco-Roman culture, Bava Qamma 85a advises one not to use a wandering or foreign physician, since he would not be familiar with the local environmental conditions important for effective healing. This implies an acceptance of the Greco-Roman medical theory that the environment plays a key role in the potency of pharmacology, as well as its influence on disease etiology. Yet it is not clear whether this is a convergent evolution of Jewish and Greco-Roman medical theories or whether the training/working of Jewish physicians in places like Alexandria created the theoretical overlap.

This same tractate (Bava Qamma 85a) requires that a physician be licensed by the local court of justice;[106] it is not clear whether this licensing

102. Shabbat 133b and Sanhedrin 99b.

103. Berakhot 1, 3a; and Ohalot 4:2.

104. Samuel Kottek, "Amra Li Em: La Transmission de la Médecine Populaire par les Femmes dans le Talmud," *Revue des études juives* 169 (2010): 419–37.

105. Yoma 84a.

106. Bava Qamma 85a.

means merely paying a fee or otherwise obtaining government acknowledgment for the individual's practice. No official course of study or examination process was necessary to obtain the license. The physician did have to obtain permission from his neighbors to open up his home as a place healing. There is no evidence that Jewish physicians worked in a market or other public place. According to Philo, the Essenes would pay for the healing of a sick person out of the community's funds. This argues against the idea that the Essenes were predominantly healers.[107] The community "health insurance" seems on the surface necessary, since they did not hold private property to pay for a physician, yet such a practice of communal care is not unusual for the ancient world, given the use of physicians on Egyptian work sites, Greek cities, and the Roman army. Delineation of payment by a community rather than the community assuring the availability of a physician does seem unique.

Not much has survived to give an account of how patients understood or viewed the healing practices within the Jewish communities. No votives or *iamata*, as in Greece and Rome, were produced. Yet, throughout the Talmud, numerous references to the ailments of Rabbi Judah HaNasi may allow one to reconstruct the patient experience for at least those of considerable high status within the community. Much more work needs to be done on the cultural context of healing in the early rabbinic community.

107. Kottek, "Essenes and Medicine," 81–99.

# 11. Persian Medicine

## Location and History

The region of ancient Persia occupied what is known today as the Iranian Plateau. Contrary to its name, the Iranian Plateau is not particularly flat. It actually contains five different mountain ranges, with the Caspian Sea bordering to the northwest, the Persian Gulf in the south, and the Indus River to the east. It covers the modern countries of Afghanistan, Iran, and northwestern Pakistan, as well as parts of Armenia, Azerbaijan, Turkmenistan, Uzbekistan, and Kurdistan. This geographical placement puts the inhabitants of the Iranian Plateau at a crossroads between the ancient Near East and the Indian subcontinent. Conquests and interaction with the Mediterranean world introduced Greco-Roman ideas and practices. Yet modern tensions make it difficult to fully investigate the history and archaeology. English-language scholarship, therefore, tends to group historical studies by regions, such as northwest or southwest. This is also influenced by political divisions that correspond to modern nation-states willing to work cooperatively with European and North American powers.

Although we often refer to ancient Persia, the plateau was not a cohesive political entity for much of the area's history. Various political groups of Elamites controlled the region, starting in 3200 BCE, with its major city of Susa frequently acting as the capital. The strongest empires divide into three periods: the Old Elamite Kingdom (2700–1600 BCE), Middle Elamite (1500–1000 BCE), and the overlapping Neo-Elamite (1500–539 BCE). Throughout the second and first millenniums, the Elamites engaged in continual warfare with the Assyrian and Babylonian Empires.

During the tenth century BCE, an Indo-European group known as the Medes migrated into the northwestern portion of the Iranian Plateau. Constant fighting with Assyrian forces drove the Medes into the southwest, where they settled at Pārsa, which then brought them into conflict with the

Elamites. The Medes briefly ruled until the rise of the Achaemenid Dynasty (559–330 BCE). The Achaemenid dynasty started with Cyrus I as a vassal of the Assyrians and his son Cambyses I as king under the Medes. The independence of the Achaemenids began with the next king, Cyrus II (590–530 BCE). Major cities of the Achaemenids were Susa, Persepolis, and Pasargadae. Most often when people speak of ancient Persia, they are referring to this Achaemenid dynasty, which was eventually brought to an end by the invasion of Alexander the Great and ruled by the Seleucids.

Arsaces I successfully rebelled against the Seleucids, creating the Parthian Empire (247 BCE–224 CE); thus, it is also known as the Arsacid Empire. Culturally, the Parthians were heavily influenced by the Seleucids and Hellenism, though they frequently fought against the Romans. The Sasanian Empire (226–651 CE) rose under Ardashir I, creating a more centralized government, with the Zoroastrian religion as a cornerstone, legitimizing the ruling dynasty. They had extensive relations with the Roman and Byzantine Empires, as well as trade contacts through India and as far as China, with the Han and Tang dynasties. In 651 CE, the Sasanians fell to the forces of Umar al-Faruq of the Rashidun Caliphate. Zoroastrianism did not end with the Sasanian Empire but is still a thriving religion in modern Iran and India.

Adhami divides Persian medicine into three periods:[1] (1) the Indo-European period, described by the three functional categories of knife, herbs, and mantras, paralleling the social divisions of warriors, shepherds/farmers, and the priests; (2) the Imperial period, which includes the Achaemenid, Seleucid, Parthian, and Sasanian dynasties; and (3) the Islamic period. Most studies on Persian medicine focus on the more famous physicians, such as Avicenna from the Islamic period. Instead, this chapter will address medicine and health care in these first and second periods.

## Religion and Culture

Several different religions were practiced across the Iranian Plateau, but the most dominant was Zoroastrianism under the Sasanians. Other populations also practiced Buddhism, Hinduism, Manichaeism, and Gnosticism[2] during

1. Siamak Adhami, "Two Pahlavi Chapters on Medicine," *Early Science and Medicine* 16 (2011): 331–51.

2. Although secondary sources often refer to Gnosticism, mostly it was the Nestorian form of Christianity.

the first millenniums BCE and CE. The "Magian tradition" from western Iran is considered a pre-Zoroastrian religion practiced by the Elamites, but texts and artifacts, such as liver-divination models, from those kingdoms demonstrate a religious tradition in keeping with the Mesopotamians as well. Likely, the different polities on the Iranian Plateau experienced a blending of religious traditions rather than a confrontation between them. Zoroastrian dominance occurred because of royal backing, originally by the Achaemenids,[3] that became more prominent with the Sasanians.

Zoroastrianism developed from the teachings of Zarathustra.[4] According to nineteenth-century scholars, he was a sixth-century BCE prophet who preached reforms in five *gāthās*, or songs/hymns, but the historical accuracy of claims about Zarathustra and his life are highly debated.[5] These *gāthās* likely existed in oral form as early as 1000 BCE but did not have a written form until the Sasanian Empire around 600 CE. The *Avesta* contains the *gāthās* as well as other hymns and liturgical texts used during the *yasna* ceremony. Also in the *Avesta* are the *Vespirad*, which are invocations of different deities and legal texts concerning purity, called the *Vendidad* (Rules for Keeping Bad Old Gods[6] Away). Pollution presented a constant threat especially to rivers, so river washing did not figure prominently in the religion. This will impact medical practices, especially in comparison to the other cultures of the ancient Near East and Mediterranean. Priests spent a considerable amount of time determining pollution sources. To avoid pollution by dead things, bones were picked clean by birds and then elevated from the ground, with a roof to prevent rain hitting them but allowing light to come through. Light has a positive cosmological significance in Zoroastrianism. Finally, a container of stone and plaster stored the bones. The oldest known copies of the *Avesta* date to the thirteenth or fourteenth century CE.

3. Philip G. Kreyenbroek, "Zoroastrianism under the Achaemenians: A Non-Essentialist Approach," in *The World of Achaemenid Persia: History, Art, and Society in Iran and the Ancient Near East*, ed. John Curtis and St John Simpson (London: I. B. Tauris, 2010), 103–9.

4. Zoroaster is the Greek form of his name.

5. Abolala Soudavar, "The Formation of Achaemenid Imperial Ideology and Its Impact on the Avesta," in *The World of Achaemenid Persian History, Art, and Society in Iran and the Ancient Near East*, ed. John Curtis and St John Simpson (London: I. B. Tauris, 2010), 111–38; S. K. Mendoza Forrest, *Witches, Whores, and Sorcerers: The Concept of Evil in Early Iran* (Austin: University of Texas Press, 2011), 11.

6. The term for "bad old gods" is *daēwas*, which is often translated as "demons." This is misleading, since their qualification as "bad" stems from being deceived by The Lie. They are not inherently bad, as is commonly thought of demons, but rather their state depends on context.

Recognizing that the religion predates Zarathustra, some secondary sources refer to the religion as Mazdeism after the principle god Ahura Mazda.

## Cosmology

The cosmology of Zoroastrianism espouses a dualistic worldview, with good and evil existing for eternity. The god Ahura Mazda, or the Wise Lord, represents good, while Angra Mainyu, or the Hostile Spirit, signifies the bad. Good means the upholding of the cosmic order, both between humans and gods, as well as among the gods—that is, community cohesion. Bad is then the converse, a breaking down of the cosmic order/community cohesion. Ahura Mazda and Angra Mainyu are sometimes portrayed as twin brothers in the womb of Time (Druva), who is an eternal cosmic entity along with Firmament and Empty Space. In some texts, only the Hostile Spirit is the child of Druj,[7] meaning the Lie. Unlike the polytheistic religions of the rest of the ancient Near East and Mediterranean, these opposing Zoroastrian gods do not work in cooperation or form a council but always struggle against each other. The earthly world is a mixture, because in one version of creation the Hostile Spirit attacked the good creation of the Wise Lord. Another version, more in keeping with Manichaeism, has the Hostile Spirit making the world, but the Wise Lord infused light/goodness into humans, thus creating a soul. Some books in the *Avesta* describe the creation of the present world and how it will end when good finally defeats evil. Plutarch's *On Isis and Osiris* attests to such dualism and mentions Zoroaster, "who lived five thousand years before the Trojan War," though his dating is considerably inaccurate.

According to the *Avesta*, the cosmos exists in two parts. There is This World, made up of bones and living things. The second world is called the Other World, consisting of gods, demons, and thoughts. Ahura Mazda is an omniscient lord with divine entities that help him maintain cosmic order. Mithra, the morning star, is one of them, who prepares the path for the sun.[8] There is more evil the further west one goes. Mithra became a popular god in his own right, among the lower ranks of the Roman army. Although the gods under Ahura Mazda work together, such cooperation is never seen between the sides of good and evil. A "good god" will not use an "evil demon" to send

7. Some older translations use the spelling Druz.

8. Many of the qualities of Mithra become grafted on to the image of Jesus Christ.

a message to humans. Meanwhile, normal human perception cannot see the Other World, but their souls can reach it.

In this cosmology, Ahura Mazda gave the kings royal command so that they may establish and maintain order, which in turn provided happiness for the people. Following this ordered system allowed them to be among the chosen after death. Those who uphold the cosmic order are referred to as the "once dead,"[9] in contrast to those still suffering under the cosmic deception, which is thought of as the demonic entity, The Lie. The Achaemenid king Darius I promoted his conquests as upholding the cosmic order at the behest of Ahura Mazda, while his opponents were deceived by The Lie. The Sasanians made a more explicit connection between the king's actions in This World, paralleling Ahura Mazda in the Other World. The description of the enemy as deceived by The Lie functioned as internal propaganda to bolster the king, as just yet it did not galvanize the masses to action against an enemy. In practice, ancient empires of the Iranian Plateau, including the Achaemenid and Sasanian dynasties, tolerated other religions. The Cyrus Cylinder demonstrates such religious acceptance. Written in Akkadian, it describes Cyrus II's religious policy in Babylonia but says nothing of his personal or the official practices in Persia proper. The ancient societies of the Iranian Plateau balanced this good/bad dualism with the need for an intra- and inter-community cohesion. This idea of humans needing to maintain a cosmic order (human-human and human-divine communities) influenced the approach to medicine practiced by the various cultures of ancient Persia.

Accessing the power and order of the cosmos, commonly referred to as magical practices, centered on dream interpretation, divination, and soul travel. Rituals to control evil usually fell into the two categories of apotropaic and exorcistic. Scholars understand the oral rite as the most important aspect to Persian religion as well as medicine. Physical rites for the side of Good were typically carried out at dawn or during the day, whereas rituals for the Bad were done at night. In each of these, practitioners did the exact same ritual acts, only the intent behind them determined whether they propagated the Good or the Bad. Many of these rituals included sacrifice with fire and the drinking of a mixture from the *haoma* or *soma* plant, signs of obedience to the gods. An underlying concept to the sacrifices is that the libations poured into the fire represent the sacrifice of the worshiper's body and soul

9. Prods Oktor Skjærvø, "Avesta and Zoroastrianism under the Achaemenids and Early Sasanians," in *The Oxford Handbook of Ancient Iran*, ed. D. T. Potts (Oxford: Oxford University Press, 2013), 546–65.

without having to be physically sacrificed. To the ancient Persians, the body has symbolic substitutes, which impacts how anatomy and physiology function in a medical context. The following is a brief list of deities that oversee human health and medical practices.

## Persian Gods and Goddesses of Disease and Healing

### *Ahura Mazda*

As the supreme Good god, Ahura Mazda has the ability to heal and is often referred to as simply The Healer, as is the prophet Zarathustra. He appears frequently in the prayers used in medical cases. No stories exist, though, of him healing a specific incident of disease, as seen with other deities, such as the Mesopotamian Enlil.

### *Airyaman*

The god Airyaman is a personification of the concept of harmonic union and thus represents friendship and acts as a healing deity. He is specifically designated as the power behind the *materia medica* and the one who can heal the 99,999 diseases created by The Hostile Spirit.[10] He is also the one who shows humans how to perform the proper purification rituals to treat disease. His popularity as a healing deity lasted into the third century CE, when he became syncretized with Jesus Christ, particularly by the Manichaeans.

### *Anahita*

The goddess Anahita is a personification of the divine water associated with wisdom, fertility, and healing. The Aredvi Sura Anahita is a heavenly river said to purify the semen and wombs of humans and makes milk flow. The worship of Anahita likely predates Zoroastrianism and became part of the pantheon under the Achaemenids, who also equated her with Ištar. She became synonymous with Artemis/Diana under the influence of Hellenism. Although numerous temples were dedicated to her, they do not appear to

10. *Greater Bundahishn* 26.97–98.

have served as specific healing shrines. The most important rituals in Zoroastrianism are dedicated to her, and by the reign of Artaxerxes II (452–358 BCE), she became part of a divine triad with Ahura Mazda and Mithra.

### *Azi Dahaka*

The deity Azi Dahaka, a son of the Hostile Spirit, represents snakes and other venomous animals. Scholarship in the nineteenth century claimed that as he caused serpent attacks, Azi Dahaka would then be invoked as a cure. This ideology holds true for most ancient medical cultures but directly contradicts the idea of good and evil struggling against each other that underlies Zoroastrianism. No primary sources account for a force of evil working for the side of good.[11] We should then be cautious looking at Azi Dahaka as a healing deity, since that perspective is likely a modern corruption by overzealous comparative ethnology. More likely, he is a source of injury rather than a healer.

### *Druva*

Elamite texts from Persepolis mention the Persian deity Druva, which may be either a male or female deity of healing. The name could also refer to the masculine personification of eternal Time. Interestingly, it is this masculine personification of Time that carried the twins Ahura Mazda and Angra Mainyu in its womb, according to one creation story. As the god Time, Druva should not be confused with the goddess Druj (The Lie), who is the mother of the Hostile Spirit/Angra Mainyu.

### *Fravashis*

The Fravashis are immortals who act as protective spirits for individual humans. In this capacity, they can be invoked for healing purposes. Creation stories attribute to them the role of midwife both for the birth of the cosmos and human children. Among the Fravashis are the concepts of *airyaman*, which is harmonic union and healing, and *amertatat* or "non-dyingness,"

11. *Yasht* 23.131, cited as the source of Azi Daharak curing snakebites, does not actually support such a claim but mentions the deity only as a cause of them.

meaning not passing before one's appointed time, as well as being free of blemish and defects. The concept of an appointed time for dying points to a different system of relationships. Rather than humans negotiating changing relations due to individual wills, every entity whether mortal or supernatural has a fixed role; thus, relationships become almost mechanistic and predictable. Although the texts refer to Fravashis as female, their iconography depicts a male figure superimposed over a solar disc.

### *Mithra*

Mithra oversees all forms of contracts, from the typical business deal to the cohesiveness of communities between people, as well as between humans and gods. In this capacity, he upholds the cosmic order. Mithra ensures the sanctity of contracts, even if formed under the misguidance of The Lie. Soldiers invoked Mithra as the enforcer of contracts to help them in battle against those who broke treaties. As a warrior himself, he battles evil and The Lie, clearing a path for the sun, which is the All-Seeing Eye. One text describes Mithra in this role as "vitalizing strength," who surveys the "healing settlement of the Gawas."[12] Although not explicitly referred to as a healer, Mithra's place in a triad with Ahura Mazda and his status as the enforcer of contracts that ultimately govern health make him an important deity for understanding the medical culture in ancient Persia.

## Sources

Unlike the sources from most other ancient societies, many of our documents for Persia come through Arabic translations from Old and Middle Persian rather than from the primary texts themselves. The oldest copies of the *Avesta* do preserve the ancient languages of Avestan and Pahlavi. The collective name *Avesta* for the texts comes from the oldest form of language in them. The passages related to healing are found in the younger, Pahlavi sections. The rarity of texts containing the entire ritual process presents another problem for researching medicine in ancient Persia. Zoroastrian priests purposefully refrained from writing out complete rituals, because of the danger of them falling into the wrong hands and being used for evil.

12. *Yasht* 10.13–16; see Forrest, *Witches, Whores, and Sorcerers*, 16.

The Elamite Fortification and Treasury tablets from the fifth century BCE describe the religion but have yet to be published and translated, so their value to medicine is unknown. Written records from the Seleucid and Parthian periods are rare, whereas a considerable amount from the Sasanians, especially for the high priest Kerdīr (fl. 240–293 CE), are available. The *Acts of the Religion* (a ninth-century CE encyclopedia) contains passages touching on ancient medical topics, but the work is a compilation of older sources, including the *Avesta*.

Old Persian inscriptions start with Darius I (r. 522–486 BCE), a rather late date for the history of the Iranian Plateau. Therefore, scholars must look outside Persia for sources, such as the texts of Herodotus (484–425 BCE) and Xenophon (431–354 BCE). Yet this compounds the problem, because they are not only late as well but from the perspective of an outsider to the culture.

## Texts

To date, no explicit medical texts have surfaced from the Elamite archives or the Achaemenid and Sasanian dynasties. Cases of a medical nature for the Achaemenids and Sasanians can be found in the Zoroastrian *Avesta*. This lack of dedicated medical texts means scholars must mine the literary and religious sources, as well as court documents and letters, to understand ancient Persian medical culture.

The *Vendidad*, as noted earlier from the *Avesta*, takes the format of questions to Ahura Mazda, who then answers them. This reads much like it is trying to answer the basic eight questions popular in early Greek medical texts.[13] Some of the answers have a commonality with Hippocratic treatises. It is not clear whether Zoroastrian healers simply observed the same phenomena or they directly borrowed from the Greek epistemological traditions about medicine. The use of Greek loan words, the late date of the written sources, and the fact that healers were exchanged between Persian and Greek cultures would indicate a textual borrowing perhaps reinforced by the personal observations of Zoroastrian healers.

Another important Zoroastrian text is the *Greater Bundahishn*, a creation story. There are two recensions of the creation, with one coming from India and the other, a longer one, coming from Iran. It is this latter text that

13. The eight questions originally formulated by Diogenes of Apollonia (ca. 425 BCE) centered on the formation of semen and embryonic development; see chapter 6 on Greek medicine.

is known as the *Greater Bundahishn*. This text also shows Hippocratic and Aristotelian influences, such as cold/wet attributes for females and hot/dry for males. Additionally, the text's use of the term "mixture" follows more an Aristotelian sense of balanced substances rather than the Zoroastrian connotation of the struggle between light and dark forces in humans, which could indicate Hellenistic influences on the conception of anatomy and physiology.

## Archaeology

Unfortunately, the political and economic fortunes of the modern nations on the Iranian Plateau make archaeological studies extremely difficult. A few sites are known to us through textual sources, but adequate surveys and excavations using modern techniques have yet to be carried out on a significant scale. Archaeologists from these nations or neighboring powers, such as Russia, may be conducting research, but their findings have yet to be published beyond their respective borders. Two important sites that do have some available information are Gondishapur and Samarkand.

Shapur II (309–379 CE) made the city Gondishapur his capital, located in the southwest of present-day Iran. As a cosmopolitan city, this became the center of medical sciences for several centuries and hosted the Academy of Gondishapur, considered the first teaching hospital in the history of medicine.[14] During late antiquity, scholars of philosophy and medicine made the academy their base of operations not only for clinical practice but also for the translation into Pahlavi of medical texts from the Hellenistic world as well as India and China. The history of this city is known mostly from texts, since the area has not been significantly excavated. Roughly thirty tells have been identified, but sixteen of them were still under cultivation by local farmers as of 2007. Archaeologists estimate that nearly 90 percent of possible finds have been obliterated by the area's farming activity.

The ancient city of Samarkand, famed for learning and healing, lies in modern Uzbekistan. Most likely the city was founded in the eighth century BCE along the Silk Road between China and the Mediterranean. During the Achaemenid dynasty, it served as the capital of the Sogdian satrapy. It is this area that the *Avesta* refers to when describing Mithra as surveying "the area

14. Mohammadali M. Shoja and Tubbs R. Shane, "The History of Anatomy in Persia," *Journal of Anatomy* 210 (2007): 359–78; Roy J. Shephard, *An Illustrated History of Health and Fitness from Pre-History to Our Post-Modern World* (New York: Springer, 2014), 261–62.

where the Gawas dwell, the healing settlements of the Gawas."[15] Although this city has had numerous excavations, they focus on either the period of its foundation or much later. So far, most discoveries relating to medicine date to the medieval period rather than the Bronze and Iron Ages.

## Cultural Concepts

### Anatomy and Physiology

The overarching concept to Zoroastrian cosmology is the struggle between good and evil; the human body then is one location for this fight. Although some tales of creation mark the material world as the work of the Hostile Spirit, the *Greater Bundahishn* explicitly outlines the formation of the human body as a work of the Wise Lord and therefore as inherently good. "I established sons in the wombs of their mothers and protected them, gave them individually hair, skin, nails, blood, sinews, eyes, ears, and the . . . limbs . . . I shall call the bones from the earth in the world of thought, the blood from the water, the hair, from the plants, the soul from the wind, as they received them at the original creation."[16] So each person's conception and birth is a reenactment of the moment of creation of the good world. It is important to note that material for the fetus comes from "the world of thought," intimately linking human anatomy and physiology with the Other World, the realm of the god Ahura Mazda, thus inherently separating humans from the material world of the Hostile Spirit. Taking care of the body, then, is taking care of what is Good rather than perpetuating the Bad of the (material) This World.

Shoja and Tubbs note that every individual represents a microcosm, with their anatomy having a counterpart in the universe, or macrocosm.[17] This is easily seen when comparing the above passage to one describing the creation of the first human: "The skin is like the sky, the flesh is like the earth, the bones are like the mountains, the veins are like the rivers, the blood in the body is like the water in the sea, the hair is like the plants, the hairier parts are like the forests."[18] In this description, scholars understand the

15. This is an ethnic designation for Sogdians and not a term for healers.

16. *Greater Bundahishn* 34.5; see Forrest, *Witches, Whores, and Sorcerers*, 127.

17. Shoja and Tubbs, "History of Anatomy in Persia," 359–78.

18. Cyril Elgood, *A Medical History of Persia and the Eastern Caliphate from the Earliest Times to the Year A.D. 1932* (Cambridge: Cambridge University Press, 1951).

seven parts of the material world as matching human marrow, blood, veins, sinews, bones, flesh, and hair of man and also corresponding to the Bounteous Immortals (Amesha Spenta).[19] When looking at the relationship between anatomy and the two worlds, the body parts are not fully human or This World but share in the Other World of gods, spirits, and thought, with the possibility of forming its own relationships in that Other World. It is unclear to what extent anatomy has the ability of independent will apart from the individual human and how much it forms a community with the gods apart from humans. Since parts of the body, such as blood, carry impurity even when inside a person who is considered pure, it seems as if they do form a distinct community, even if it is at times with the evil side of the Other World. In some respects, anatomy is then symbiotic, but its communicative function shifts between Good and Evil by almost a mechanistic, predictable process.

Any phenomenon that alters the body is the work of the Hostile Spirit and his minions. This means that anything coming from the body can be used by demons. So even things supposedly as inconsequential as nail clippings would need to be protected by special rites and spells and then deposited in a hole some distance from the community.[20] These spells for hair and nails return them to the plants and earth so demons cannot use them. Such trimmings can also turn into pests, such as lice.[21] So, although anatomy stems from the Wise Lord, individual body parts are essentially neutral and can be corrupted. The body is much like the rituals; good or bad is imparted to them by use rather than being an inherent characteristic.

## Disease Etiology

Unlike the other cultures of the ancient Near East and Mediterranean that see illness as a message from any of the gods, the dualistic ideology of Zoroastrianism understands good health as coming from the Wise Lord (Ahura Mazda), while illness comes from the Hostile Spirit (Angra Mainyu). Illness is not a warning message about disruptions to community cohesion/Cosmic Order but an active attempt to destroy it.

19. These are emanations from Ahura Mazda, who helps him fight Angra Mainyu.

20. James Darmesteter, *The Zend-Avesta: The Vendîdâd* (Westport, CT: Greenwood, 1972), lxxviii.

21. Darmesteter, *Zend-Avesta*, 190.

As part of the eternal struggle, The Hostile Spirit created the Azi Dahaka (the Dragon/Serpent), spittle and phlegm, the exposure and burning of corpses, sorcerers and magicians, and untimely or long-lasting (more than nine days) menses.[22] All of these are avenues by which humans can become ill. Some passages describe Angra Mainyu as directly creating 99,999 diseases, which need healing by prayers to the Holy Word or Airyaman, one of the Bounteous Immortals.[23] Ultimately, illness comes from the fact that the Hostile Spirit has no body and thus must try to inhabit the human body as a matter of survival. The final victory of Good over Evil occurs when all bodies are in a state of perfection, impervious to the predations of Angra Mainyu.

The *Vendidad* organizes cases either by symptoms, like pain and fever, or by the name of the demons causing the illness, such as Kurugha, which equates to the Evil Eye. According to the *Greater Bundahishn*, a demon called Nasush, in the form of a fly, can cause disease by first having contact with dead matter or menstrual blood and then landing on people.[24] Similarly, hair and nail clippings can be a conduit. This demon had contaminated the first humans, as well as animals and plants, bringing death into the world for the first time. Some scholars refer to Nasush as a female demon, but that is because the word itself is feminine; there is no iconography of the entity to discern its gender one way or the other. As we have seen with Druva and the Fravashis, gender is neither strictly binary nor permanent for supernatural entities.

According to Forrest, the god Verthragna stands as an exception to the rule that the deities under Ahura Mazda do not cause illness. The name essentially means "victory," and texts describe the god as one "who strides between the ordered battle lines back and forth, consulting with Mithra and Rashnu . . . sickness and destruction."[25] This text is not explicit that Verthragna causes disease but instead depicts an acknowledgment that Evil will strike some people. Other sources directly highlight his ability to heal as his being one of the Bounteous Immortals.

These disease etiologies show an inherent tension in that some things necessary for life have an inherent Evil. For example, the Hostile Spirit lies behind the impurity of menses, but the process itself signifies the fertility of a woman, which comes from Ahura Mazda. Yet this inherent tension was

22. Forrest, *Witches, Whores, and Sorcerers*, 42.

23. *Vendidad* 22.1–2.

24. *Greater Bundahishn* 4.10.

25. *Yasht* 14.47; see Forrest, *Witches, Whores, and Sorcerers*, 49.

not always present. Zoroastrian texts claim that Yima, the first king, reigned when there was no disease, old age, and death. At this time, Yima and his father looked fifteen years old, the peak of strength and beauty.[26] With the introduction of disease and death, they aged another thirty years. Although this indicates a Persian value on youth, it should not be taken as an indication that the average life span was only forty-five years.

Apart from these supernatural causes, human activity can also bring illness, through the simple act of bad magic. Rituals that access power were inherently neutral; the intent of the practitioner determined their results of disease or healing. This ability to switch sides makes humans different from the gods, who by nature are only either Good or Evil.

## Restoration of Health

According to Zoroastrian beliefs, Ahura Mazda created a healing plant for people that could be either consumed or smeared, indicating that it could be used for both diseases and trauma, "so that the evil, damage, and discomfort from the striking might be less. It immediately became weak and sick, and its milk came out, and it passed away."[27] This illustrates several key points for the concept of healing among the ancient Persians. First, healing is possible only with the help of the gods, particularly those on the side of Good. Second, a physical rite with a specially charged substance is part of healing. Third, illness is an entity in its own right.

An important aspect of human health as the battle ground for Good and Evil is the concept of purity. Disease makes one impure; therefore, those suffering an illness are barred from the wider community. In this context, impurity means that it is not acceptable to be in the presence of the Good human community rather than the divine. For the duration of the illness, the afflicted must reside in a separate room or building (*armest-gah*) and is referred to as "one who is unfit for work."[28] The phrasing indicates a shift from normally fulfilling one's social role to taking on the transient sick role. The Zoroastrians regarded the state of impurity as a "temporary death," so like the dead body, the afflicted must be removed from the presence of the community. This separation is not based on the modern idea of a contagious

26. *Yasna* 9.5; see Forrest, *Witches, Whores, and Sorcerers*, 45.
27. Forrest, *Witches, Whores, and Sorcerers*, 46.
28. Darmesteter, *Zend-Avesta*, 65.

germ but the idea that impurity itself is contagious. This is evident by the fact that women are also separated, especially after a stillbirth. The woman does not reside in the typical *armest-gah* but in a place called "*dakhma* for the living." *Dakhman* normally refers to the tower or platform that keeps a dead body elevated. The practice of body disposal by exposure, instead of cremation or burial in either the ground or water, prevented offending and polluting the elements of fire, earth, and water.

Help of the Good gods is necessary to remove the impurity caused by the Evil origins of the illness and the Evil entity that is the illness. Being ill essentially meant that one was possessed by a demon; therefore, healers used therapies to exorcise the demons/illnesses based on their own priestly power, while also invoking the help of the gods. Spells in the *Vendidad* take the form of direct commands for the ailment to leave, while other spells invoke Ahura Mazda to give strength to smite and drive away the illness.[29] Spells to aid childbirth invoke the goddess Anahita, because water acted as a conduit for the powers of healing. Although the sick should not bathe in rivers for fear of pollution, rain itself could be used as a healing agent. Additionally, light is therapeutic and achieved through the sun, moon, and stars, so the healing prayers were often said three times for each celestial entity. Healing magic often had a retaliatory character that returned the Evil to the one who originally sent it, whether to a human practitioner working under The Lie or to the Evil gods, like Angra Mainyu himself. Incantations often were general in nature rather than targeting specific diseases, such as, "Diseases, run away! Destructions runaway! Demons, run away! Adversaries, run away! Unorderly obscurantist, run away! Men who are tyrants, run away!"[30] Use of spells and rituals demonstrated obedience on the part of the patient, while the response of the Good gods to help shows their consideration. Like the Greco-Roman ideology of natural order informing their medical practices, the consideration of the Zoroastrian Good gods depends on the strict adherence to the employment of oral and physical rites and charged substances. There is a blend of predictable and unpredictable aspects to Persian medicine that would allow the importation of healing techniques from Hellenistic cultures.

Often, physical rites accompanied these healing prayers or spells as part of the exorcism of the evil spirits, and they reintegrated the afflicted with the human community. The rite of *barashnûm* originally cleansed a person

29. Darmesteter, *Zend-Avesta*, 228–29.

30. *Yasht* 3.7; see Forrest, *Witches, Whores, and Sorcerers*, 172.

who had come into contact with the dead, but eventually its use expanded to curing diseases. This ritual lasted nine days and began with the cleansing of the head and worked its way down the body. These rituals signify to both the Good gods and the human community that the afflicted is obedient to the forces of Good, that is, not deceived by The Lie, and that the Good gods accept the person back into the religious community. This acceptance then allows for their reintegration with the human community, the removal of the sick role. As Williams notes, health and purity are synonymous, and the rites of purification were "of *public* concern, and infringement of them resulted in nothing less than social ostracization and public ignominy."[31]

Some scholars assess Persian healing on a hierarchy of resort, with spells and rituals being more important than somatic treatments with *materia medica*.[32] Yet the texts show that the physical rite of a somatic treatment had equal importance. The healing of a woman after a stillbirth involved the eating and drinking of purifying substances, as well as washing. There is no stated hierarchy to treatments in the Zoroastrian texts themselves. Some scholars assume that healers tried herbal remedies first, with surgeries and incantations as a last resort if they considered the offending demon too powerful for the drug therapy.[33] Like the scholarly descriptions of Azi Dahaka, this is a forced conclusion in order to make Persian medicine fit a model known from other cultures.

Some scholars on ancient Persian medicine follow the early twentieth-century social-linguist Benveniste, who claimed that the three forms of healing in prayers, drugs, and surgery match the three classes of society. But we have no evidence that in ancient Persia anyone other than priests practiced healing.[34] Perhaps these three forms do not indicate different healers but were used to target the different social roles of the patients. Scholars also speculate that surgery removed the demon, or the damaged part, but it is not clear how the priest circumvented the risk of exposure to the impure blood produced by surgery. This perspective assumes that the ancient surgeon cuts into the body like a modern practitioner rather than simply sets bones. If the healer stitches up wounds, including debriding, this may have required the typical purification after coming into contact with blood, but this is not

31. Alan Williams, "Zoroastrianism and the Body," in *Religion and the Body*, ed. Sarah Coakley (Cambridge: Cambridge University Press, 1997), 155–66.

32. Darmesteter, *Zend-Avesta*, lxxx.

33. Forrest, *Witches, Whores, and Sorcerers*, 114.

34. Forrest, *Witches, Whores, and Sorcerers*, 116.

explicitly mentioned. Interestingly, the texts also do not mention how one is purified after contact with blood during battle.

Any hierarchy of resort for treatment measures would depend really on how the healer first perceived the disease. Spells may have been a first recourse if the healer thought the demon was particularly powerful and the afflicted was a normally pure person, like a priest. In the struggle between good and evil, it would be a greater victory for a demon to possess the cautious person rather than the one who easily becomes polluted.

Although some of the *materia medica* are charged through rituals, others naturally possess such powers. The *haoma* plant[35] falls into the category of naturally charged substances, since it is the "plant of life" given to humans by the Wise Lord. This *haoma* plant is the basis for all sacrificial rituals in Zoroastrianism and not just for healing. It is interesting, though, that the spiritual keeper of the *haoma* plant is Thrita, the first recognized healer in Zoroastrianism. The converse is that some things naturally lose their powers over time. The impurity caused by a corpse dissipates after a year. Similarly, the demon Drui Nasu has considerable power when first summoned, but it wanes over time, making his defeat easier. The overlap of rituals for healing with those of purification highlights the fact that health in itself means being pure or free from the evil of The Lie and the Hostile Spirit.

## Illness

We do not have significant paleopathological studies for ancient Persia to determine whether certain diseases were more prevalent, especially as an epidemic, along the Iranian Plateau, with the exception of the Armenian Plateau. Although journals from the University of Tehran do publish such studies particular to Iran, they tend to focus on skeletal remains from the medieval period rather than the ancient world.

Bodies from a number of cemeteries in present-day Armenia, which date to the Bronze Age and from the first century BCE to third century CE, have been analyzed for the use of trephination and for the intentional molding of the skull and teeth as social markers. These bodies indicate that healers used trephination to cure a variety of diseases, as well as trauma that caused swellings within the head. The trephination holes were similar in character to ones found in skulls from Anatolia and the Levant, showing that ancient

35. This plant appears in Vedic texts as *soma*.

Persia shared in this therapy as part of a greater ancient Near Eastern and Mediterranean medical culture. The cranial modifications occurred in early childhood, so they may have been initiated by midwives but are likely due to the actions of the families rather than healers. They seem to have held no medical significance even as an apotropaic measure.

The cemetery at Lchashen in Armenia contained the largest number of bodies, with substantial grave goods from the Late Bronze to the Early Iron Age. These burials were then compared to smaller cemeteries throughout the rest of Armenia, dating to the same time frame. This extensive study covers both disease processes and incidents of trauma, with the goal of giving an overall assessment of health for the population around Lchashen.[36]

### Disease

The Armenian skeletons show a number of infections, either bacterial or fungal, that likely were introduced through minor traumas. In particular, a number of serious sinus infections were noted, which likely started from infections in badly worn teeth. Poor nutrition for the population as a whole contributed to the number of people adversely affected by infections. Hansen's disease is also present, which is significantly earlier than its appearance in the Levant or further west, supporting the idea that Alexander the Great's troops originally encountered it in the Iranian Plateau or along the Indus River. No other infectious disease was noted as frequently. When looking at the cemeteries over centuries, they did have periods of increased burials, but this is due to an overall increase in the population at those times, as opposed to a sudden epidemic.

### Trauma

The majority of skeletal remains from Armenia exhibiting signs of trauma indicate that most of the wounds came from interpersonal confrontations rather than warfare. Paleo-osteologists came to this conclusion based on the higher rate of blunt force causing the trauma and the small area of the body affected, as well as signs of medical intervention. Trauma from war-

36. Anahit Khudaverdyan, "Pattern of Disease in 2nd-1st Millennium BC Necropolis from Lchashen, Armenia," *Anthropologie* 48 (2010): 239–54.

fare would not only have a higher incidence of edged-weapon use but also affect a larger part of the body and cause a more rapid death, not allowing for medical intervention. Another ubiquitous type of injury comes from repetitive use, such as worn dentition and jaw fractures in women who used their mouths as a work tool. This seems to dovetail with the higher rate of sinus infections from worn teeth.

## Disability

According to the *Yasht*,[37] certain disabilities can carry pollution; thus, the afflicted cannot be part of the sacrifices: someone with fever, fat, pimples, leprosy (Hansen's disease as well as general skin disorders), women who do not perform the *gāthās*, the blind, the deaf, the epileptic, men with blocked semen, a whore in menopause, a child, or a virgin. The *Videvdad* prohibits sacrifice by one who drivels, by a deceitful person, or by one with a hump, pustules, crooked or irregular teeth, or blotches or other marks. These marks of Evil were not considered a moral sin; Zoroastrianism does not blame the sufferer, but the afflictions show that the person has a connection to the Evil, although it may have been inadvertent. These signs are just the condition of living in the world that the Hostile Spirit has invaded.

## Conditional States

The ancient Persians did not medicalize the conditional states of puberty, pregnancy, and geriatrics as modern societies do. The onset of puberty was marked by initiation and purification rituals, with no mention of it in the *Avesta* passages focusing on medical issues. In keeping with this, Zoroastrianism holds the belief that fertility is a gift from the god Ahura Mazda.[38] Menses, when following a normal process, is Good, although the blood itself causes impurity. An exception comes in the disruption of menses, such as infertility or a prolonged menstrual cycle, which indicates contamination by the Hostile Spirit or other evil force.

Similarly, pregnancy itself does not necessitate medical intervention for the Persians, although later passages in the *Videvdad* adopted Greek

37. The *Yasht* is a subsection of the *Avesta*.

38. Williams, "Zoroastrianism and the Body," 155–66; Darmesteter, *Zend-Avesta*, lxxix.

philosophical positions on the medical science behind conception and development of the fetus. According to Forrest, priests could not treat women who were menstruating or had any related issues. She then argues that the isolation of women from sacrifices and the rest of the community during menses possibly created a peripheral group of female healers, which would then give rise to ideas about witches.[39] Since priests did not have to treat pregnancy itself as a medical concern, any complications during it would have been addressed by midwives. It would be a natural or logical progression for midwives, thus supporting the claim that a peripheral group of female healers existed and were possibly targeted by the priesthood in certain cultural power struggles. Zoroastrianism considered women who performed abortions with herbs as supporting evil, usually being referred to as an "Old Woman," the term for a sorceress.

Geriatrics also straddled the line between Good and Evil. Zoroastrianism taught that old age was not a polluting condition, but the Hostile Spirit caused the degradation of the body as part of the aging process. Yet it existed, like menses, as a manifestation of Good.

## Healers

As far as existing documents attest, the only indigenous healers recognized by Zoroastrianism and ruling dynasties were the priests. This stems from the tradition that Zarathustra was the first good magician. Ahura Mazda endowed him to combat the Hostile Spirit. Only those from the line of Zarathustra had the ability to properly perform rituals. It is not clear whether this tradition followed a true biological lineage or it just became a way of culturally designating the priestly class. The unclear historicity of Zarathustra reinforces the idea of descent as a cultural marker rather than a true genealogy for the priests.

Zarathustra had asked Ahura Mazda, "Who was the first healer?" not only in terms of sickness but in trauma; the god answered with the name Thrita. He is credited with the first use of herbal medicine, identifying up to ten thousand healing plants that grew around the tree of life.[40] Although given a lineage with the Sama family, Thrita appears to be a mythical personage existing in an "age of heroes." The name has linguistic connections

39. Forrest, *Witches, Whores, and Sorcerers*, 80.
40. Darmesteter, *Zend-Avesta*, 225–26.

with Thraetaona, who appears in Vedic medical texts. Similar to Thraetaona, Thrita is said to have slain the dragon-demon Azi Dahaka, reinforcing his healing character. Additionally, the god Khshathra Vairya revealed the medical uses of the knife to Thrita. Khshathra Vairya is one of the Bounteous Immortals representing good thoughts; thus, he is linked to the power within each person to care for other people. Various gems inscribed with the name Thrita have been found throughout the Iranian Plateau and likely served as medical amulets.

Apart from the mythical beginnings of the priestly tradition of healing through physical and oral rites, little is known of the actual clinical practices of healers in the Iranian Plateau. We do have texts addressing the remuneration of healers, who received payment according to the socioeconomic status of the patient. The most common type of payment was oxen of varying degrees of value. Sheep stood as the lowest form of payment, while a chariot with a team of horses served as the highest fee.[41]

It can be safely assumed that healers typically learned their craft through a form of apprenticeship that taught them all their priestly duties. The *Avesta* advises that, when first learning the medical arts, the healer must practice on non-Zoroastrians. "If he treats with the knife for the third time a worshiper of the *daêvas*[42] and he dies, he is unfit [as a healer] for ever and ever."[43] A clinical division between Zoroastrians and other religious groups appears also in texts advising Zoroastrian healers how to adopt new techniques from other cultures by first practicing it on the nonbelievers.[44] Given the tendency of Persian royalty to hire healers from areas like Greece, a system of adoption that does not tip the scales toward Evil becomes necessary. These practices protect the authority of the Zoroastrians, because the standard of "no bad healers" must be (ideally) maintained within the community. This is important given the connection between health, purity, and the struggle between Good and Evil. Anyone falsely purporting to perform purification/exorcism can be beheaded since these actions actually promote illness by promoting Lies.

41. Darmesteter, *Zend-Avesta*, 86–87.

42. An Avestan term for "false gods," a way of designating non-Zoroastrians.

43. Darmesteter, *Zend-Avesta*, 85.

44. Adhami, "Two Pahlavi Chapters on Medicine," 331–51.

# *Bibliography*


Abusch, Tzvi. "Witchcraft Literature in Mesopotamia." In *The Babylonian World*, edited by Gwendolyn Leick, 373–85. New York: Routledge, 2007.

———. *The Witchcraft Series Maqlû*. Atlanta: Society of Biblical Literature, 2015.

Adams, Francis, trans. *The Medical Works of Paulus Aegineta*. London: Sydenham Society, 1861.

Adams, Winthrop Lindsay. "The Hellenistic Kingdoms." In *The Cambridge Companion to the Hellenistic World*, edited by Glenn R. Bugh, 28–51. Cambridge: Cambridge University Press, 2006.

Adamson, P. B. "Human Diseases and Deaths in the Ancient Near East." *Die Welt Des Orients* 13 (1982): 5–14.

Adhami, Siamak. "Two Pahlavi Chapters on Medicine." *Early Science and Medicine* 16 (2011): 331–51.

Andorlini, Isabella, ed. *Greek Medical Papyri I*. Firennze: Instituto Papirologico, 2001.

———. *Greek Medical Papyri II*. Firenze: Istituto Papirologico, 2009.

Aparaschivei, Dan. "Healthcare in the Roman Province of Moesia Inferior." *Mankind Quarterly* 53 (2012): 110–29.

Archi, Alfonso. "Kamrusepa and the Sheep of the Sun-God." *Orientalia* 62 (1993): 404–9.

Arda, Berna, and Murat Aksu. "What the Hittites' Tablets Tell Us? A Short Historical View of Deafness on the Basis of Genetics." *Turkish Journal of Medical Sciences* 34 (2004): 357–58.

Arnott, Robert. "Disease and the Prehistory of the Aegean." In *Health in Antiquity*, edited by Helen King, 12–31. London: Routledge, 2005.

Austin, Ann E. "Accounting for Sick Days: A Scalar Approach to Health and Disease at Deir el-Medina." *Journal of Near Eastern Studies* 74 (2015): 75–85.

Avalos, Hector. *Illness and Health Care in the Ancient Near East: The Role of the Temple in Greece, Mesopotamia and Israel*. Atlanta: Scholars Press, 1995.

Avalos, Hector, Sarah J. Melcher, and Jeremy Schipper, eds. *This Abled Body:*

*Rethinking Disabilities in Biblical Studies*. Atlanta: Society of Biblical Literature, 2007.

Bagnall, R. S., and P. Derow, eds. and trans. *The Hellenistic Period: Historical Sources in Translation*. Malden, MA: Blackwell, 2004.

Bahrani, Zainab. "The Babylonian Visual Image." In *The Babylonian World*, edited by Gwendolyn Leick, 155–70. New York: Routledge, 2007.

———. *The Graven Image: Representation in Babylon and Assyria*. Philadelphia: University of Pennsylvania Press, 2003.

Baker, Patricia A. *The Archaeology of Medicine in the Greco-Roman World*. Cambridge: Cambridge University Press, 2013.

Baker, Patricia A., Han Nijdam, and Karine van 't Land, eds. *Medicine and Space: Body, Surroundings, and Borders in Antiquity and the Middle Ages*. Leiden: Brill, 2011.

Balberg, Mira, and Moulie Vidas. "Impure Scholasticism: The Study of Purity Laws and Rabbinic Self." *Prooftexts* 32 (2012): 312–56.

Battini, Laura, and Pierre Villard, eds. *Médecine et médicins au Proche-Orient ancien*. Oxford: British Archaeological Reports, 2006.

Beckman, Gary. "From the Cradle to the Grave: Women's Role in Hittite Medicine and Magic." *Journal of Ancient Civilizations* 8 (1993): 25–39.

———. "Hittite Religion." In *Cambridge History of Religions in the Ancient World*, edited by Michele Renee Salzman, 85–101. Cambridge: Cambridge University Press, 2012.

Belser, Julia Watts. "Disability, Animality, and Enslavement in Rabbinic Narratives of Bodily Restoration and Resurrection." *Journal of Late Antiquity* 8 (2015): 288–305.

Betz, Hans Dieter, ed. *The Greek Magical Papryi in Translation, Including the Demotic Spells*. 2nd ed. Chicago: University of Chicago Press, 1992.

Biggs, Robert D. "The Human Body and Sexuality in the Babylonian Medical Texts." In *Médecine et médecins au Proche-Orient ancient*, 39–52. Oxford: British Archaeological Reports, 2006.

Böck, Barbara. *The Healing Goddess Gula: Towards an Understanding of Ancient Babylonian Medicine*. Boston: Brill, 2014.

Boorse, Christopher. "Health as a Theoretical Concept." *Philosophy of Science* 44 (1977): 555.

Borghouts, J. F. "Witchcraft, Magic, and Divination in Ancient Egypt." In *Civilizations of the Ancient Near East*, edited by Jack Sasson, 1783–84. Peabody, MA: Hendrickson, 2000.

Bottéro, Jean. "Magic and Medicine." In *Everyday Life in Ancient Mesopotamia*,

edited by Jean Bottéro, 162–82. Baltimore: Johns Hopkins University Press, 1992.
———. *Mesopotamia: Writing, Reasoning, and the Gods*. Chicago: University of Chicago Press, 1992.
Boyarin, Daniel. "Hellenism in Jewish Babylonia." In *The Cambridge Companion to the Talmud and Rabbinic Literature*, edited by Charlotte Elisheva Fonrobert and Martin S. Jaffee, 336–64. Cambridge: Cambridge University Press, 2007.
Boyle, Marjorie O'Rourke. "The Law of the Heart: The Death of a Fool (1 Samuel 25)." *Journal of Biblical Literature* 120 (2001): 401–27.
Bradley, Mark. "Obesity, Corpulence and Emaciation in Roman Art." *Papers of the British School at Rome* 79 (2011): 1–41.
Brain, Peter. *Galen on Bloodletting: A Study of the Origins, Development, and Validity of His Opinions, with a Translation of the Three Works*. Cambridge: Cambridge University Press, 1986.
Breasted, James Henry. *The Edwin Smith Surgical Papyrus*. Chicago: University of Chicago Press, 1991.
Brothwell, Don R., and A. T. Sandison, eds. *Diseases in Antiquity: A Survey of Disease, Injuries, and Surgeries of Early Populations*. Springfield: C. C. Thomas, 1967.
Bryce, Trevor. *Life and Society in the Hittite World*. Oxford: Oxford University Press, 2004.
Bugh, Glenn R., ed. *The Cambridge Companion to the Hellenistic World*. Cambridge: Cambridge University Press, 2006.
Bynum, William. *A History of Medicine*. Oxford: Oxford University Press, 2008.
Campbell, Ian. "The 'Minerva Medica' and the Schola Medicorum: Pirro Ligorio and Roman Toponymy." *Papers of the British School of Rome* 79 (2011): 299–328.
Canby, Jeanny Vorys. "Hittite Art." *Biblical Archaeologist* 52 (1989): 109–29.
Carella, Michael Jerome. *Matter, Morals, and Medicine: The Ancient Greek Origins of Science, Ethics, and the Medical Profession*. New York: Peter Lang, 1991.
Carr, Gillian. "A Time to Live, a Time to Heal, and a Time to Die: Healing and Divination in Later Iron Age and Early Roman Britain." In *Practitioners, Practices and Patients: New Approaches to Medical Archaeology and Anthropology*, 58–73. Oxford: Oxbow, 2002.
Carrick, Paul J. *Medical Ethics in the Ancient World*. Washington, DC: Georgetown University Press, 2001.
Cathcart, Kevin J. "The Phoenician Inscriptions from Arslan Tash and Some Old Testament Texts." In *On Stone and Scroll: Essays in Honour of Graham Ivor*

*Davies*, edited by James K. Aitken, Katharine J. Dell, and Brain A. Mastin, 87–99. Boston: de Gruyter, 2011.

Charney, Leon H., and Saul Mayzlish. *Battle of the Two Talmuds: Judaism's Struggle with Power, Glory, & Guilt*. Fort Lee, NJ: Barricade, 2010.

Cherpion, Nadine. "The Human Image in Old Kingdom Non-Royal Reliefs." In *Egyptian Art in the Age of the Pyramids*, 103–15. New York: Metropolitan Museum of Art, 1999.

Ciaraldi, Marina. "Drug Preparation in Evidence? An Unusual Plant and Bone Assemblage from the Pompeian Countryside, Italy." *Vegetation History and Archaeobotany* 9 (2000): 91–98.

Cohen, Chaim, and Daniel Sivan. *The Ugaritic Hippiatric Texts: A Critical Edition*. New Haven: American Oriental Society, 1983.

Cokayne, Karen. *Experiencing Old Age in Ancient Rome*. New York: Routledge, 2003.

Cole, Steven W., Peter Machinist, and Simo Parpola, eds. *Letters from Priests to the Kings Esarhaddon and Assurbanipal*. State Archives of Assyria. Helsinki: Helsinki University Press, 1998.

Collins, Terence. "The Physiology of Tears in the Old Testament." *Catholic Biblical Quarterly* 33 (1971): 18–38, 185–97.

Collins, Timothy. "Natural Illness in Babylonian Medical Incantations." PhD diss., University of Chicago, 1999.

Collon, Dominique. "Neo-Assyrian Gula in the British Museum." In *Beschreiben und Deuten in der Archäologie des Alten Orients: Feschrift für Ruth Mayer-Opificius*, edited by M. Dietrich and O. Loretz, 43–48. Münster: Ugarit, 1994.

Compton, Michael T. "The Association of Hygieia with Asklepios in Graeco-Roman Asklepieion Medicine." *Journal of the History of Medicine and Allied Sciences* 57 (2002): 312–29.

Coogan, Michael David. *Stories from Ancient Canaan*. Louisville: Westminster John Knox, 2012.

Craik, E. M. "Dogmatism, Medical." In *The Encyclopedia of Ancient History*, edited by Roger S. Bagnall, Kai Brodersen, Craige B. Champion, Andrew Erskine, and Sabine R. Huebner. London: Blackwell, 2013.

Cronier, Marie. "Diocles of Karystos." In *The Encyclopedia of Ancient History*, edited by Roger S. Bagnall, Kai Brodersen, Craige B. Champion, Andrew Erskine, and Sabine R. Huebner. London: Blackwell, 2013.

Cruse, Audrey. *Roman Medicine*. Gloucestershire: Tempus, 2004.

Dalley, S., C. B. F. Walker, and J. D. Hawkins, eds. *The Old Babylonian Tablets from Tell al Rimah*. London: British School of Archaeology in Iraq, 1976.

Dalley, Stephanie. "Evolution of Gender in Mesopotamian Mythology and

Iconography with a Possible Explanation of ša rēšēn, 'The Man with Two Heads.'" In *Sex and Gender in the Ancient Near East*, edited by S. Parpola and R. M. Whiting, 117–22. Helsinki: The Neo-Assyrian Text Corpus Project, 2002.

———. *Myths from Mesopotamia*. New York: Oxford University Press, 2008.

Darmesteter, James. *The Zend-Avesta: The Vendîdâd*. Oxford: Clarendon, 1895.

Deacy, Susan. "'Famous Athens, Divine Polis': The Religious System at Athens." In *A Companion to Greek Religion*, edited by Daniel Ogden, 221–35. London: Blackwell, 2007.

Debru, Armelle. "Physiology." In *The Cambridge Companion to Galen*, edited by R. J. Hankinson, 263–82. Cambridge: Cambridge University Press, 2008.

Deines, H. von, and W. Westerndorf, eds. *Worterbuch der medizinischen Texte, Erste Halfte*. Grundiss der Medizin der altem Ägypter. Berlin: Akademie-Verlag, 1961.

Depauw, Mark. "Notes on Transgressing Gender Boundaries in Ancient Egypt." *Zeitschrift für Ägyptische Sprache und Altertumskunde* 130 (2003): 49–59.

Dietrich, M., and O. Loretz. "Baal RPU in KTU 1.108, 1.113 und Nach 1.17 VI 25–33." *Ugarit-Forschungen* 12 (1980): 171–82.

Dillon, M. P. J. "The Didactic Nature of the Epidaurian Iamata." *Zeitschrift für Papyrologie und Epigraphik* 101 (1994): 239–60.

Disler, Caroline. "Oxyrhynchus 1381." *Target: International Journal of Translation Studies* 24 (2012): 225–52.

Douglas, Mary. *Purity and Danger: An Analysis of the Concepts of Pollution and Taboo*. London: Routledge, 2002.

Draycott, Jane. *Approaches to Healing in Roman Egypt*. BAR International Series. Oxford: Archaeopress, 2012.

———. "Reconstructing the Lived Experience of Disability in Antiquity: A Case Study from Roman Egypt." *Greece & Rome* 62 (2015): 189–205.

Ebbell, B. *The Ebers Papyrus*. Copenhagen: Levin and Munksgaard, 1937.

Ebeling, Erich. *Keilschrifttexte medizinischen Inhalts*. Berlin: Selbstverlag, 1916–1923.

Edelstein, E. J., and L. Edelstein. *Asclepius: A Collection and Interpretation of the Testimonies I–II*. Baltimore: Johns Hopkins University Press, 1998.

Edelstein, Ludwig. *Ancient Medicine: Selected Papers of Ludwig Edelstein*. Edited by Oswei Temkin and C. Lilian Temkin. Baltimore: Johns Hopkins University Press, 1967.

Eijk, Philip J. van der. *Diocles of Carystus: A Collection of Fragments with Translation and Commentary*. Boston: Brill, 2000.

———. "Therapeutics." In *The Cambridge Companion to Galen*, edited by R. J. Hankinson, 283–303. Cambridge: Cambridge University Press, 2008.

Ekroth, Gunnel. "Heroes and Hero-Cults." In *A Companion to Greek Religion*, edited by Daniel Ogden, 100–114. London: Blackwell, 2007.

Elgood, Cyril. *A Medical History of Persia and the Eastern Caliphate from the Earliest Times to the Year A.D. 1932*. Cambridge: Cambridge University Press, 1951.

Erskine, Andrew, ed. *A Companion to the Hellenistic World*. Oxford: Blackwell, 2003.

Estes, J. Worth. *The Medical Skills of Ancient Egypt*. Canton, MA: Science History, 1993.

Faulkner, Raymond O., trans. *The Ancient Egyptian Book of the Dead*. London: British Museum, 1985.

Feder, Yitzhaq. "Defilement, Disgust, and Disease: The Experiential Basis of Hittite and Akkadian Terms for Impurity." *Journal of the American Oriental Society* 136 (2016): 99–116.

Ferngren, Gary B. *Medicine and Health Care in Early Christianity*. Baltimore: Johns Hopkins University Press, 2009.

Ferngren, Gary B., and Ekaterina N. Lomperis. *Essential Readings in Medicine and Religion*. Baltimore: Johns Hopkins University Press, 2017.

Fitzmyer, Joseph A. "The Aramaic Inscriptions of Sefire I and II." *Journal of American Oriental Society* 81 (1961): 178–222.

Flemming, Rebecca. *Medicine and the Making of Roman Women*. Oxford: Oxford University Press, 2000.

Forrest, S. K. Mendoza. "Empires of Knowledge: Medicine and Health in the Hellenistic World." In *A Companion to the Hellenistic World*, edited by Andrew Erskine, 449–63. Oxford: Blackwell, 2003.

———. *Witches, Whores, and Sorcerers: The Concept of Evil in Early Iran*. Austin: University of Texas Press, 2011.

Foster, Benjamin. *The Epic of Gilgamesh*. New York: W. W. Norton, 2001.

———. *Before the Muses: An Anthology of Akkadian Literature*. Bethesda: CDL, 2005.

Fredrick, David, ed. *The Roman Gaze: Vision, Power, and the Body*. Baltimore: Johns Hopkins University Press, 2002.

Friedman, R. E. *Who Wrote the Bible?* New York: Harper Collins, 1987.

Garland, Robert. "Disability." In *The Encyclopedia of Ancient History*, edited by Roger S. Bagnall, 2156–57. London: Blackwell, 2013.

———. *The Eye of the Beholder: Deformity and Disability in the Graeco-Roman World*. London: Bristol Classical, 2010.

Gasperetti, Matthew Alexander, and Susan G. Sheridan. "Cry Havoc: Interpersonal Violence at Early Bronze Age Bab Edh-Dhra." *American Anthropologist* 115 (2013): 388–410.

Gaster, Theodore H. "The Magical Inscription from Arslan Tash." *Journal of Near Eastern Studies* 6 (1947): 186–88.

Geller, Markham J. *Ancient Babylonian Medicine Theory and Practice*. Oxford: Wiley-Blackwell, 2010.

———. *Babylonisch-assyrische Medizin: Renal and Rectal Disease Texts*. Berlin: de Gruyter, 2005.

———. "Bloodletting in Babylonia." In *Magic and Rationality in Ancient Near Eastern and Greco-Roman Medicine*, edited by John Scarborough, Philip J. vander Eijk, Ann Hanson, and Nancy Siraisi, 305–24. Boston: Brill, 2004.

Genz, Hermann, and Dirk Paul Mielke. "Research on the Hittites: A Short Overview." In *Insights into Hittite History and Archaeology*, edited by Hermann Genz and Dirk Paul Mielke, 1–29. Walpole, MA: Peeters, 2011.

Ghalioungui, Paul. *The Physicians of Pharaonic Egypt*. Cairo: Al-Ahram Center for Scientific Translations, 1983.

Gibson, Craig A. "Doctors in Ancient Greek and Roman Rhetorical Education." *Journal of the History of Medicine and Allied Sciences* 68 (2013): 529–50.

Gilfillan, S. C. "Lead Poisoning and the Fall of Rome." *Journal of Occupational Medicine* 7 (1965): 53–60.

Giusfredi, Federico. "The Akkadian Medical Text KUB 37.1." *Altorientalische Forschungen* 39 (2012): 49–63.

Glueck, Nelson. *Exploration in Eastern Palestine II*. New Haven: American Schools of Oriental Research, 1935.

Goebs, Katja. "Kingship." In *The Egyptian World*, edited by Toby Wilkinson, 275–95. New York: Routledge, 2010.

Good, Byron J. *Medicine, Rationality, and Experience: An Anthropological Perspective*. Cambridge: Cambridge University Press, 1994.

Gorteman, Claire. "Médecins de cour dans l'Égypte du IIIe siècle avant J.-C." *Chronique d'Égypte* 32 (1957): 313–36.

Graumann, Luts Alexander. "Monstrous Births and Retrospective Diagnosis: The Case of the Hermaphrodites in Antiquity." In *Disabilities in Roman Antiquity: Disparate Bodies* a Capite ad Calcem, edited by Christian Laes, C. F. Goodey, and M. Lynn Rose, 181–209. Boston: Brill, 2013.

Gray, Kimberly Calnan. "The Health Status of Bronze Age Greek Women." *American Journal of Archaeology* 98 (1994): 340.

Griffith, F. Ll., and Herbert Thompson, eds. *The Leyden Papyrus: An Egyptian Magical Book*. New York: Dover, 1974.

Grummond, Nancy Thomson de. *Etruscan Myth, Sacred History, and Legend*. Philadelphia: University of Pennsylvania Museum, 2006.

Grummond, Nancy Thomson de, and Erika Simon, eds. *The Religion of the Etruscans*. Austin: University of Texas Press, 2006.

Gurney, O. R. "The Sultantepe Tablets V: The Tale of the Poor Man of Nippur." *Anatolian Studies* 6 (1956): 145–64.

Gurney, O. R., and J. J. Finkelstein, eds. *The Sultantepe Tablets I*. London: British Institute of Archaeology at Ankara, 1957.

———, eds. *Sultantepe Tablets II*. London: British Institute of Archaeology at Ankara, 1964.

Güterbock, Hans G. "Hittite Medicine." *Bulletin of the History of Medicine* 36 (1962): 109–13.

Haas, Volkert. *Materia Magica et Medica Hethitica*. New York: de Gruyter, 2003.

Halioua, Bruno, and Bernard Ziskind. *Medicine in the Days of the Pharaohs*. Cambridge, MA: Belknap, 2005.

Halivni, David Weiss. *The Formation of the Babylonian Talmud*. Translated by Jeffrey L. Rubenstein. Oxford: Oxford University Press, 2013.

Hallo, William W., and K. Lawson Younger Jr., eds. *The Context of Scripture: Archival Documents*. Boston: Brill, 2003.

———, eds. *The Context of Scripture: Canonical Compositions*. Boston: Brill, 2003.

Hankinson, R. J. "The Man and His Work." In *The Cambridge Companion to Galen*, edited by R. J. Hankinson, 1–33. Cambridge: Cambridge University Press, 2008.

Hanson, Ann Ellis. "Greek Medical Papyri from the Fayum Village of Tebtunis: Patient Involvement in a Local Health-Care System?" In *Hippocrates in Context: Papers Read at the XIth International Hippocrates Colloquium*, edited by Philip J. van der Eijk, 387–402. Leiden: Brill, 2005.

Harris, William V., ed. *Mental Disorders in the Classical World*. Leiden: Brill, 2013.

———, ed. *Popular Medicine in Graeco-Roman Antiquity: Explorations*. Leiden: Brill, 2016.

Haynes, Sybille. *Etruscan Civilization: A Cultural History*. Los Angeles: J. Paul Getty Museum, 2000.

Heeßel, Nils P. *Babylonisch-assyrische Diagnostik*. Alter Orient und Altes Testament. Münster: Ugarit-Verlag, 2000.

———. "The Babylonian Physician Rabâ-Ša-Marduk: Another Look at Physicians and Exorcists in the Ancient Near East." In *Advances in Mesopotamian*

*Medicine from Hammurabi to Hippocrates*, edited by Annie Attia, Gilles Buisson, and Markham J. Geller, 13–28. Boston: Brill, 2009.

Helman, Cecil G. *Culture, Health, and Illness*. Boston: Butterworth Heinemann, 2000.

Henrichs, Albert. "What Is a Greek God?" In *The Gods of Ancient Greece: Identities and Transformations*, edited by Jan N. Bremmer and Andrew Erskine, 19–39. Edinburgh: Edinburgh University Press, 2010.

Hesiod. *Theogony and Works and Days*. Translated by M. L. West. Oxford: Oxford University Press, 1988.

Hezser, Catherine. "Representations of the Physician in Jewish Literature from Hellenistic and Roman Times." In *Popular Medicine in Graeco-Roman Antiquity*, edited by William V. Harris, 173–97. Leiden: Brill, 2016.

Hirschberger, Martina. *Gynaikôn Katalogos und Megalai Ehoiai: Ein Kommentar zu den Fragmenten zweier hesiodeischer*. Boston: de Gruyter, 2004.

Hoffner, Harry A. *Hittitte Myths*. Atlanta: Scholars Press, 1998.

———. "Paskuwatti's Ritual against Sexual Impotence." *Aula Orientalis* 5 (1987): 271–87.

Horstmanshoff, Manfred, Helen King, and Claus Zittel, eds. *Blood, Sweat, and Tears: Changing Concepts of Physiology*. Leiden: Brill, 2012.

Hughes, Jessica. "Fragmentation as Metaphor in the Classical Healing Sanctuary." *Social History of Medicine* 21 (2008): 217–36.

Israelowich, Ido. *Society, Medicine and Religion in the Sacred Tales of Aelius Aristides*. Boston: Brill, 2012.

Jackson, R. P. J. "Roman Medicine: The Practitioners and Their Practices." *ANRW* 37.1:79–101. Part 2, *Principat*, 37.1. Edited by H. Temporini and W. Haase. New York: de Gruyter, 1993.

Jackson, Ralph. "An Ancient British Medical Kit from Stanway, Essex." *The Lancet* 350 (1997): 1471–73.

———. "A Set of Roman Medical Instruments from Italy." *Britannia* 17 (1986): 119–67.

Jacob, Irene, and Walter Jacob. *The Healing Past: Pharmaceuticals in the Biblical and Rabbinic World*. Leiden: Brill, 1993.

Jacobsen, Thorkild. "Mesopotamia." In *The Intellectual Adventure of Ancient Man*, edited by Henri Frankfort, H. A. Frankfort, John A. Wilson, Jacobsen Thorkild, and William A. Irwin, 125–219. Chicago: University of Chicago Press, 1977.

Jannot, Jean-René. *Religion in Ancient Etruria*. Madison: University of Wisconsin Press, 2005.

Janowski, Bernd, and D. Schwemer. *Texte aus der Umwelt des Alten Testaments.* Gütersloh: Gütersloh Verlagshaus, 2011.
Jouanna, Jacques. *Greek Medicine from Hippocrates to Galen.* Boston: Brill, 2012.
———. *Hippocrates.* Translated by M. B. DeBevoise. Baltimore: Johns Hopkins University Press, 1999.
Kalmin, Richard. *Jewish Babylonia Between Persia and Roman Palestine: Decoding the Literary Record.* Oxford: Oxford University Press, 2006.
Kapparis, Konstantinos A. *Abortion in the Ancient World.* London: Duckworth Academic, 2002.
Keyser, Paul T., and Georgia Irby-Massie. "Science, Medicine, and Technology." In *The Cambridge Companion to the Hellenistic World*, edited by Glenn R. Bugh, 241–64. Cambridge: Cambridge University Press, 2006.
Khudaverdyan, Anahit. "Pattern of Disease in 2nd-1st Millennium BC Necropolis from Lchashen, Armenia." *Anthropologie* 48 (2010): 239–54.
King, Helen. *Health in Antiquity.* New York: Routledge, 2005.
Kinnier Wilson, J. V. "Two Medical Texts from Nimrud." *Iraq* 18 (1956): 130–46.
Kleinman, Arthur. *Patients and Healers in the Context of Culture.* Berkeley: University of California Press, 1980.
Knoll, K. L. "Canaanite Religion." *Religion Compass* 1 (2007): 61–92.
Kotsonas, Antonis. "Phoenicia." In *The Encyclopedia of Ancient History*, edited by Roger S. Bagnall, Kai Brodersen, Craige B. Champion, Andrew Erskine, and Sabine R. Huebner. Oxford: Wiley-Blackwell, 2012.
Kottek, Samuel. "Amra Li Em: La Transmission de la Médecine Populaire par les Femmes dans le Talmud." *Revue des études juives* 169 (2010): 419–37.
———. "The Essenes and Medicine: A Comparative Study of Medical and Para-Medical Items with Reference to Ancient Jewish Lore." *Clio Medica* 18 (1983): 81–99.
———. "Hygiene and Healing among the Jews in the Post-Biblical Period: A Partial Reconstruction." *ANRW* 37.3:2843–65. Part 2, *Principat*, 37.3. Edited by H. Temporini and W. Haase. New York: de Gruyter, 1996.
Köcher, Franz. *Babylonisch-assyrische Medizin in Texten und Untersuchungen.* Berlin: de Gruyter, 1963–1980.
Kotzé, Zacharias. "Humoral Theory as Motivation for Anger Metaphors in the Hebrew Bible." *Southern African Linguistics and Applied Language Studies* 23 (2005): 205–9.
Kreyenbroek, Philip G. "Zoroastrianism under the Achaemenians: A Non-Essentialist Approach." In *The World of Achaemenid Persia: History, Art, and Society in Iran and the Ancient Near East*, edited by John Curtis and St John Simpson, 103–9. London: I. B. Tauris, 2010.

Küchler, Friedrich. *Beitrage zur Kenntnis der assyrisch-babylonischen Medizin.* Leipzig: J. C. Hinrichs, 1904.

Kühn, Karl Gottlob, ed. and trans. *Opera Omnia.* Leipzig: C. Cnobloch, 1821–1833.

Künzl, E. "Aesculapius in the Valetudinarium, or: The Hitherto Existing Interpretation of Roman Military Hospital Is Furthermore Valid." *Würzburger Medizinhistoriche Mitteilungen* 24 (2005): 99–109.

Labat, René. *Traité akkadien de diagnostics et prognostics médicaux.* Paris: Académie internationale d'histoire de sciences, 1951.

Laes, Christian. "Silent Witness: Deaf-Mutes in Graeco-Roman Antiquity." *Classical World* 104 (2011): 451–73.

Laes, Christian, C. F. Goodey, and M. Lynn Rose. "Approaching Disabilities *a Capite ad Calcem*: Hidden Themes in Roman Antiquity." In *Disabilities in Roman Antiquity: Disparate Bodies* a Capite ad Calcem, edited by Christian Laes, C. F. Goodey, and M. Lynn Rose, 1–15. Boston: Brill, 2013.

Lajtar, Adam. *Deir El-Bahari in the Hellenistic and Roman Periods: A Study of an Egyptian Temple Based on Greek Sources.* Warsaw: Institute of Archaeology, Warsaw University, 2006.

Lambert, W. G. "The Gula Hymn of Bullutsa-Rabi." *Orientalia* 36 (1967): 105–32.

Lang, Philippa. *Medicine and Society in Ptolemaic Egypt.* Boston: Brill, 2013.

Langslow, David, and Brigitte Maire, eds. *Body, Disease, and Treatment in a Changing World.* Lausanne: BHMS, 2010.

Larsen, Mogens Trolle. *Ancient Kanesh: A Merchant Colony in Bronze Age Anatolia.* Cambridge: Cambridge University Press, 2015.

Larson, Jennifer. *Ancient Greek Cults: A Guide.* London: Routledge, 2007.

Le Bay, Frédéric. "Pneumatism in Seneca: An Example of Interaction between Physics and Medicine." In *"Greek" and "Roman" in Latin Medical Texts: Studies in Cultural Change and Exchange in Ancient Medicine*, edited by Brigitte Maire, 63–76. Boston: Brill, 2014.

Leftwich, Gregory V. "Polykleitos and Hippokratic Medicine." In *Polykleitos, the Doryphoros, and Tradition*, edited by Warren G. Moon, 38–51. Madison: University of Wisconsin Press, 1995.

Letts, Melinda. "Rufus of Ephesus and the Patient's Perspective in Medicine." *British Journal for the History of Philosophy* 22 (2014): 996–1020.

Levin, S. S. "Eshmun, Healing of God of Sidon." *Adler Museum Bulletin* Special Issue (1983): 39–42.

Lewis, Naphtali. "The Romanity of Roman Egypt: A Growing Consensus." In *On Government and Law: Collected Essays of Naphtali Lewis*, 298–305. Atlanta: American Society of Papyrologists, 1995.

Lewis, Theodore J. "'Athtartu's Incantations and the Use of Divine Names as Weapons." *Journal of Near Eastern Studies* 70 (2011): 207–27.

———. "The Shaʿtiqatu Narrative from the Ugaritic Story about the Healing of King Kirta." *Journal of Ancient Near Eastern Religions* 13 (2013): 188–211.

Livingstone, A. "The Isin 'Dog House' Revisited." *Journal of Cuneiform Studies* 40 (1988): 54–60.

Lloyd, G. E. R. *Greek Science after Aristotle*. New York: W. W. Norton, 1973.

Longrigg, James. *Greek Rational Medicine: Philosophy and Medicine from Alcmaeon to the Alexandrians*. London: Routledge, 1993.

Löwisch, Ingeborg. *Trauma Begets Genealogy: Gender and Memory in Chronicles*. Sheffield: Sheffield Phoenix, 2015.

Majno, Guido. *The Healing Hand: Man and Wound in the Ancient World*. Cambridge, MA: Harvard University Press, 1975.

Manley, Bill. "Anaximander of Miletos." In *The Encyclopedia of Ancient History*, edited by Roger S. Bagnall, Kai Brodersen, Craige B. Champion, Andrew Erskine, and Sabine R. Huebner. London: Blackwell, 2013.

Marganne, Marie-Hélène. *La chirurgie dans l'Égypte Gréco-Romaine d'après les papyrus littéraires Grecs*. Boston: Brill, 1998.

Marganne, Marie-Hélène, and Magali de Haro Sanchez. "At the Crossroads of Greek and Roman Medicine: The Contribution of Latin Papyri 1. Medical Texts; 2. Iatromagical Papyri." In *"Greek" and "Roman" in Latin Medical Texts: Studies in Cultural Change and Exchange in Ancient Medicine*, edited by Brigitte Maire, 92–116. Boston: Brill, 2014.

Marino, Katherine R. "Setting the Womb in Its Place: Toward a Contextual Archaeology of Graeco-Egyptian Uterine Amulets." PhD diss., Brown University, 2010.

Markoe, Glenn E. "The Emergence of Phoenician Art." *Bulletin of the American Schools of Oriental Research* 279 (1990): 13–26.

Martin, Geoffrey T. *The Sacred Animal Necropolis at Saqqâra: The Southern Dependencies of the Main Temple Complex*. London: Egyptian Exploration Society, 1981.

Mattern, Susan P. *Galen and the Rhetoric of Healing*. Baltimore: Johns Hopkins University Press, 2008.

———. *The Prince of Medicine: Galen in the Roman Empire*. Oxford: Oxford University Press, 2013.

May, Margaret Tallmadge. *Galen on the Usefulness of the Parts of the Body*. Ithaca, NY: Cornell University Press, 1968.

McCaffrey, Kathleen. "Reconsidering Gender Ambiguity in Mesopotamia: Is a Beard Just a Beard?" In *Sex and Gender in the Ancient Near East*, edited by

Simo Parpola and R. M. Whiting, 379–91. Helsinki: The Neo-Assyrian Text Corpus Project, 2002.

Meier, G. *Die assyrische Beschwörungssammlung Maqlû*. Berlin: AfO Beiheft, 1937.

Melcher, Sarah J., Mikeal C. Parsons, and Amos Young. *The Bible and Disability: A Commentary*. Waco: Baylor University Press, 2017.

Melfi, Milena. "Lost Sculptures from the Asklepieion of Lebena." *Creta Antica* 10 (2009): 607–18.

Michaelids, Demetrios, ed. *Medicine and Healing in the Ancient Mediterranean World*. Philadelphia: Oxbow, 2014.

Mikalson, Jon D. "Greek Religion: Continuity and Change in the Hellenistic Period." In *The Cambridge Companion to the Hellenistic World*, edited by Glenn R. Bugh, 208–22. Cambridge: Cambridge University Press, 2006.

Milgrom, Jacob. *Leviticus 1–16: A New Translation with Introduction and Commentary*. New York: Doubleday, 1991. Repr., New Haven: Yale University Press, 2009.

Milne, J. Grafton. "The Sanatorium of Dêr el-Baḥri." *Journal of Egyptian Archaeology* 1 (1914): 96–98.

Mitchell, Alexandre G. "Disparate Bodies in Ancient Artefacts: The Function of Caricature and Pathological Grotesques among Roman Terracotta Figurines." In *Disabilities in Roman Antiquity: Disparate Bodies* a Capite ad Calcem, edited by Christian Laes, C. F. Goodey, and M. Lynn Rose, 275–97. Boston: Brill, 2013.

Mitchell-Boyask, Robin. *Plague and the Athenian Imagination: Drama, History, and the Cult of Asclepius*. Cambridge: Cambridge University Press, 2008.

Moran, William L., ed. and trans. *The Amarna Letters*. Baltimore: Johns Hopkins University Press, 1992.

Moss, Candida R., and Joel S. Baden. *Reconceiving Infertility*. Princeton: Princeton University Press, 2015.

Münnich, Maciej. "The Cult of Bronze Serpents in Ancient Canaan and Israel." In *IGGUD: Selected Essays in Jewish Studies, Volume 1: The Bible and Its World, Rabbinic Literature and Jewish Thought, and Jewish Law*, edited by Baruch J. Schwartz, Abraham Melamed, and Aharon Shemesh, 39–56. Jerusalem: World Union of Jewish Studies, 2008.

Nerlich, Andreas G., Albert Zink, Ulrike Szeimies, and Hjalmar G. Hagedorn. "Ancient Egyptian Prosthesis for the Big Toe." *Lancet* 356 (2000): 2176–79.

Newmyer, Stephen. "Talmudic Medicine and Greek Sources." *Ḳorot* 9 (1985): 34–57.

———. "Talmudic Medicine and Greco-Roman Science: Crosscurrents and

Resistance." *ANRW* 37.3:2895–911. Part 2, *Principat*, 37.3. Edited by H. Temporini and W. Haase. New York: de Gruyter, 1996.

Nijhuis, Karin. "Greek Doctors and Roman Patients: A Medical Anthropological Approach." In *Ancient Medicine in Its Socio-Cultural Context*, edited by Philip van der Eijk, H. F. J. Horstmanshoff, and P. H. Schrijvers, 49–67. Atlanta: Rodopi, 1995.

Nunn, John. *Ancient Egyptian Medicine*. Norman: University of Oklahoma Press, 1996.

Nutton, Vivian. *Ancient Medicine*. 2nd ed. New York: Routledge, 2013.

———. "The Medical Meeting Place." In *Ancient Medicine in Its Socio-Cultural Context*, edited by Philip J. van der Eijk, H. F. J. Horstmanshoff, and P. H. Schrijvers, 3–25. Atlanta: Rodopi, 1995.

———. "Physiology from Galen to Jacob Bording." In *Blood, Sweat, and Tears: Changing Concepts of Physiology*, edited by Manfred Horstmanshoff, Helen King, and Claus Zittel, 27–40. Leiden: Brill, 2012.

Oberhelman, Steven M. "Melampus." In *The Encyclopedia of Ancient History*, edited by Roger S. Bagnall, Kai Brodersen, Craige B. Champion, Andrew Erskine, and Sabine R. Huebner. London: Blackwell, 2013.

Olyan, Saul M. *Disability in the Hebrew Bible*. Cambridge: Cambridge University Press, 2008.

Ortner, Donald J., and Bruno Frohlich. *The Early Bronze Age I Tombs and Burials of Bâb-Edh-Drhâ', Jordan*. Lanham, MD: AltaMira, 2008.

Ozturk, S. "Description of Painful Neuropathy in Hittite Tablets." *European Journal of Neurology* 13 (2006): 139.

Papagrigorakis, Manolis, Christos Yapijakis, Philippos N. Synodinos, and Effie Baziotopoulou-Valavani. "DNA Examination of Ancient Dental Pulp Incriminates Typhoid Fever as the Probable Cause of the Ancient Plague of Athens." *International Journal of Infectious Disease* 10 (2006): 206–14.

Parpola, Simo. *Letters from Assyrian Scholars to the Kings Esarhaddon and Assurbanipal*. Winona Lake, IN: Eisenbrauns, 2007.

Peterson, Jane. *Sexual Revolutions: Gender and Labor at the Dawn of Agriculture*. Walnut Creek, CA: AltaMira, 2002.

Petridou, Georgia, and Chiara Thumiger, eds. *Homo Patiens: Approaches to the Patient in the Ancient World*. Leiden: Brill, 2016.

Pfeiffer, Robert. *State Letters of Assyria*. New Haven: American Oriental Society, 1935.

Philip, Tarja S. *Menstruation and Childbirth in the Bible*. New York: Peter Lang, 2006.

Pleket, H. W. "The Social Status of Physicians in the Graeco-Roman World." In

*Ancient Medicine in Its Socio-Cultural Context*, edited by Philip van der Eijk, H. F. J. Horstmanshoff, and P. H. Schrijvers, 27–34. Atlanta: Rodopi, 1995.

Pollard, Elizabeth Ann. "Amulets, Greece and Rome." In *The Encyclopedia of Ancient History*, edited by Roger S. Bagnall, Kai Brodersen, Craige B. Champion, Andrew Erskine, and Sabine R. Huebner, 388–89. London: Blackwell, 2013.

Porter, Roy. *The Greatest Benefit to Mankind: A Medical History of Humanity*. W. W. Norton, 1999.

Preuss, Julius. *Biblical and Talmudic Medicine*. Edited and translated by Fred Rosner. Northvale, NJ: Jason Aronson, 1993.

Pringle, Jackie. "Hittite Birth Rituals." In *Images of Women in Antiquity*, edited by Avril Cameron and Amélie Kuhrt, 128–41. London: Croom Helm, 1983.

Prioreschi, Plinio. *A History of Medicine: Greek Medicine*. Omaha: Horatius, 1996.

Pritchard, James B. *Ancient Near Eastern Texts Relating to the Old Testament*. Princeton: Princeton University Press, 1969.

———. "Atra-Ḫasis." In *Ancient Near Eastern Texts Relating to the Old Testament*, 104–6. Princeton: Princeton University Press, 1969.

———. "The Code of Hammurabi." In *Ancient Near Eastern Texts Relating to the Old Testament*, 163–80. Princeton: Princeton University Press, 1969.

———. "A Cosmological World Incantation: The Worm and the Toothache." In *Ancient Near Eastern Texts Relating to the Old Testament*, 100–101. Princeton: Princeton University Press, 1969.

Quirke, Stephen. *Ancient Egyptian Religion*. New York: Dover, 1997.

Richer, Nicholas. "The Religious System at Sparta." In *A Companion to Greek Religion*, edited by Daniel Ogden, 236–52. London: Blackwell, 2007.

Riddle, John M. *Contraception and Abortion from the Ancient World to the Renaissance*. Cambridge, MA: Harvard University Press, 1992.

———. "High Medicine and Low Medicine in the Roman Empire." *ANRW* 37.1:102–20. Part 2, *Principat*, 37.1. Edited by H. Temporini and W. Haase. New York: de Gruyter, 1993.

Ritner, Robert. "The Famine Stela." In *The Literature of Ancient Egypt*, edited by William Kelly Simpson, 386–91. New Haven: Yale University, 2003.

———. "Magic." In *The Oxford Encyclopedia of Ancient Egypt*, 326. New York: Oxford University Press, 2001.

Rocca, Julius. "Anatomy." In *The Cambridge Companion to Galen*, edited by R. J. Hankinson, 242–62. Cambridge: Cambridge University Press, 2008.

———. "Empiricism, Medical." In *The Encyclopedia of Ancient History*, edited by Roger S. Bagnall, Kai Brodersen, Craige B. Champion, Andrew Erskine, and Sabine R. Huebner. London: Blackwell, 2013.

Roehrig, Catharine. "Reserve Heads: An Enigma of Old Kingdom Sculpture." In *Egyptian Art in the Age of the Pyramids*, 73–81. New York: Metropolitan Museum of Art, 1999.

Rosner, Fred. *Medicine in the Bible and Talmud: Selections from Classical Jewish Sources*. Hoboken: Yeshiva University Press, 1995.

Rowling, J. Thompson. "Hernia in Egypt." In *Diseases in Antiquity*, edited by Don R. Brothwell, A. T. Sandison, and Warren R. Dawson, 444–49. Springfield: Bannerstone House, 1967.

Salazar, Christine F. *The Treatment of War Wounds in Graeco-Roman Antiquity*. Leiden: Brill, 2000.

Sanchez, Gonzalo M., and Edmund S. Meltzer. *The Edwin Smith Papyrus: An Updated Translation of the Trauma Treatise and Modern Medical Commentaries*. Atlanta: Lockwood, 2012.

Sauneron, Serge. *The Priests of Ancient Egypt*. Ithaca: Cornell University Press, 2000.

———. *Une traité égyptien d'ophiologie*. Le Caire: Institut française d'archéologie orientale, 1989.

Scarborough, John. *Roman Medicine*. Ithaca: Cornell University Press, 1969.

———. *Pharmacy and Drug Lore in Antiquity: Greece, Rome, Byzantium*. Burlington: Ashgate, 2010.

Scheid, John. *An Introduction to Roman Religion*. Bloomington: Indiana University Press, 2003.

Schipper, Jeremy. *Disability Studies and the Hebrew Bible: Figuring Mephibosheth in the David Story*. New York: T&T Clark, 2006.

Schmitz, Philip C. "Phoenician-Punic Religion." In *The Cambridge History of Religions in the Ancient World*, edited by Michele Renee Salzman, 205–34. Cambridge: Cambridge University Press, 2013.

Schroer, Silvia, and Thomas Staubli. *Body Symbolism in the Bible*. Collegeville, MN: Liturgical, 2001.

Schwartz, Seth. "The Political Geography of Rabbinic Texts." In *The Cambridge Companion to the Talmud and Rabbinic Literature*, edited by Charlotte Elisheva Fonrobert and Martin S. Jaffee, 75–96. Cambridge: Cambridge University Press, 2007.

Scott, Nora E. "The Metternich Stela." *Metropolitan Museum of Art Bulletin* 9 (1951): 201–17.

Scurlock, JoAnn. *Magico-Medical Means of Treating Ghost-Induced Illnesses in Ancient Mesopotamia*. Boston: Brill, 2006.

———. "Physician, Exorcist, Conjurer, Magician: A Tale of Two Healing Professions." In *Mesopotamian Magic: Textual, Historical, and Interpretative Perspectives*, edited by Tzvi Abusch and Karel van der Toorn, 69–79. Groningen: Styx, 1999.

———. *Sourcebook for Ancient Mesopotamian Medicine*. Atlanta: Society of Biblical Literature, 2014.

Scurlock, JoAnn, and Burton R. Andersen. *Diagnoses in Assyrian and Babylonian Medicine: Ancient Sources, Translations, and Modern Medical Analyses*. Urbana: University of Illinois Press, 2005.

Shephard, Roy J. *An Illustrated History of Health and Fitness from Pre-History to Our Post-Modern World*. New York: Springer, 2014.

Sherwin-White, Susan M. *Ancient Cos: An Historical Study from the Dorian Settlement to the Imperial Period*. Göttingen: Vandenhoeck & Ruprecht, 1978.

Shoja, Mohammadali M., and R. Shane Tubbs. "The History of Anatomy in Persia." *Journal of Anatomy* 210 (2007): 359–78.

Siegel, Rudolph E. *Galen's System of Physiology and Medicine*. New York: S. Karger, 1968.

Simpson, William Kelly, ed. *The Literature of Ancient Egypt: An Anthology of Stories, Instructions, Stelae, Autobiographies, and Poetry*. New Haven: Yale University Press, 2003.

Skehan, Patrick W., and Alexander A. di Lella. *The Wisdom of Ben Sira: A New Translation and Commentary*. Anchor Bible. New York: Doubleday, 1987.

Skjærvø, Prods Oktor. "Avesta and Zoroastrianism under the Achaemenids and Early Sasanians." In *The Oxford Handbook of Ancient Iran*, edited by D. T. Potts, 546–65. Oxford: Oxford University Press, 2013.

———. *Introduction to Zoroastrianism*. 2005. https://sites.fas.harvard.edu/~iranian/Zoroastrianism/Zoroastrianism1_Intro.pdf.

Snowden, Frank M., Jr. *Blacks in Antiquity: Ethiopians in the Greco-Roman Experience*. Cambridge, MA: Belknap, 1970.

Soudavar, Abolala. "The Formation of Achaemenid Imperial Ideology and Its Impact on the Avesta." In *The World of Achaemenid Persian History, Art, and Society in Iran and the Ancient Near East*, edited by John Curtis and St John Simpson, 111–38. London: I. B. Tauris, 2010.

Staden, Heinrich von. "Body and Machine: Interactions between Medicine, Mechanics, and Philosophy in Early Alexandria." In *Alexandria and Alexandrianism*, 85–106. Malibu, CA: J. Paul Getty Museum, 1996.

———. *Herophilus: The Art of Medicine in Early Alexandria*. Cambridge: Cambridge University Press, 2007.

Stedman, Thomas. *Stedman's Medical Dictionary*. 27th ed. Baltimore: Lippincott Williams and Wilkins, 2012.

Steiner, Richard C. *Disembodied Souls: The Nefesh in Israel and Kindred Spirits in the Ancient Near East, with an Appendix on the Katumuwa Inscription*. Atlanta: SBL, 2015.

———. "Northwest Semitic Incantations in an Egyptian Medical Papyrus of the Fourteenth Century B.C.E." *Journal of Near Eastern Studies* 51 (1992): 191–200.

Steuer, R. O. *Aetiological Principle of Pyemia in Ancient Egyptian Medicine*. Baltimore: Johns Hopkins University Press, 1948.

Stol, Marten. *Epilepsy in Babylon*. Groningen: Styx, 1993.

———. *Birth in Babylonia and the Bible: Its Mediterranean Setting*. Groningen: Styx, 2000.

Strathern, Paul. *A Brief History of Medicine*. New York: Carroll & Graf, 2005.

Stucky, Rolf A. *Das Eschmun-Heiligtum von Sidon*. Basel: Vereinigung der Freunde antiker Kunst, 2005.

Taracha, Piotr. "Sculptures of Alacahöyük: A Key to Religious Symbolism in Hittite Representational Art." *Near Eastern Archaeology* 65 (2012): 108–15.

Taub, Liba. "Physiological Analogies and Metaphors in Explanations of the Earth and the Cosmos." In *Blood, Sweat, and Tears: Changing Concepts of Physiology*, edited by Manfred Horstmanshoff, Helen King, and Claus Zittel, 41–64. Leiden: Brill, 2012.

Thomas, Angela. *Anatomical Idiom and Emotional Expression: A Comparison of the Hebrew Bible and the Septuagint*. Sheffield: Sheffield Phoenix, 2014.

Thompson, R. Campbell. "An Assyrian Incantation against Rheumatism." *Proceedings for the Society of Biblical Archaeology* 30 (1908): 63–69, 145–52, 245–51.

———. *Assyrian Medical Texts*. London: Oxford University Press, 1923.

———. "Assyrian Medical Texts." *Proceedings of the Royal Society of Medicine* 17 (1924): 1–34.

———. "Assyrian Medical Texts." *Proceedings of the Royal Society of Medicine* 19 (1926): 29–78.

———. "Assyrian Prescriptions for Diseases of the Head." *American Journal of Semitic Languages and Literatures* 24 (1907): 1–6.

———. "Assyrian Prescriptions for Diseases of the Head." *American Journal of Semitic Languages and Literatures* 24 (1908): 323–53.

———. "Assyrian Prescriptions for the Head." *American Journal of Semitic Languages* 53, no. 4 (1937): 217–38.

———. "Assyrian Prescriptions for the Head." *American Journal of Semitic Languages and Literatures* 54, no. 1 (1937): 12–40.

———. "Assyrian Prescriptions for Treating Bruises or Swellings." *American Journal of Semitic Languages and Literatures* 47 (1930): 1–25.

Tomlin, R. S. O. "'Sede in Tuo Loco': A Fourth-Century Uterine Phylactery in Latin from Roman Britain." *Zeitschrift für Papyrologie und Epigraphik* 115 (1997): 291–94.

Tomlinson, Richard A. *Epidauros*. London: Granada, 1983.

———. "From Houses to Tenements: Domestic Architecture in Hellenistic Alexandria." *British School at Athens Studies* 15 (2007): 307–11.

Toorn, K. van der. *Sin and Sanction in Israel and Mesopotamia*. Maastrich: Van Gorcum, 1985.

Toorn, K. van der, Bob Becking, and Pieter Willem van der Horst, eds. "Resheph." In *Dictionary of Deities and Demons in Bible*. Grand Rapids: Eerdmans, 1999.

Torri, Giulia. "A Hittite Magical Ritual to Be Performed in an Emergency." *Journal of Ancient Near Eastern Religions* 4 (2004): 129–41.

Touwaide, Alain. "Disease, Conceptions of." In *The Encyclopedia of Ancient History*, edited by Roger S. Bagnall, Kai Brodersen, Craige B. Champion, Andrew Erskine, and Sabine R. Huebner. London: Blackwell, 2013.

Trentin, Lisa. "Exploring Visual Impairment in Ancient Rome." In *Disabilities in Roman Antiquity: Disparate Bodies* a Capite ad Calcem, edited by Christian Laes, C. F. Goodey, and M. Lynn Rose, 89–114. Boston: Brill, 2013.

———. *The Hunchback in Hellenistic and Roman Art*. London: Bloomsbury Academic, 2013.

Trevisanato, Siro Igino. "The 'Hittite Plague' an Epidemic of Tularemia and the First Record of Biological Warfare." *Medical Hypotheses* 69 (2007): 1371–74.

Uehlinger, Christoph. "Anthropomorphic Cult Statuary in Iron Age Palestine and the Search for Yahweh's Cult Images." In *The Image and the Book: Iconic Cult, Aniconism, and the Rise of Book Religion in Israel and the Ancient Near East*, edited by Karel van der Toorn, 97–155. Leuven: Peeters, 1997.

Ullinger, Jamie M., Susan G. Sheridan, and Donald J. Ortner. "Daily Activity and Lower Limb Modification at Bab Edh-Dhra', Jordan, in the Early Bronze Age." In *Bioarchaeology and Behavior: The People of the Ancient Near East*, edited by Megan A. Perry, 180–201. Gainesville, FL: University Press of Florida, 2012.

Vallance, John. "The Medical System of Asclepiades of Bithynia." *ANRW* 37.1:693–727. Part 2, *Principat*, 37.1. Edited by H. Temporini and W. Haase. New York: de Gruyter, 1993.

Van De Mieroop, Marc. *A History of the Ancient Near East ca. 3000–323 BC.* Malden, MA: Blackwell, 2007.

Versnel, H. S. *Coping with the Gods: Wayward Readings in Greek Theology*. Boston: Brill, 2011.

Wainwright, Elaine M. *Women Healing/Healing Women: The Genderization of Healing in Early Christianity*. London: Equinox, 2006.

Wente, Edward F., trans. *Letters from Ancient Egypt*. Atlanta: Scholars Press, 1990.

Westendorf, Wolfhardt. "Götter, androgyne." In *Lexikon der Ägyptologie*, edited by Wolfgang Helck and Wolfhardt Westendorf, 634–35. Wiesbaden: Otto Harrassowitz, 1977.

Wickkiser, Bronwen. *Asklepios, Medicine, and the Politics of Healing in Fifth-Century Greece: Between Cult and Craft*. Baltimore: Johns Hopkins University Press, 2008.

Wildung, Dietrich. *Imhotep und Amenhotep: Gottwerdung im alten Ägypten.* Munich: Deutscher Kunstverlag, 1977.

Wilfong, T. G. "Gender and Sexuality." In *The Egyptian World*, edited by Toby Wilkinson, 205–17. New York: Routledge, 2010.

Wilkinson, Toby, ed. *The Egyptian World*. New York: Routledge, 2010.

Williams, Alan. "Zoroastrianism and the Body." In *Religion and the Body*, edited by Sarah Coakley, 155–66. Cambridge: Cambridge University Press, 1997.

Wolff, Hans Walter. *Anthropology of the Old Testament*. London: SCM, 1981.

Wolters, Al. "Untying the King's Knots: Physiology and Wordplay in Daniel 5." *Journal of Biblical Literature* 110 (1991): 117–22.

World Health Organization. "Constitution." In *The First Ten Years of the World Health Organization*. Geneva: WHO, 1958.

Worthington, Martin. "Edition of UGU 1 (=BAM 480 Etc.)." *Le Journal des Médecines Cunéiformes* 5 (2005): 6–43.

———. "Some Notes on Medical Information outside the Medical Corpora." In *Advances in Mesopotamian Medicine from Hammurabi to Hippocrates*, 47–77. Boston: Brill, 2009.

Wright, David P. "Syro-Canaanite Religions." In *The Cambridge History of Religions in the Ancient World*, edited by Michele Renee Salzman, 129–50. Cambridge: Cambridge University Press, 2013.

Yener, K. Aslihan, and Harry A. Hoffner, eds. *Recent Developments in Hittite Archaeology and History: Papers in Memory of Hans G. Guterböck*. Winona Lake, IN: Eisenbrauns, 2002.

Yon, Marguerite. *The City of Ugarit at Tell Ras Shamra*. Winona Lake, IN: Eisenbrauns, 2006.

Zimmer-Vorhaus, Caroline. "Hittite Temples: Palaces of the Gods." In *Insights into Hittite History and Archaeology*, edited by Herman Genz and Dirk Paul Mielke, 195–218. Walpole, MA: Peeters, 2011.

Zucconi, Laura M. "Can No Physician Be Found?" PhD diss., University of California San Diego, 2005.

———. *Can No Physician Be Found? The Influence of Religion on Medical Pluralism in Ancient Egypt, Mesopotamia, and Israel*. Piscataway: Gorgias, 2013.

———. "From the Wilderness of Zin Alongside Edom: Edomite Territory in the Eastern Negev During the Eighth-Sixth Centuries B.C.E." In *Milk and Honey: Essays on Ancient Israel and the Bible in Appreciation of the Judaic Studies Program at the University of California, San Diego*, edited by Sarah Malena and David Miano, 241–56. Winona Lake, IN: Eisenbrauns, 2007.

# Index of Authors

# Index of Subjects

# Index of Scripture and Other Ancient Texts

## Hittite Literature



## Zoroastrian Works



## Papyri and Tablets